Date due

Solid State Biophysics

SOLID STATE BIOPHYSICS

APPLICATIONS OF ELECTRON SPIN RESONANCE,
DIELECTRIC MEASUREMENTS, THE MÖSSBAUER
EFFECT, AND LASERS TO BIOLOGY AND MEDICINE

Edited by

S. J. Wyard

Physics Department
Guy's Hospital Medical School
London

McGraw-Hill Book Company

New York   St. Louis   San Francisco   Toronto   London   Sydney

Solid State Biophysics

72148

1 2 3 4 5 6 7 8 9 0   M A M M   7 6 5 4 3 2 1 0 6 9

PREFACE

There is a continuing need for books which describe the application of newly devised physical techniques to problems in medicine and biology. This book is an attempt to meet the need in one rapidly developing area of the field. The topics chosen form a coherent group, because each technique has several features in common with the others, but they have not yet been defined by a commonly accepted name.

For these reasons one of the most difficult tasks in the preparation of this book was the choice of the title. *Solid State Biophysics* was chosen because most of the techniques are used in solid state physics laboratories, and are familiar to solid state physicists. However, the topics are on the borders of traditional subjects and inevitably overlap them, so that physics must be understood to include chemistry, and solid must be understood not to exclude liquid. A more precise title would be *Applied Solid State Biophysics*, distinguishing the present book from a possible companion volume called *Theoretical Solid State Biophysics*, in which the ideas of solid state physics, i.e., the extension of quantum mechanics to systems involving many atoms, would be applied to the still more complex biological systems. But I do not think the time is ripe for the companion volume, so no confusion should arise.

The book was planned to meet the needs primarily of graduate and research students. It is hoped that it will also be of use to more seasoned scientists in the fields of medical research, biology, biochemistry, biophysics, and physics, who wish to know what has been done already and also what might be done by applying these new techniques to their own problems. So as to give the student an authentic picture of research in progress, the authors were chosen from among those who had made a personal contribution to the topics they describe. An attempt has been made throughout the book to avoid aspects that seem to be merely fashionable or unduly speculative, and to concentrate on whatever hard facts are available.

The scope of the book is something between a textbook, a review, and an original research contribution, combining some of the qualities of all three. Each author was asked to write an introduction to his subject, followed by a brief review, then an account in some detail of his own recent research, and finally to suggest possibilities for future work. The introductions are not as complete as would be required for a textbook, since this would have made the book far too long; but they should make each topic understandable to any newcomer to it who possesses a normal science background. The review sections are mostly not complete, in the sense of covering every paper on the subject, but they do include all the work which in the opinion of the authors is essential to an understanding of the subject; and they are supplemented by rather full lists for further reading.

More than half the book is devoted to electron spin resonance spectroscopy, covering every major application of this technique in medicine and biology with the exception of enzyme reactions and photosynthesis. The first was omitted because an excellent review by Beinert and Palmer (referred to in the text) appeared while this book was in preparation; the second was omitted because although there have been several hundred papers on ESR and photosynthesis it has apparently not been established what role, if any, the free radicals observed by ESR play in the photosynthetic process. Separate chapters give an elementary introduction to ESR for newcomers to this topic (chapter 1), and an account of more sophisticated techniques which are likely to be useful in biological and medical applications (chapter 2). The other topics—dielectric measurements, the Mössbauer effect and the laser—are each covered in a single chapter but, it is believed, adequately.

ACKNOWLEDGEMENTS

I have been greatly assisted in the preparation of this book by criticism and advice from numerous colleagues, especially from those at Guy's Hospital Medical School, Stanford University, and the University of California, Berkeley.

I am particularly indebted to Professor C. A. Tobias for suggesting this book and persuading me to undertake it.

I also wish to acknowledge my debt to my students, past and present, from whom I have learnt many things.

SIDNEY J. WYARD

J. M. Baker, The Clarendon Laboratory, Oxford, England.

M. S. Blois, Jr., Department of Dermatology, School of Medicine, Stanford University, Stanford, California, U.S.A.

J. B. Cook, Haileybury and Imperial Service College, Hertford, England. (Previously, Physics Department, Guy's Hospital Medical School, London, England.)

E. H. Grant, Department of Physics, Queen Elizabeth College, London, England.

T. E. Gunter, Donner Laboratory, University of California, Berkeley, California, U.S.A.

T. Henriksen, Fellow of the Norwegian Cancer Society, Norsk Hydro's Institute for Cancer Research, Montebello, Norway.

J. E. Maling, Biophysics Laboratory, Stanford University, Stanford, California, U.S.A.

R. C. Smith, Department of Electronics, The University, Southampton, England.

M. Weissbluth, Biophysics Laboratory, Stanford University, Stanford, California, U.S.A.

S. J. Wyard, Physics Department, Guy's Hospital Medical School, London, England.

CONTENTS

Solid State Biophysics

CHAPTER ONE

ELECTRON SPIN RESONANCE SPECTROSCOPY

S. J. Wyard

*Physics Department, Guy's Hospital Medical
School, London, England*

1.1 INTRODUCTION

1.1.1 SCOPE

This chapter has been written for the newcomer to electron spin resonance spectroscopy, either physicist or chemist, biologist or medical scientist; and its aim is to bring him to the point where he can follow the other chapters which deal with the same subject (chapters 2–8). The approach is practical rather than theoretical and emphasizes the aspects of the subject which so far have had the widest biological and medical applications. Thus solid samples are considered rather than liquids, free radicals rather than paramagnetic ions; and particular attention is paid to methods of measuring the number of radicals present in a sample and of identifying the radicals from their spectra.

1.1.2 PRELIMINARY SURVEY

Electron spin resonance spectroscopy is a form of absorption spectroscopy having some features in common with the more familiar optical, ultraviolet, and infrared spectroscopies. In each case, electromagnetic radiation is passed through the sample, and one measures the frequencies at which maximum absorption occurs. One then deduces the energy levels within the sample, from the quantum energies of the photons that were absorbed, by the familiar equation

$$hv = E_2 - E_1. \tag{1.1}$$

The special feature of electron spin resonance spectroscopy is that the absorption takes place when the sample is subjected to a magnetic field. This indicates that the absorption is connected with the presence of magnetic dipoles in the sample. It is well known that many atomic nuclei possess an intrinsic magnetic moment which, together with the associated angular momentum, is described by the term 'spin'. Electrons also possess an intrinsic magnetic moment and angular momentum and, in addition, there is usually a magnetic moment associated with the orbital motion of the electron. All of these magnetic moments can give rise to magnetic resonance. There is an important difference that the nuclear magnetic moment (which varies from nucleus to nucleus) is about 1000 times smaller than the electronic magnetic moment, and this has resulted in two branches of magnetic resonance: nuclear magnetic resonance (NMR) and electron spin resonance (ESR). Both the techniques used and the results obtained are rather different for the two branches of spectroscopy, and we shall not deal specifically with NMR. However, much of the basic theory is common to both branches and in fact it is the presence of nuclear magnets which gives ESR much of its interest and usefulness.

Although electrons are ubiquitous and all possess spin, yet it is well

3

known that most materials are diamagnetic, and that this is because the electrons go in pairs so that there is no net magnetic moment. Diamagnetic materials will not give a spectrum, and this is a great convenience in ESR spectroscopy, since it means that extensive preparation and purification of the sample is often unnecessary. Paramagnetic impurities in the sample, or sample holder or associated apparatus, can however produce spectra which give rise to confusion, and one has to watch out for these.

For a material to give an ESR spectrum, there must be unpaired electrons in it. Materials which contain unpaired electrons fall into two broad classes: first, paramagnetic ions from the transition groups of the periodic table, which contain partly filled electron shells; and, second, free radicals and radical ions, where the unpaired electron is a valence electron that normally takes part in chemical binding. Both paramagnetic ions and free radicals are present, or can be made to appear, in biological materials, and both have been studied by magnetic resonance. Up to the present, considerably more attention has been paid to the free radicals, and we shall largely concentrate on these in this chapter. For the sake of completeness we should also mention triplet state molecules, conduction electrons, and charge-transfer complexes, all of which can give ESR spectra.

Historically, the development of paramagnetic resonance in the transition groups came first, beginning with Zavoisky (1945). When, a few years later, free radicals were studied in chemical and biological systems, the theory and techniques developed for paramagnetic salts were taken over, and adapted and extended as necessary. Much of the work on paramagnetic salts was done at the Clarendon Laboratory, Oxford, where the subject was generally referred to as paramagnetic resonance. Some authors use the title electron paramagnetic resonance (EPR) in order to differentiate it from nuclear magnetic resonance (NMR). The use of the title ESR appears to be gaining ground at present, and we shall adhere to it in this book. The title ESR is certainly justified for free radicals, where, as we shall see, the magnetic moment is almost entirely due to the spin of the electron, the orbital motion making very little contribution.

In the space of a single chapter we can only present a simplified version of ESR. For further reading there are very many review papers and quite a few textbooks, although not, as yet, a comprehensive book on ESR. The best single book, in the present author's opinion, is by Pake (1962); this goes into the theory of paramagnetic resonance in some detail but has not much to say on either the experimental techniques or the applications of the method. This book can be supplemented by the collection of articles edited by Blois, et al. (1961) which deal with applications in biological systems, and by the book by Ingram (1958) which contains much information of practical use for the experimenter. There are also two very good books on NMR by Andrew (1958) and by Abragam (1961). These cover much the same ground, the second far more extensively than the first, and both contain much that is applicable to ESR. Finally, one should look at the authoritative review by Bleaney and Stevens (1953), and not only for historical reasons.

1.2 BASIC THEORY

1.2.1 THE RESONANCE CONDITION

To begin in the most elementary way possible, if a magnetic dipole is placed in a uniform magnetic field, its potential energy is

$$E = - \boldsymbol{\mu} \cdot \mathbf{H}. \tag{1.2}$$

We now consider what is known as a 'free electron', i.e., an unpaired electron which is only influenced by the external magnetic field, and whose magnetic moment is entirely due to its spin, with no contribution from any orbital motion. We know from quantum theory that the electron has a spin of $\frac{1}{2}$, and that when placed in an external magnetic field it is aligned with its magnetic moment μ_s either parallel or anti-parallel to the field direction. The corresponding magnetic quantum numbers are $m = -\frac{1}{2}$ and $m = +\frac{1}{2}$. If a circularly polarized magnetic field in the plane perpendicular to the steady magnetic field H is also applied, transitions are possible in which m changes by ± 1. In ESR jargon, the electron spin is said to have 'flipped over' in the magnetic field. The condition for this to occur is that the quantum energy of the photon which provides the circularly polarized magnetic field should be equal to the energy difference of the two states, i.e., to $2\mu_s H$. The spin magnetic moment of the electron is known from both theory (Sommerfield, 1957) and experiment (Wilkinson and Crane, 1963) to be equal to $1.0011596 \, \beta$, where β is the Bohr magneton, or $eh/4\pi mc$. Thus for a free electron, transitions can occur when

$$h\nu = 2.00232\beta H. \tag{1.3}$$

In equation (1.3), h is Planck's constant, equal to 6.6256×10^{-27} erg sec and β is equal to 9.2732×10^{-21} erg/Oe (Cohen and Du Mond, 1965). Equation (1.3) shows that the absorption of electromagnetic radiation in this case is a resonant phenomenon, since it occurs at a particular frequency; it shows that resonance will occur for any value of the external magnetic field; and it shows that the resonant frequency is proportional to the magnetic field. The situation is illustrated in Fig. 1.1.

Putting in the values of the constants β and h in equation (1.3) we obtain

$$\nu = 2.8025H \tag{1.4}$$

where v is in MHz and H is in oersted. ESR has been performed at a number of frequencies but for reasons of practical convenience and of sensitivity, which will be discussed later, measurements are most commonly made close to 9000 MHz, with a corresponding magnetic field of 3200 Oe.

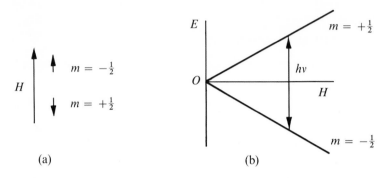

Fig. 1.1   (a) Alignment of electron spin in a magnetic field. (b) Energy levels for spin $\frac{1}{2}$; $E = \pm\ \mu_s H$.

So far we have considered the idealized case of a free electron. In actual cases, the unpaired electron will be part of an atom, ion, or radical, or trapped in a solid in some way, so that it is subject to other forces besides the external magnetic field. This has the effect of shifting the position of resonance. The resonance condition is now written

$$hv = g\beta H \qquad (1.5)$$

where g is called the 'spectroscopic splitting factor', or simply the 'g-factor'. The g-factor is not to be confused with the Landé splitting factor, which applies to free atoms, but is purely an empirical term, defined by equation (1.5). The g-value for a free electron is written g_e.†

Of course, there are always reasons why the resonance is not perfectly sharp—as equations (1.3), (1.4), and (1.5) would imply—but spreads over a range of frequencies, giving a bell-shaped absorption curve with a certain line width. Line widths vary a great deal in ESR and will be discussed later. At present, we state that, although sometimes the lines are so broad that no resonance can be detected, they are very often sufficiently narrow for well resolved lines to be obtained. The g-factor is then measured from the frequency at the center of the resonance.

† Strictly speaking, both β and g are negative. However, we follow the usual practice and use the moduli of these values.

1.2.2 THE ABSORPTION OF POWER

The quantum theory of radiation tells us that at the frequencies with which we are concerned spontaneous emission is negligible, and absorption and stimulated emission, corresponding to transitions up and down in energy, are equally likely. Hence a net absorption of radiation must depend on a difference of population between the numbers of spins (unpaired electrons) in the two states. In the absence of radiation the populations are determined by Boltzmann statistics, which state that the probability of finding an electron in a state with energy E is proportional to $\exp(-E/kT)$, where k is Boltzmann's constant and T the absolute temperature. Before proceeding further, we must justify the use of Boltzmann statistics when talking about electrons which, having a spin of $\frac{1}{2}$ and being indistinguishable, obey Fermi–Dirac statistics. The reason is that, although it is convenient to talk about the electrons in a graphic manner, since their spin is almost entirely responsible for the resonance, we are really dealing with the atoms, ions, or radicals of which the electrons are a part. These entities, although identical among themselves, are located at fixed points in the sample material, and are therefore distinguishable by virtue of their positions. Provided the interaction energy between the magnetic dipoles is sufficiently small—and this is the case for radicals and paramagnetic ions at ordinary temperatures—it is correct to apply Boltzmann statistics. For further discussion of this point see a standard work on statistical mechanics, e.g., that by Davidson (1962). Exceptions to Boltzmann statistics do occur, for example in ferromagnetism or in conduction electrons. Such cases can also occur in biological materials, and use of the wrong statistics can give rise to confusion.

Considering the case where Boltzmann statistics do apply, and where there are just two energy levels, we have for the population difference

$$\frac{N_- - N_+}{N_- + N_+} = \frac{e^{\mu H/kT} - e^{-\mu H/kT}}{e^{\mu H/kT} + e^{-\mu H/kT}} \qquad (1.6)$$

where N_- and N_+ are the number of spins in the sample in the lower and upper energy levels. Writing $N = N_- + N_+$ for the total number of unpaired electrons, and $n = N_- - N_+$ for the population difference between the two levels we have

$$n = N \tanh(\mu H/kT). \qquad (1.7)$$

The ratio n/N is called the 'polarization'.

To get an idea of the magnitude of the polarization, we put in the values of the constants and find that at room temperature $kT = 4.14 \times 10^{-14}$ ergs, while $\mu H = 2.96 \times 10^{-17}$ ergs for electron spins in a field of 3200 Oe. Since $\mu H/kT$ is a small number, we can simplify equations (1.6) and (1.7) by expanding the exponentials and neglecting the higher terms.   This gives

$$n = N\frac{\mu H}{kT} = \frac{Ng\beta H}{2kT}.$$ (1.8)

Even at $4.2°K$, which is the lowest temperature normally used in ESR, the value of $\mu H/kT$ is still sufficiently small (0.051 for electron spins in a field of 3200 Oe) for equation (1.8) to be a good approximation; the error involved in using equation (1.8) in this case is 1 part in 1000, which would be quite undetectable in an ESR measurement.

We saw that the net absorption of radiation depends on the population difference between the two levels.   Equation (1.8) shows that, other things remaining equal, the absorption can be increased, and the sensitivity improved, by going to higher magnetic fields and to lower sample temperatures.   However, the sample temperature is usually decided by other considerations; and there are many other factors involved in the sensitivity, which will be discussed later.   Making measurements over a range of temperatures provides a method for distinguishing between free radicals and paramagnetic ions on the one hand, for which the absorption is proportional to T^{-1}, and conduction electrons and ferromagnetic samples on the other hand, for which the absorption is independent of temperature.

It is worthwhile to write down at this point the expression for the static magnetic susceptibility χ_0, defined as the magnetic moment of the sample divided by the field producing it.   Each of the excess electrons in the lower energy level has a resolved magnetic moment in the direction of the applied field equal to μ (the other electrons cancel each other out), so the net magnetic moment $M = n\mu = N\mu^2 H/kT$, from equation (1.8); and

$$\chi_0 = \frac{M}{H} = \frac{N\mu^2}{kT}.$$ (1.9)

The dependence of χ_0 on T in equation (1.9) is the well known Curie law.

We note here that measurements of magnetic susceptibility, which can be made very sensitive, provide another method of measuring N, the number of unpaired electrons in the sample.   This is a useful alternative to the ESR method for determining N, especially when the absorption lines are so broad that the ESR method cannot be used.

The power absorbed by the sample depends on the rate at which the spins are flipped between the two energy levels by the electromagnetic radiation.   We must take account of the fact that the energy levels, and hence the absorption line, have a certain width, and this is done by introducing the line-shape function $f(v - v_0)$.   The line-shape function is normalized so that $\int_0^\infty f(v - v_0)\,dv = 1$; it has a maximum value at v_0, the resonant frequency; and for lines of the same shape the maximum value is inversely proportional to the line width Δv (Fig. 1.2). Two shapes to which the absorption line commonly approximates are the Gaussian and Lorentzian defined in equations (1.32) and (1.33). For these, the product of maximum absorption and line width is $2(\ln 2/\pi)^{1/2}$ and $2/\pi$ respectively. It then

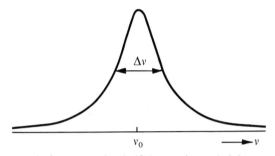

Δv is measured at half the maximum height.

Fig. 1.2   Line shape function for ESR absorption line.

follows from radiation theory (see Abragam (1961) for a full discussion) that for a spin of $\frac{1}{2}$ the transition probabilities per unit time due to the radiation are

$$P_{1/2 \to -1/2} = P_{-1/2 \to 1/2} = P = \frac{(\gamma H_1)^2}{16} f(v - v_0) \qquad (1.10)$$

where H_1 is the amplitude of a linearly polarized radiofrequency or microwave magnetic field, oscillating in a plane perpendicular to the external field H_0 and γ is the gyromagnetic ratio, equal to the angular frequency at resonance divided by the external magnetic field. For a free spin

$$\gamma = \frac{g_e e}{2mc} = 1.7608 \times 10^7 \text{ radians sec}^{-1} \text{ Oe}^{-1} \qquad (1.11)$$

from equations (1.3) and (1.4). In section 1.2.1, we said that transitions are produced by a circularly polarized magnetic field. Linearly oscillating fields are generally used, and are equivalent to two circular fields each with amplitude $H_1/2$, rotating in opposite directions. Only one of these circular fields is effective in inducing transitions. There is some confusion in the literature between those who use H_1 as the amplitude of the linear field and those who use it as the amplitude of the circular field.

A transition up absorbs a quantum of energy hv; a transition down emits a quantum hv. Hence the net power absorption is the product of hv

with expressions (1.10) and (1.8), i.e.,

$$A = \tfrac{1}{16}\gamma^2 H_1^2 f(v - v_0)\frac{Nh^2 v v_0}{2kT} \qquad (1.12)$$

where we have substituted hv_0 for $g\beta H$ using the resonance condition.

Two important consequences follow from equation (1.12). First, the maximum power absorbed is inversely proportional to the line width, with only a small dependence on the line shape. Second, whatever the line shape and line width, $\int_0^\infty A\, dv$, or the area under the absorption line, equals $\tfrac{1}{16}\gamma^2 H_1^2 (Nh^2 v_0^2/2kT)$, and is proportional to N, the number of spins. However, this result has only been proved for free spins, and may need modification in other cases (see chapter 3, section 3.2.3A).

From the macroscopic point of view the sample can be regarded as possessing a complex magnetic susceptibility $\chi = \chi' - j\chi''$. The power absorbed by the sample is then $\pi v \chi'' H_1^2$. Equating this expression with the right-hand side of equation (1.12), and using the expression for χ_0 from equation (1.9), we have

$$\chi'' = \frac{\pi}{2}\chi_0 f(v - v_0)v_0. \qquad (1.13)$$

The maximum value of χ'', at the centre of the line, is $\chi_0(v_0/\Delta v)$, exactly for a Lorentzian line shape, and approximately for other line shapes (see equations (1.32)–(1.35)). We note at this point that, since absorption is always accompanied by dispersion, it is possible to detect the resonance by means of the dispersion. However, this is rarely done in ESR, and one's concern with dispersion is usually only to avoid it, so as not to distort the shape of the absorption line.

1.2.3 SATURATION

So far we have considered the spins present in the sample to be free in the sense that they interact only with the magnetic field and with the microwave radiation. If this were really the case, the effect of the microwave radiation would be to make the populations in the two energy levels the same, and when this happened absorption would cease. In fact, there are always ways in which the spins can change from one energy level to the other without assistance from the microwave radiation. Processes by which the spin populations return to their state of thermal equilibrium after being disturbed are called 'relaxation processes'.[†] The process in which energy absorbed by the spins from the microwave radiation is handed over to the rest of the sample

† The existence of relaxation processes was in fact implied by the statement in section 1.2.2 that in the absence of radiation the populations are determined by Boltzmann statistics.

is called 'spin-lattice relaxation'. We are not concerned here with the mechanism of the process, but we need to know how relaxation affects the absorption line. Furthermore, measurements of relaxation may help in identifying the species which contains the unpaired electron.

Suppose that in the absence of microwave radiation the transition probabilities between the two levels per unit time are W_+, for a transition down, and W_- for a transition up. In equilibrium, the numbers of transitions up and down are equal, so

$$N_{eq-} \, W_- = N_{eq+} \, W_+ . \tag{1.14}$$

Now suppose the system has departed from thermal equilibrium so that N_+ and N_- are not determined by the Boltzmann condition. To find the rate at which equilibrium is restored we have

$$\frac{dn}{dt} = 2N_+ W_+ - 2N_- W_-$$

$$= (2N_+ - 2N_{eq+})W_+ - (2N_- - 2N_{eq-})W_- \tag{1.15}$$

using equation (1.14). The factor 2 arises because each transition transfers a spin from one level to the other. Writing $W = \frac{1}{2}(W_- + W_+)$ for the mean transition probability, and remembering that the total number of spins remains constant, we obtain

$$\frac{dn}{dt} = 2W(n_{eq} - n) \tag{1.16}$$

which gives on integration

$$n - n_{eq} = (n_0 - n_{eq}) \, e^{-2Wt}. \tag{1.17}$$

Thus the spin system approaches equilibrium exponentially with a time constant $1/2W$. This is the situation, for example, when the magnetic field H is turned on or off. The time constant $1/2W$ is written T_1, and is called the 'spin-lattice relaxation time'.

We now consider the sample in the magnetic field and also absorbing microwave radiation. This modifies the conditions of equilibrium, so that equation (1.16) becomes

$$\frac{dn}{dt} = \frac{n_{eq} - n}{T_1} - 2nP. \tag{1.18}$$

When equilibrium is reached, $dn/dt = 0$, and under these new conditions the population difference

$$n_s = \frac{n_{eq}}{1 + 2PT_1}. \tag{1.19}$$

Taking the value of P from equation (1.10) we have

$$\frac{n_s}{n_{eq}} = \frac{1}{1 + \frac{1}{8}\gamma^2 H_1^2 f(v - v_0)T_1}.$$ (1.20)

The ratio n_s/n_{eq} is written Z, and is called the 'saturation factor' (Pake, 1962). For large values of H_1, Z becomes small, and the sample is then said to be 'saturated'. Equation (1.20) shows that saturation is greatest at the resonant frequency, and this results in a broadening of the absorption line. By defining $\frac{1}{2}[f(v - v_0)]_{max}$ as T_2 (since the line-shape function is normalized, T_2 is a measure of the line width) we have for the saturation factor at the line center

$$Z_0 = \frac{1}{1 + \frac{1}{4}\gamma^2 H_1^2 T_1 T_2}.$$ (1.21)

It will be shown later that the absorption signal is proportional to $Z_0 H_1$. Hence as the microwave power is increased from zero the absorption signal increases to a maximum and then decreases again. There is a limit to the power which can be absorbed by the sample, which is determined by the rate at which the spins can hand on the power to the bulk of the sample, i.e., by the spin-lattice relaxation time. The maximum signal is found by differentiating the expression for $Z_0 H_1$ and occurs when

$$H_1 = 2/\gamma(T_1 T_2)^{1/2}.$$ (1.22)

However, in ESR one generally keeps the power sufficiently low to prevent saturation, and thus one avoids distortion of the line shape. It must be pointed out that the saturation behavior discussed in this section is a somewhat idealized case, seldom met in practice. This point will be taken up again later.

1.2.4   THE SPECTRUM: GENERAL CONSIDERATIONS

Up to now we have considered an unpaired electron which is affected by an external fixed magnetic field, and by an oscillating magnetic field, and which can exchange energy with the lattice, but which is otherwise free. In this case, the spectrum would consist of a single line centered at $g = 2.00232$, and the only information we could obtain would be the number of spins in the sample and the spin-lattice relaxation time. Fortunately, the spectrum is nearly always more complicated than this, and the information which can be obtained from it is correspondingly greater.

If we were to approach the problem from a purely theoretical point of view, we would consider the unpaired electron moving in an orbit in some species, e.g., free radical or paramagnetic ion, which is held in position by forces between it and its neighbors. (We assume at present that we are dealing with a solid sample.) Following the methods of quantum mechanics we would write down the Hamiltonian by adding terms from all the interactions with the unpaired electrons, both electric and magnetic in character, e.g., with the nuclei, with the electron spins and orbits, with the electric fields present in the material of the sample, and with the external magnetic fields (fixed and oscillating). From the Hamiltonian we could obtain the frequencies at which absorption occurred, and also the transition probabilities. This approach would not take us very far, partly because the Hamiltonian would be too complicated, and partly because many of the constants required, which are properties of the material of the sample, are not known. The approach which has proved very successful is to write down an 'effective spin-Hamiltonian' where only those terms appear which are important in predicting the shape of the spectrum, and where the constants appear in a semi-empirical form. If the spectrum fits the Hamiltonian, one can deduce these constants. Thus most of the information contained in the spectrum can be described by a few constants; and from these one can hope to identify the free radical, for example, if this is not known, and to obtain information such as the orbit in which the unpaired electron moves, and the bonding of the free radical to the other molecules in the sample. A number of forms of the spin-Hamiltonian have been worked out, and these are described in the references given in section 1.1. These were all derived for particular paramagnetic salts, but some of them have been found to be suitable for the free radicals with which we are mostly concerned in this chapter. When choosing a Hamiltonian to which to fit the spectrum, one naturally takes the simplest form which will account for the main features of the spectrum, and only introduces complications such as second order effects or so-called forbidden transitions when these are found to be necessary. (The Hamiltonian is discussed in more detail in chapter 4.)

The features of the ESR spectrum which are generally observed are (a) a shift in the position of the center of resonance from $g = 2.00232$, known as 'g-value variation'; (b) a splitting of the line into a number of components symmetrically disposed about the center, known as 'hyperfine splitting'; (c) changes in line width and line shape. Spectra from free radicals differ from spectra from paramagnetic ions in two ways: first, the g-value variation is small, generally less than 1%, whereas in paramagnetic ions g-values of 6 and higher are not uncommon; second, there is an absence of the 'fine structure' which can only appear in ions with spin greater than $\frac{1}{2}$. We shall discuss features (a), (b), and (c) in turn, attempting to give a physical insight into these effects and only giving enough theory to account for the main experimental results. Before doing so, there are two general observations to make.

The first observation is that the features of the spectrum are usually dependent on the direction between the applied magnetic field and a set of axes fixed in the radical or in the matrix in which the radical is embedded. As the radical, or the matrix, is rotated about the magnetic field direction, in general the whole spectrum shifts in frequency, the components move together or apart, and the line width alters.   The result is that, if the radicals have random orientation, as in a powder or polycrystalline sample, the details of the spectrum are usually smeared out, resulting in a poorly resolved line from which one can deduce little more than the number of spins present. There are exceptions to this rule, and cases are discussed in chapters 5 and 6 where considerable information was obtained from polycrystalline samples.   Still, it remains true that for good resolution one needs single crystals, and that from polycrystalline samples one can seldom identify the species giving rise to the spectrum.   The case is different for liquid samples, which will be discussed later.

The second observation is that the ESR spectrum, and the constants in the spin-Hamiltonian, depend not only on the ion or radical, but also on the matrix in which it is embedded.   Naturally, this makes identification of an unknown radical from its ESR spectrum more difficult; but fortunately, as we shall see, there are a number of general rules which make identification possible in many cases.

The effective spin-Hamiltonian most frequently used to describe ESR spectra from free radicals may be written

$$\mathcal{H} = \beta \mathbf{S} \cdot g \cdot \mathbf{H} + \mathbf{S} \cdot A \cdot \mathbf{I} \qquad (1.23)$$

where g and A are second rank tensors.   The first term represents the interaction between the electron and the magnetic field, and gives the g-value variation; the second term represents the interaction between the electron and the nucleus, and gives the hyperfine splitting.

1.2.5 g-VALUE VARIATION

For a free spin the value of g in equation (1.23) would be a constant (2.00232). However, experiment shows that the g-value in general differs from the free spin value, and moreover varies with the angle between the magnetic field and the crystal axes.   This departure from the free spin value is due to coupling between the magnetic moments of the spin and the orbit of the electron.   This spin-orbit coupling alters the energy levels by an amount which can be calculated from the Hamiltonian.   The effect can be pictured by assigning to the unpaired electron a spin—the 'effective spin'—which differs from the free spin.   However, it must be remembered that the value of the effective spin varies as the crystal is rotated in the magnetic field.

In equation (1.23), g is a symmetric tensor.   If the magnetic field has direction cosines l_1, l_2, l_3 with respect to a set of axes fixed in the crystal, the square of the corresponding g-value is given by an expression of the form

$$g^2 = \sum_{i,\,j=1}^{3} A_{ij}l_il_j, \, (A_{ij} = A_{ji}) \tag{1.24}$$

where the coefficients A_{ij} depend on the choice of reference axes.   The matrix A may be diagonalized by a suitable choice of axes, to give the 'principal g-values' g_1, g_2, g_3.   With this choice of axes

$$g^2 = l^2g_1{}^2 + m^2g_2{}^2 + n^2g_3{}^2 \tag{1.25}$$

where direction cosines are now denoted by l, m, n.   Methods for determination of the principal g-values have been discussed by Schonland (1959).

The magnitude of the departure of g from the free spin value is given by

$$g - g_e \simeq \frac{\lambda}{\Delta} \tag{1.26}$$

where g_e is the free spin value, λ is the spin-orbit coupling, and Δ is the energy separation between the electronic ground state and the excited state being admixed by the spin-orbit coupling. λ can be either positive or negative, giving g-values either larger or smaller than g_e.   For free radicals, the spin-orbit coupling is generally small and positive, so that g is close to and slightly greater than the free spin value.

g-Values can be measured with an accuracy of 1 part in 10^5, or even better in favorable cases (Blois, Brown, and Maling, 1961; Segal, et al., 1965).   However, the information needed to calculate g-values from the Hamiltonian is generally lacking, so not much can be done with such precise measurements.   In particular, it is not possible to identify a free radical from g-value measurements, especially as these also depend on the matrix.   Nevertheless, g-value measurements are helpful as a guide to the nature of the radical, and its location in the matrix.   In some cases, the g-value is axially symmetric, or very nearly so.   We then write $g_1 = g_2 = g_\perp$; $g_3 = g_\parallel$; and equation (1.25) becomes

$$g^2 = g_\parallel^2 \cos^2\theta + g_\perp^2 \sin^2\theta \tag{1.27}$$

where θ is the angle between the magnetic field and the axis of symmetry.   In this case, the orientation of the axis of symmetry can be derived from the ESR spectrum.   This method was used by Smith and Wyard (1961) to study preferred orientation of molecules and radicals in samples of H_2O_2–H_2O frozen into quartz tubes.

Another example of the use of g-value measurements comes from the work of Känzig and Cohen (1959) and Känzig (1962). By diffusing oxygen into alkali halides, an ESR spectrum was produced which was attributed to O_2^-. The principal g-values were measured at 9.3 GHz and $11°K$, and are given in Table 1.1. The limit of error was ± 0.0002.

Table 1.1

	g_1	g_2	g_3
KCl	1.9512	1.9551	2.4359
KBr	1.9268	1.9314	2.5203
KI	1.9370	1.9420	2.4859

It will be noted that in each matrix, g_1 is nearly equal to g_2, and also that the g-values differ slightly in the different crystals. The principal g-values were also calculated from the spin-Hamiltonian as

$$g_x = g_e\left(\frac{\Delta^2}{\lambda^2 + \Delta^2}\right)^{1/2} - \frac{\lambda}{E}\left[-\left(\frac{\lambda^2}{\lambda^2 + \Delta^2}\right)^{1/2} - \frac{\Delta}{(\lambda^2 + \Delta^2)^{1/2}} + 1\right] \quad (1.28)$$

$$g_y = g_e\left(\frac{\Delta^2}{\lambda^2 + \Delta^2}\right)^{1/2} - \frac{\lambda}{E}\left[\left(\frac{\lambda^2}{\lambda^2 + \Delta^2}\right)^{1/2} - \frac{\Delta}{(\lambda^2 + \Delta^2)^{1/2}} - 1\right] \quad (1.29)$$

$$g_z = g_e + 2\left(\frac{\lambda^2}{\lambda^2 + \Delta^2}\right)^{1/2} l \quad (1.30)$$

where λ is the effective spin-orbit coupling of the molecular ion in the crystal, Δ and E are separations between particular energy levels, and l represents a correction to the angular momentum due to the crystal field. The axes were chosen so that z is the internuclear axis and x is the direction of the $p\pi$ orbital. From these equations and the results in Table 1.1, Känzig and Cohen deduced the orientation of the O_2^- ion in the crystal, and obtained values for λ/Δ, λ/E, and l.

g-Values in π-electron radicals have been calculated in general terms by McConnell and Robertson (1957). The g-tensor is expected to be approximately axially symmetric, with the axis of symmetry (z-axis) perpendicular to the plane of the aromatic ring. The predictions are that g_z will be very close to g_e, and that g_x and g_y will be slightly greater. Table 4.6 in chapter 4 lists a number of π-electron radicals, for which these predictions are borne out. For these radicals, g_z lies between 2.0017 and 2.0037, and g_x and g_y between 2.0026 and 2.0078.

A theoretical treatment of g-tensors in aromatic molecules has been presented by Stone (1963a, b). Segal, et al. (1965) have measured average

g-values for twenty aromatic free radicals in solution with an accuracy approaching 1 part in 10^6, and obtained excellent agreement with Stone's theory.

1.2.6   HYPERFINE SPLITTING

Hyperfine splitting provides most of the detail in ESR spectra from radical species, and most of the evidence from which the radical can be identified, if this is possible.   The basic features of hyperfine splitting are very simple.

Hyperfine splitting arises from the interaction between the magnetic moment of the electron (the spin) and any nuclei in the sample which have magnetic moments.   Distant nuclei give a very small interaction, which shows up as a broadening of the absorption line.   This will be discussed in the next section; here we shall be concerned with nuclei which are close to the spin, particularly those which are in the same radical.

We can begin by forming a picture in which we think of the magnetic nucleus, which will be oriented by the external magnetic field H, producing its own local field at the site of the unpaired electron.   Thus the electron experiences a field which differs slightly from H, so that the resonance frequency is correspondingly shifted from the free spin value.   To take a definite example, suppose the unpaired electron interacts with a proton. Since the proton has a spin $I = \frac{1}{2}$, it will have two possible orientations in the magnetic field, and from the Boltzmann statistics the populations in these two orientations will be almost exactly equal.   Thus half the unpaired electrons in the sample will experience a field slightly greater than H, and half will experience a field slightly smaller than H.   The result will be to split the absorption line into two lines, shifted to higher and lower frequencies by equal amounts, each line being half the height of the unsplit line.   In general, a nucleus with a spin I splits the absorption line into $(2I + 1)$ equally spaced lines, symmetrically disposed about the unsplit line, and with height $1/(2I + 1)$ of the unsplit line.   For example, the nitrogen nucleus, which is often present in biological samples, has $I = 1$, giving a triplet for the hyperfine structure.

A slightly more complicated case occurs when the unpaired electron interacts with more than one magnetic nucleus.   The nuclei are all oriented independently in the magnetic field, and the number of lines in the hyperfine spectrum is equal to the number of possible combinations of orientation of the nuclei.   Thus interaction with two protons, each of which gives a different splitting, gives rise to 2×2 or 4 lines.   A proton and a nitrogen nucleus gives 2×3 or 6 lines, and so on.   In such cases, the lines all have equal height.   It can also happen that the unpaired electron interacts with a number of 'equivalent nuclei', each of which produces the same splitting.

In this case, some of the individual components are superimposed, resulting in fewer lines and with unequal heights. Thus n equivalent protons give $(n + 1)$ lines with heights given by the binomial coefficients $1, n, [n(n - 1)]/2$, ..., since these give the relative probabilities of a particular spin finding $0, 1, 2, \ldots$ nuclei oriented parallel to the magnetic field.

To put our physical picture on a firm basis, and to put some numbers in it, we return to the spin-Hamiltonian, using the form given in equation (1.23). Quoting results to be found in the references given in section 1.1, it turns out that, provided the g-value variation is small, as it is for free radicals, and provided the magnetic field is large compared to the magnitude of the hyperfine splitting, expressed in oersted, then our simple picture gives the correct result.

The expression for the energy of interaction between an electron spin and a single nucleus can be written

$$\mathcal{H}' = \frac{8\pi g\beta\gamma}{3}\,\psi^2(0)\mathbf{S} \cdot \mathbf{I} + g\beta\gamma\left[\frac{3(\mathbf{S} \cdot \mathbf{r})(\mathbf{I} \cdot \mathbf{r})}{r^5} - \frac{\mathbf{S} \cdot \mathbf{I}}{r^3}\right] \quad (1.31)$$

where γ is the gyromagnetic ratio of the nucleus, $\psi^2(0)$ is the electronic density at the nucleus, and r is the distance of the electron from the nucleus. The first term in this expression is isotropic and is called the Fermi or contact term, since it has a value only when the electron has a non-zero density at the nucleus. The second term is anisotropic, and arises from the classical interaction between the electron and the nucleus regarded as bar magnets; this has to be averaged over the orbital of the unpaired electron. Now the first term of equation (1.31) is zero, except for s-electrons; while, for s-electrons, the second term comes out to be zero when the averaging is done. However, it is found experimentally that in free radicals the hyperfine splitting usually contains both isotropic and anisotropic contributions. This is because the electron is in a molecular orbital with contributions from both p- and s-wave functions.

If the wave functions were known, the numerical values of the hyperfine splitting could be calculated from equation (1.31). The isotropic hyperfine splitting can be calculated from the term $(8\pi g\beta\gamma/3)\psi^2(0)$ where values of $\psi^2(0)$ are available for s-orbitals of various nuclei. The anisotropic splitting can also be calculated for p-orbitals, and includes the directional term $(3 \cos^2 \theta - 1)$, where θ is the angle between the magnetic field and principal axis of the radical. The combination of the two splittings results in a symmetric tensor. From experimental measurements of the hyperfine splitting constant the tensor elements can be determined, giving separately the isotropic and anisotropic terms, and the directions of the principal axes referred to axes fixed in the crystal. (The method of doing this is discussed in chapter 4.)   These can then be compared with the calculated values to give the amounts of p and s character for the nuclei which are involved.

Since the wave functions are in general not known for the free radicals, but are determined from the ESR measurements, the value of the hyperfine splitting constant will not usually suffice to identify a radical. However, there is by now enough data for comparison for the value of the hyperfine splitting constant to be a useful aid in identification.   The problem is also complicated by the 'matrix effect', i.e., by the fact that for a given radical the hyperfine splitting varies for different matrices, because the wave functions are perturbed.   Thus Jen, et al. (1958) measured the hyperfine splitting constants of hydrogen and nitrogen atoms trapped in matrices of solid H_2, A, N_2, and CH_4.   For hydrogen atoms, where the wave function is almost entirely s-character, the splitting constants were all within 0.66% of the value calculated for a free atom.   For nitrogen atoms, on the other hand, where the wave functions are mainly p-character, deviations of nearly 30% from the value calculated for a free atom were found.

Finally, we mention two effects which sometimes complicate the simple picture we have considered so far.   We have tacitly assumed that, when a microwave photon is absorbed, the unpaired electron flips over, but all the nuclei remain as they were; and this is usually the case.   It is possible, however, for an absorbed photon to flip over an electron and a nucleus simultaneously.   Such an event is sometimes called a 'forbidden transition' because the probability of its occurrence is normally much smaller than that of the 'allowed transitions' which we have discussed so far.   Still, forbidden transitions can be observed under suitable conditions, causing extra lines to appear in the spectrum.   This point will be taken up again in chapter 4.

The second point is that, when the hyperfine splitting, expressed in oersted (the conversion from frequency to oersted uses equation (1.4)), is comparable with the external magnetic field, our assumption that the splitting is independent of the field strength is no longer correct.   The energy levels must be calculated from the spin-Hamiltonian.   The solution is given by the Breit–Rabi formula (Breit and Rabi, 1931; Nafe and Nelson, 1948).   When working at the usual field strength of 3000 Oe the approximation is sufficiently accurate except for the hydrogen atom, which has a hyperfine splitting of 500 Oe.

As an example of hyperfine splitting Fig. 1.3 shows the spectrum of the peroxylamine disulfonate ion $\dot{O}N (SO_3)_2^{2-}$ in solution.†   The unpaired electron is located mainly on the oxygen atom but has a small interaction with the nitrogen nucleus giving a hyperfine splitting of 13 Oe.   The rapid

† This is a first derivative recording; see section 1.2.7 and Fig. 1.4.

tumbling motion of the ion in solution averages out the anisotropic parts of both the g-value and the hyperfine splitting (section 1.2.8) and is responsible for the simple and well resolved spectrum.   Figure 1.3(a) was recorded at a

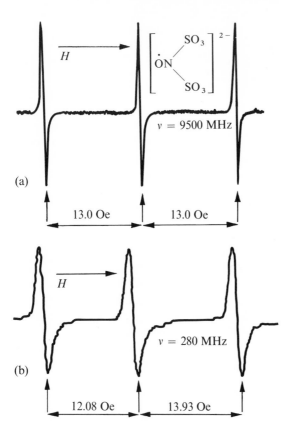

Fig. 1.3   Absorption spectra for peroxylamine disulfonate in solution, first derivative presentation.   (a)
Recorded at 9500 MHz; (b) Recorded at 280 MHz.

frequency of 9000 MHz, where the 'high-field approximation' of equal splittings is sufficiently accurate.   Figure 1.3(b) shows the spectrum of the same sample recorded at a frequency of 280 MHz, where the splittings are noticeably different.   At this frequency the Breit–Rabi formula predicts splittings of 12.1 and 13.95 Oe, in agreement with the experimental values.

The subject of hyperfine structure is taken up again in chapter 2.

1.2.7 LINE WIDTH

The third feature of the spectrum, the shape and width of the absorption line, is not calculated directly from the spin-Hamiltonian. Instead, the various contributions to the line width are discussed separately, and then an attempt is made to combine them together. The information which can be obtained from the line width is not very specific, and often one is interested only in ways of reducing the line width so that the hyperfine structure can be resolved. There are occasions, however, when the line width gives hints as to the identity of the radical, or its situation in the matrix. As an example, the line width can be used to determine the 'local concentration' of radicals (Wyard, 1965). This is discussed again in chapter 5.

For the sake of mathematical convenience the line shape is usually discussed in terms of either the Gaussian or the Lorentzian functions. In the normalized form used in section 1.2.2, these may be written

$$f(v) = \frac{1}{a\sqrt{(2\pi)}} \exp\left\{\frac{-(v - v_0)^2}{2a^2}\right\} \quad \text{(Gaussian)} \qquad (1.32)$$

$$f(v) = \frac{a}{\pi} \frac{1}{a^2 + (v - v_0)^2} \quad \text{(Lorentzian).} \qquad (1.33)$$

The line widths for these curves, defined as the frequency difference between points where the signal has fallen to half the maximum, are

$$\Delta v = 2a\sqrt{(2\ln 2)} = 2.36a \quad \text{(Gaussian)} \qquad (1.34)$$
$$\Delta v = 2a \quad \text{(Lorentzian).} \qquad (1.35)$$

The expressions for the separation between points of maximum slope, written $\Delta v_{\text{m.sl.}}$, are useful, since the spectrometer often records a first derivative curve, so that $\Delta v_{\text{m.sl.}}$ can be read off directly. The expressions are

$$\Delta v_{\text{m.sl.}} = 2a \quad \text{(Gaussian)} \qquad (1.36)$$
$$\Delta v_{\text{m.sl.}} = \frac{2a}{\sqrt{3}} \quad \text{(Lorentzian).} \qquad (1.37)$$

Figure 1.4 shows a Lorentzian line shape, together with its first and second derivatives.

A full discussion of line shapes and line widths would be too lengthy here, so we content ourselves with quoting results and citing the references given in section 1.1 for justification and amplification.

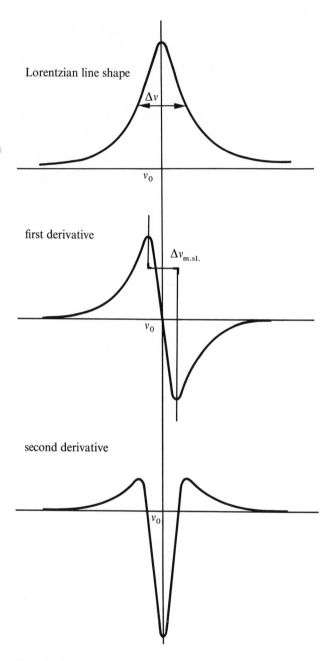

Fig. 1.4   Lorentzian line shape, together with first and second derivatives.

A. *LINE WIDTH DUE TO SPIN-LATTICE RELAXATION*

In common with all spectral lines, the line width is affected by the lifetime of the states between which transitions take place. This is a result of the Uncertainty Principle. It gives a line approximating to a Lorentzian shape, with Δv equal to $1/\pi T_1$. Consequently, a very short relaxation time would give lines so broad that hyperfine structure could not be resolved, and possibly the line could not be detected at all. The spin-lattice relaxation time increases as the temperature of the sample is lowered, so this gives an experimental possibility for sharpening the lines. The spin-lattice relaxation time also depends on the spin-orbit coupling; and when this is small, as it is for free radicals, long relaxation times are obtained. Consequently, the spin-lattice relaxation time is seldom a limiting factor in the line width of ESR spectra from free radicals in solids.

In some cases, the lifetime of the states is limited not by relaxation but by other processes such as chemical reactions. This gives a line width $1/\pi \tau$, where τ is the resultant lifetime, so that measurement of the line width gives the rate constant of the chemical reaction. Ward and Weissman (1954) used this technique to measure the rate constant for the transfer of an electron from a radical ion in solution. A similar effect would occur in the detection of short lived radicals (lifetime less than a microsecond) produced by radiation.

B. *LINE WIDTH DUE TO DIPOLAR BROADENING BY LIKE SPINS*

By 'like spins' are meant those which have the same resonant frequency. This form of broadening can be reduced by keeping the spins far apart (there are cases, however, where a high concentration of spins results in a so-called 'exchange-narrowed' line). For radical species produced by irradiation, broadening by like spins gives an approximately Lorentzian line shape, with a line width, expressed in oersted, of the order of $2 \times 10^{-19} N$, where N is the number of spins per ml (Wyard, 1965). This form of broadening is not usually serious in radical studies.

C. *LINE WIDTH DUE TO DIPOLAR BROADENING BY UNLIKE SPINS*

In free radical studies the unlike spins are usually magnetic nuclei present in the sample. The effect can also be regarded as unresolved hyperfine splitting. When the broadening is due to protons, which is the most common magnetic nucleus in samples of biological interest, an estimate of the line width in oersted may be obtained from the formula $10^{-22} N$, where N is the number of protons per ml (Wyard, 1965). However, the width varies considerably with the arrangement of the protons in the immediate neighborhood of the unpaired electron. The line is approximately Gaussian in shape. This is often the main contribution to line width, and there is no way to reduce it apart from the use of special techniques, such as ENDOR, described in chapter 2.

D. LINE WIDTH DUE TO g-VALUE ANISOTROPY

This is not a cause of broadening in single crystals, where the radicals are all oriented in the same direction and have the same g-value, which varies as the crystal is rotated in the magnetic field. (The situation in a single crystal is slightly more complicated when 'site-splitting' exists, but the lines from different sites can usually be resolved; this is discussed in chapter 4.) However, in polycrystalline samples all orientations are present, and the observed spectrum is a superposition of the spectra for all the different orientations. This usually results in a broad line with very little structure to be seen.

It follows from the resonance condition (equation (1.5)) that line width due to g-value anisotropy can be reduced by going to lower magnetic fields, and occasionally the resolution can be improved in this way. However, there is usually anisotropy of the hyperfine splitting also present, and this is unaffected by the magnitude of the magnetic field.

E. LINE WIDTH DUE TO INSTRUMENTAL CAUSES

These include inhomogeneity of the magnetic field, and distortion of the line shape by the spectrometer. This form of broadening can always be made smaller than those discussed previously.

F. THE RESULTANT LINE WIDTH

There is no universal rule for combining the contributions to the line width from all the different causes. The references cited in section 1.1 give rules applicable in certain cases; and the matter is discussed more generally by Hughes and MacDonald (1961). In practice, it generally happens that one form of line broadening is predominant, and the others can be neglected. As a very rough guide we may say that for single crystals of organic molecules the line width is of the order of 3 Oe; for materials with a high proton concentration, such as water and hydrogen peroxide, the line width is of the order of 10 Oe; and for polycrystalline materials of biological interest the line width is of the order of 20–30 Oe.

1.2.8   ESR IN LIQUIDS

Although we are primarily concerned with the solid state, we shall briefly consider ESR in liquids.   This is partly because of our interest in biological samples, which generally contain a large proportion of water, and partly because much of our knowledge of ESR spectra of radicals has come from studies of liquids.   In liquids, provided the radical is tumbling about rapidly enough, which is usually the case in a non-viscous solvent, the anisotropic parts of both the g-value and the hyperfine splitting are averaged out (Weissman, 1954).   The observed g factor is an average of the diagonal values of the g-tensor

$$< g > \ = \tfrac{1}{3}(g_1 + g_2 + g_3)$$ (1.38)

and the hyperfine splitting is simply that due to the Fermi contact term. Under suitable conditions very narrow lines are observed (less than 0.1 Oe wide), and very many hyperfine components (more than 100 in some cases).

1.2.9   RADICAL PAIRS AND RADICAL CLUSTERS

In a few materials radiation produces radicals in pairs or in clusters.   Provided the separation within the pair or cluster is not too large, these distributions give rise to a particular form of ESR spectrum from which the separation distance can be determined.   First observed in hydrogen peroxide glasses (Wyard, 1962), pairs have also been found in single crystals of potassium persulfate (Atkins, *et al.*, 1963) and in single crystals of dimethyl glyoxime and related molecules (Kurita, 1964; Kurita and Kashiwagi, 1966; Kashiwagi and Kurita, 1966).   Livingston (1966) has also found pairs in single crystals of hydrogen peroxide.   Clusters of radicals have been found in hydrogen peroxide glasses (Wyard, 1965).

The simplest case to consider is that of pairs of radicals trapped in a single crystal, in such a way that the separation is the same for all pairs and the axes of all pairs have the same orientation in the crystal.   From a classical point of view each radical is affected by the magnetic field from the other radical of the pair, which either adds to or subtracts from the external magnetic field H according as the unpaired electron is parallel or antiparallel to H.   The effect is to split each absorption line into a doublet.   A quantum-mechanical calculation gives the same result but with the doublet splitting increased by a factor 3/2 in the case where the magnetic centers are identical (see, e.g., Andrew, 1958).   In this case, the splitting is given by

$$D = 3\mu_0(3 \cos^2\theta - 1)/R^3$$ (1.39)

where R is the distance between the unpaired electrons in the pair and θ is the angle which the line joining them makes with the field H.   Putting in the constants, the maximum splitting, obtained when the pair axis is parallel to H, is

$$D = 5.57 \times 10^4 R^{-3} \text{ Oe} \qquad (1.40)$$

where R is in Å. If we take the minimum splitting which can be resolved as 1 Oe, the maximum observable separation is 38 Å. A beautiful spectrum of radical pairs is shown in Fig. 1.5 (from Kurita and Kashiwagi, 1966), in which the central group of lines M_1 is due to isolated radicals, the K_1 groups are due to pairs rather closer than 5 Å, and the K_2 groups are due to other pairs having a little greater separation.

Besides splitting the normal absorption line at $g = 2$ into a doublet, the existence of pairs also gives rise to a new absorption line at $g = 4$, known as a half-field line, due to a $\Delta M = 2$ transition.† The $\Delta M = 2$ transition can be intuitively understood by considering the two unpaired electrons to be linked by their magnetic fields (like a couple of compass needles) so that they form a single system with which an incoming microwave photon can interact. Thus one photon simultaneously flips over two spins, and must therefore have twice as much energy as for the normal $\Delta M = 1$ transition. Since ESR spectrometers operate at a fixed frequency, and since the energy needed to flip over an electron is proportional to the magnetic field strength, the transition is observed in practice at half-field, for which $g = 4$. The $\Delta M = 2$ transition is said to be 'forbidden', since to a first approximation the transition probability is zero. Intuitively, one can see that the closer the spins are together the greater will be the transition probability, since the stronger are the forces linking the two spins. A calculation shows that the transition probability for $\Delta M = 2$ relative to $\Delta M = 1$ is proportional to R^{-6}. In hydrogen peroxide glasses where the value of R averaged about 6 Å, the $\Delta M = 2$ line was about 1000 times less intense than the $\Delta M = 1$ line. Hence the half-field line will not be seen unless the radicals are quite close, and also there are a sufficient number of them to give a strong signal at $g = 2$. The $\Delta M = 2$ transition is much harder to saturate than the $\Delta M = 1$ (because the relaxation time is the same, while the transition probability is much less), so it may be possible to bring out the half-field line by increasing the microwave power. Care may be necessary to avoid confusion due to paramagnetic impurities which can also give weak lines around $g = 4$.

† Also referred to as a triplet state. This description is correct from the point of view of quantum mechanics, but could be misleading, since it suggests the triplet state familiar in chemistry in which two unpaired electrons are present in the same molecule. In the chemical case, the triplet state is usually an excited and short-lived state. With a pair of radicals the triplet state is as stable as the radicals themselves. In both cases, the ESR spectrum is similar in principle and includes a half-field line, but in practice the appearance of the spectrum is quite different.

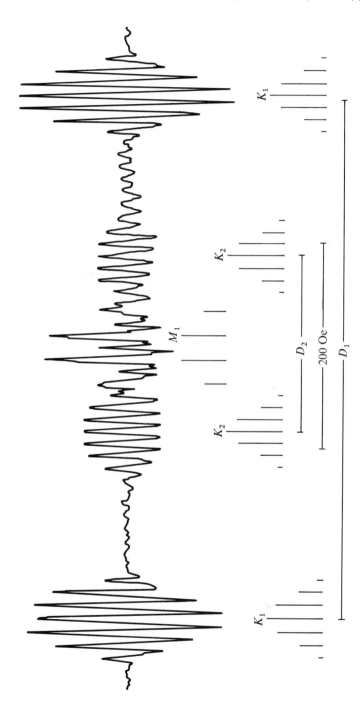

Fig. 1.5   Second derivative ESR spectrum of an X-irradiated single crystal of glyoxime at 77°K for the magnetic field at +35° from the a-axis in the ac plane.

In a powder or a glassy material, all possible orientations of the pair axis will be present.   Since the doublet splitting at $g = 2$ varies with the angle θ, as shown by equation (1.39), the spectrum of pairs of radicals trapped in glasses or powders is a line of a particular and calculable shape from which, in theory, the separation distance can be obtained.   In practical cases, g-value anisotropy and unresolved hyperfine splittings are likely to distort the line shape so that it will be difficult to estimate the separation with any accuracy.   The separation can still be obtained from the intensity of the half-field line, if it is detectable.

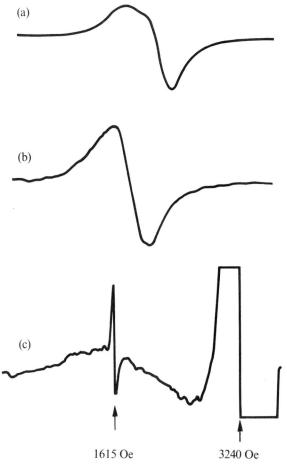

(a)

(b)

(c)

1615 Oe   3240 Oe

Fig. 1.6   50% w/w H_2O_2 in H_2O glassy sample at 77°K irradiated to 50 Mrad with 6 MeV electrons. (a) normal ESR spectrum; (b) half-field spectrum; (c) both spectra on one recording.

Clusters of radicals give rise to an absorption line at $g = 2$ of approximately Lorentzian shape. The local concentration within the cluster can be obtained from the line width (Wyard, 1965). There is a $g = 4$ line, whose intensity also gives the local concentration. There are also lines at $g = 6, 8, 10, \ldots$, but these are so weak that they are unlikely to be detectable. Figure 1.6 shows the $g = 2$ and $g = 4$ lines in a hydrogen peroxide glass. In trace C the spectrometer was swept continuously through both lines, resulting in gross overloading for the $g = 2$ line. The slight divergence of the $g = 4$ line from exactly half the field of the $g = 2$ line is due to g-value anisotropy.

1.3 SPECTROMETER DESIGN

Having discussed the main features of the ESR spectrum, we are now in a position to consider the design of the spectrometer. Since line width and hyperfine splitting are largely independent of the frequency, the choice of frequency is mainly determined by considerations of sensitivity and of practical convenience. However, when g-value anisotropy is present, measurement at a second frequency will give a different spectrum, which may assist in the interpretation. This is particularly the case when the sample is in a polycrystalline form, or when a single crystal is being studied which contains two or more radicals with overlapping spectra and different g-values.

Most ESR spectrometers operate at a frequency of 9000 MHz (free-space wavelength of 3 cm). The reasons for this choice are that the microwave components are readily available, the sample is of a convenient size (about 1 ml), magnets providing the required field of 3000 Oe, which must be uniform over the sample to within a fraction of an oersted, are also readily available, and good sensitivity can be obtained. If a measurement at another frequency is required, one generally uses 23,000 or 36,000 MHz, the choice of frequency being determined by the availability of components.

The simplest spectrometer one could imagine would consist of a source of radiation, a detector, and between the two a sample placed in a magnetic field. At microwave frequencies a klystron generator and crystal detector would be used, and the power conveyed along a waveguide. As the klystron frequency passed through the resonant frequency, the sample would absorb power, which could be recorded as a dip in the reading of a galvanometer connected to the crystal detector. This would result in an absorption spectrum as illustrated in Fig. 1.7(a).

It is more convenient to keep the klystron frequency constant and to vary the magnetic field, and this results in a similar spectrum, illustrated in Fig. 1.7(b).

It should be noted that the theory predicts the spectrum for a constant magnetic field, while most spectrometers record at a constant frequency. Since the spectra from free radicals are usually narrow compared to the central frequency, when the field is 3000 Oe or more, line widths and hyperfine splittings can be converted from a frequency to a magnetic field measurement by using the constant factor obtained from equation (1.4)

$$v/H = 2.8025 \text{ MHz Oe}^{-1}. \tag{1.41}$$

The change in the populations of the energy levels, due to the changing Boltzmann distribution, as the magnetic field is swept through the spectrum, is generally negligible, but could be significant in some cases.

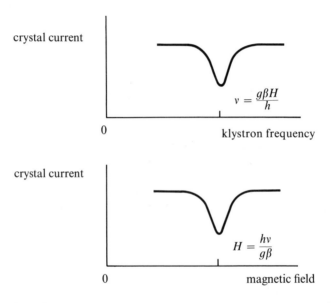

Fig. 1.7   Absorption spectra for (a) sweeping the frequency, (b) sweeping the field.

Such a simple spectrometer would have extremely poor sensitivity. To improve the sensitivity the sample is placed in a resonant cavity, and some form of narrow band amplification is used to reduce the noise from the crystal.   The main purpose of the cavity is to increase the amplitude of the microwave field H_1, since from equation (1.12) this increases the power absorbed by the sample.   It has the added advantage for a sample which has a high dielectric loss, such as an aqueous sample, that the maximum of the magnetic microwave field occurs at a node of the electric field, so that a sample placed there will have minimum loss.

There have been many descriptions of spectrometer design, and the optimum design varies considerably with the sample to be studied. Several aspects of design were discussed in a series of articles in *Laboratory Practice* of November, 1964. A simple spectrometer, which is easy to operate, has a sensitivity approaching the optimum, and is suitable for most studies of free radicals in solids, is shown in Fig. 1.8.

Power from a klystron is led into a cavity via a three-port circulator. The cavity has variable coupling to the waveguide, and this is adjusted with the sample in position so that the cavity is perfectly matched when the magnetic field is far from the resonance position. The slide screw is then adjusted so that sufficient power is reflected to the crystal to give the optimum signal-to-noise ratio. As the magnetic field is now swept through the

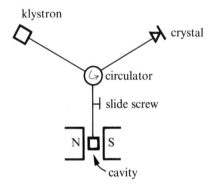

Fig. 1.8   Essential features of a micro-wave ESR spectrometer.

resonant position the sample absorbs power, upsetting the matching of the cavity, and altering the power incident on the crystal. Crystal detectors show excess noise at low frequencies, and in order to eliminate this the magnetic field is modulated at a high frequency, commonly 100 kHz, with an amplitude which is a fraction of the line width. The resultant signal from the crystal is amplified at 100 kHz with a narrow band system, and the spectrum is presented as the first derivative of the absorption curve. An automatic frequency control, not shown in the diagram, locks the klystron to the resonant frequency of the cavity. This reduces noise originating from the klystron, and also ensures that the spectrum is undistorted by any mixture of dispersion.

It was mentioned that the spectrometer usually presents the first derivative of the absorption curve. Of course, the absorption curve can be obtained by integration if required, but the first derivative is usually preferred because small differences of slope in the absorption curve are shown up, giving an apparent increase in resolution. The spectrometer can be arranged so that the second derivative is recorded, but this is used less often. For the sake of comparison, Fig. 1.9 shows a simple spectrum consisting of two Lorentzian lines with the separation between line centers equal to the line width, in all three presentations.

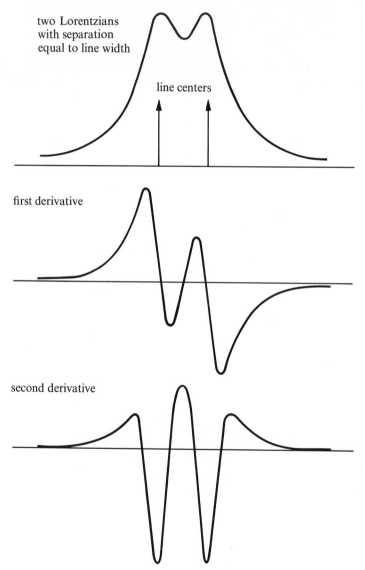

two Lorentzians
with separation
equal to line width

line centers

first derivative

second derivative

Fig. 1.9   Absorption spectrum and first and second derivatives for a Lorentzian doublet with splitting equal to the line width.

1.4 SENSITIVITY

For a spectrometer such as the one illustrated in Fig. 1.7, the theoretical limit of sensitivity is found by equating the absorption signal with the Johnson noise in the characteristic impedance of the waveguide. Calculations of this kind have been carried out by a number of authors (Bleaney and Stevens, 1953; Feher, 1957; Wilmshurst, Gambling, and Ingram, 1962). Bleaney and Stevens (1953) find that the minimum detectable value of χ'' is given by

$$\chi''_{\min} = \frac{V_{\text{eff}}}{\pi Q_0} \left(\frac{kT \, df}{P_a} \right)^{1/2} \tag{1.42}$$

V_{eff} is the 'effective volume' of the cavity, defined by the equation $V_{\text{eff}} = 1/H_s^2 \int_{\text{cavity}} H_1^2 \, dv$, where H_1 is the amplitude of the microwave magnetic field and H_s its value at the sample, the sample being assumed to be small.† Q_0 is the quality factor of the unloaded cavity. P_a is the power available from the oscillator; and df is the band width of the amplifier. From equations (1.9) and (1.13) we have $\chi'' = \chi_0 (v_0/\Delta v)$; $\chi_0 = N\mu^2/kT = N(g^2\beta^2/4kT)$, so for the minimum detectable number of spins

$$N_{\min} = \frac{4kT_{\text{sample}}}{g^2\beta^2} \left(\frac{\Delta v}{v_0} \right) \frac{V_{\text{eff}}}{\pi Q_0} \left(\frac{kT_{\text{detector}} \, df}{P_a} \right)^{1/2}. \tag{1.43}$$

The sensitivity of a spectrometer is often expressed as the minimum detectable number of spins, giving a signal equal to the noise, for a power of 1 mW, a bandwidth of 1 Hz, and a line width of 1 Oe at room temperature— probably because these are the conditions for which commercial spectrometers give their best performance. Putting the numerical values (values of V_{eff} and Q_0 are given in section 1.5) appropriate to such conditions into equation (1.43) we find $N_{\min} \simeq 7 \times 10^{10}$, for a frequency of 9 GHz. The use of a microwave circulator as shown in Fig. 1.5 increases the signal by a factor of 2 compared to earlier spectrometers which employed a magic tee (Faulkner, 1962); but with the best klystron, crystal, and amplifier the noise is some 5 times greater than the Johnson noise. Hence the minimum detectable number of spins for the conditions stated above is 2×10^{11}, with 5×10^{11} as a figure which should be achieved without too much difficulty. Commercial spectrometers are currently quoted as possessing a sensitivity

---

† Instead of V_{eff} some authors use the 'filling factor' η, defined by

$$\eta = \frac{\int_{\text{sample}} H_1^2 \, dv}{\int_{\text{cavity}} H_1^2 \, dv}.$$

For a small sample, over which H_1 may be taken as constant, $\eta = V_s/V_{\text{eff}}$, where V_s is the sample volume.

of 5×10^{10} spins under the above conditions except that the power is 200 mW; this corresponds to 7×10^{11} spins at 1 mW. It should be emphasized that the sensitivity figures apply for samples which are sufficiently small that they may be placed where the microwave H field is at a maximum, and are also 'lossless', i.e., do not absorb microwave power apart from the paramagnetic resonance absorption. The effect on sensitivity of using larger samples and 'lossy' samples is discussed in chapter 5.

If one wants better sensitivity than 5×10^{11} spins, one can look again at equation (1.43) to see what can be done. One is usually interested in measurements at a given temperature, so that T_{sample} cannot be reduced. The frequency of measurement occurs in the terms $(\Delta v/v_0)$ and V_{eff}/Q_0, and these combine to give $v^{-7/2}$, so going to a higher frequency would appear to be profitable. However, one is usually interested in the number of spins per unit volume, rather than in the detectable number of spins. The volume of sample which can be used is proportional to the volume of the cavity, i.e., to v^{-3}. Hence the gain with higher frequencies is reduced to $v^{-1/2}$; and even this is likely to be offset by poorer performance of the microwave components. An exception to this rule is when the sample volume is limited by other considerations, as, for example, the difficulty of growing single crystals, and is thus independent of frequency.

Another way of increasing the sensitivity is by increasing the microwave power. However, it is found that for the simple spectrometer of Fig. 1.7 there is little to be gained in increasing the power above about 10 mW, because of excess noise from the klystron. This difficulty can be avoided by more complicated design, and Teaney, et al. (1961) have described a spectrometer in which the power can be increased to 560 mW while the sensitivity remains only a factor of 3 below the theoretical maximum. A more fundamental limitation on the use of large powers comes from saturation. Equation (1.43) assumes that the sample is unsaturated. Free radicals, with their small spin-orbit coupling, usually saturate easily, and one often has to keep the power down to the order of a milliwatt to avoid distorting the line shape. It will be shown in the next section (equation (1.44)) that with samples that saturate, less power can be used at higher frequency; this results in N_{min} being proportional to $v^{-11/4}$ for samples of limited size, and to $v^{1/4}$ when the size is not limited.

Reducing the bandwidth of the amplifier will also improve the sensitivity, according to equation (1.43), but again it is found that for a simple spectrometer reduction much below 1 Hz often brings in extra noise (because of excess noise at very low frequencies) so that the hoped for improvement is not realized. Klein and Barton (1963) have described a way round this difficulty by averaging a large number of rapid scans of the spectrum. In this way they have improved the sensitivity by one or two orders of magnitude, and the only limitation appears to be the time one is prepared to spend on the recording.   With a bandwidth of 1 Hz, one generally requires a few minutes to record a spectrum without distortion.   The time required is proportional to the square of increase in sensitivity, so for an increase of 100 each spectrum will need a few weeks to record.

Finally, we enquire whether the sensitivity can be improved by a different detector.   Equation (1.43) already assumes a perfect detector; however, if the temperature of the cavity and waveguide were reduced below room temperature, and the effective temperature of the detector reduced by using a maser, for example, a significant improvement should be possible.   Townes (1960) has described a method where a maser is put in the same cavity as the sample, which should give even greater sensitivity. This technique does not seem to have been tried out yet.   A significant improvement in sensitivity towards the value given by equation (1.43) (but not going beyond this value) can be obtained by using a low-noise pre-amplifier before the crystal detector.   Gambling and Wilmshurst (1963) used a maser as pre-amplifier and improved the sensitivity of a 23 GHz spectrometer by a factor of 3.   Hollocher, *et al.* (1964) used a parametric amplifier as pre-amplifier and improved the sensitivity of a 9 GHz spectrometer also by a factor of 3.   In a different approach, Livingston and Zeldes (1966) replaced the standard crystal detector by a backward diode and improved the sensitivity by a factor of 2 at 9 GHz.

The conclusion of this lengthy analysis is that for most samples the best sensitivity is obtained at 9 GHz and that any improvement on 5×10^{11} ΔH spins at 1 mW and 1 second time constant, where ΔH is the line width in oersted, can only be had at considerable cost.   It should also be noted that to obtain a well resolved spectrum one requires considerably more spins than the detectable minimum.

We have not considered lossy samples so far, and water, which has a high dielectric loss, is obviously of great importance in biological studies. It can be shown (see chapters 5 and 8 for fuller discussions) that with a lossy sample the greatest sensitivity is obtained when the volume of the sample is chosen so that the cavity Q is reduced by one-third, and that at 9 GHz the corresponding volume of water is a few hundredths of a ml, resulting in a considerable loss of sensitivity.   Dielectric losses in water are reduced at lower frequencies, but it still turns out that the best sensitivity is obtained at 9 GHz.   However, there may be a case for going to lower frequencies when a biological sample is larger than a few hundredths of a ml.

1.5 SATURATION MEASUREMENTS

In this section we describe saturation measurements which can be made using a simple spectrometer such as that shown in Fig. 1.8.   Other, and possibly better, methods will be found described in the references given in section 1.1. However, these require more apparatus; and in free radical studies one's only interest in saturation is usually to avoid it. Sometimes an approximate measure of saturation will help to identify a radical, or will distinguish two radicals whose spectra overlap. For these purposes the method described here is adequate.

The method consists in recording the spectrum with a series of increasing microwave powers, until the sample becomes saturated. The height of the absorption curve (obtained from the first derivative by integration if necessary) is proportional to $\chi''\sqrt{P}$ (Bleaney and Stevens, 1953) where P is the power entering the cavity. Hence, if the absorption signal is plotted against $\sqrt{P}$, one obtains a straight line at low powers, where saturation is negligible, and the departure of the plot from this straight line is a measure of the saturation. With the spectrometer of Fig. 1.6, P is simply the power in the waveguide, since the cavity is matched to the guide; and the power can be measured with a bolometer. At very low powers, a correction may be required for the power reflected by the screw.

Under conditions of saturation χ'' is reduced, and it is convenient to define the 'experimental saturation factor' Z', as the ratio of χ'' at a given power level to the value in the absence of saturation; the measurements being made at the center of the absorption line. The value of Z' can be obtained from the graph mentioned above. When $Z' = 0.5$ the sample is said to be 50% saturated.

The theoretical discussion of saturation showed that Z' should depend on the amplitude H_1 of the microwave field (equation (1.21)). This is related to the power entering the cavity by the relation

$$H_1{}^2 = \frac{4PQ_0}{v_0 V_{\text{eff}}}$$ (1.44)

(Bleaney and Stevens, 1953). Q_0 is the unloaded Q with the sample in position, and can be measured by determining the half power points of the reflected power when the klystron frequency is varied, using the relationship

$$Q_0 = 2 \times \text{loaded } Q = \frac{2v_0}{\Delta v}.$$ (1.45)

For a rectangular H_{01} cavity of any number of half wavelengths, which is the most commonly used shape,

$$V_{\text{eff}} = \frac{1 + (d/a)^2}{4} V_c$$ (1.46)

where V_c is the actual cavity volume, d is the half-wavelength ($\lambda_g/2$) and a

is the height of the cavity. Putting in typical values for a cavity tuned to 9 GHz, with $Q_0 = 7000$, we find

$$H_1 = 0.079\sqrt{P} \tag{1.47}$$

where P is the power in milliwatts, and H_1 is measured in oersted. Thus from the saturation measurements we can obtain $H_{1/2}$, the amplitude of the microwave field which produces 50% saturation.

Since the height of the absorption curve is proportional to $\chi''\sqrt{P}$, which is also proportional to $Z'H_1$, then if Z' behaves according to equation (1.21) a saturation curve of the type we have discussed should rise to maximum, and then fall again to zero. Furthermore, in this case

$$H_{1/2} = 2/\gamma(T_1 T_2)^{1/2}. \tag{1.48}$$

The line shape should be Lorentzian, so that T_2, which was defined as $\frac{1}{2}f(v - v_0)$ is equal to $1/\pi\,\Delta v$, or $2/\gamma\,\Delta H$. This gives an expression for the spin-lattice relaxation time

$$T_1 = \frac{2\,\Delta H}{\gamma H_{1/2}^2}. \tag{1.49}$$

Portis (1953) discovered that in some cases the absorption signal did not decrease for large power, as the simple theory predicts, but tended instead to a constant value. This led him to distinguish between line width due to 'homogeneous broadening' where all the spins in the sample saturate together, and due to 'inhomogeneous broadening' where the absorption line is an envelope of a number of lines of much smaller width, each due to one 'spin packet'. The spin packets have little or no interaction with each other. Interactions such as spin-lattice relaxation and dipolar interaction between like spins, which affect all the spins equally, give homogeneous broadening; but unresolved hyperfine interactions and g-value variations, which produce spin packets with different resonant frequencies, give inhomogeneous broadening.

Free radicals in solid samples generally show some degree of inhomogeneous broadening, since the line width is often largely due to unresolved hyperfine interactions. The behavior is generally intermediate between the two cases considered by Portis which were (a) pure homogeneous broadening and (b) the case where the line width is almost entirely due to causes which produce inhomogeneous broadening. For the intermediate case T_1 cannot be obtained directly from the saturation measurements. Castner (1959) gives a method whereby T_1 can be obtained in this case, provided there is sufficient power to produce a high degree of saturation.

There are some precautions to observe when making saturation measurements of this kind. The sample should be located at the position of maximum microwave field. For a large sample, where this is not possible, corrections are given by Castner (1959). Any dielectric material in the cavity, e.g., a sample holder, will distort the microwave field and cause H_1 to differ from the value given by equation (1.44) (so-called 'lens effect'). This effect can be checked by observing the change in the signal when the dielectric is removed, since in the absence of saturation the signal is proportional to H_1. The effect can be quite large; for example, a quartz dewar was found to increase H_1 by a factor of 2. The discussion of saturation given above assumes a steady state (so-called 'slow passage'). If the sample is brought into saturation conditions in a time comparable with T_1, the equations are altered. This can happen with the spectrometer of Fig. 1.7, because modulation of the magnetic field brings the sample in and out of resonance. The condition for slow passage is

$$\omega_m H_m < H_1/T_1 \tag{1.50}$$

where ω_m and H_m are the angular frequency and amplitude of the magnetic field. Thus fast passage effects can always be avoided by keeping H_m small. Finally we mention that some discussions of saturation in the literature contain expressions and equations apparently differing from those given here. This is mainly because different authors use different definitions for the terms V_{eff}, Q, H_1, and ΔH. It is believed that the expressions given here are correct, and consistent with the definitions employed.

REFERENCES

Abragam, A., 1961, *The Principles of Nuclear Magnetism* (Oxford: Clarendon Press).

Andrew, E. R., 1958, *Nuclear Magnetic Resonance* (Cambridge: University Press).

Atkins, P. W., Symons, M. C. R., and Trevalion, P. A., 1963, *Proc. chem. Soc.*, 222.

Bleaney, B., and Stevens, K. W. H., 1953, *Rep. Prog. Phys.*, 16, 108–59.

Blois, M. S., Jr., Brown, H. W., Lemmon, R. M., Lindblom, R. O., and Weissbluth, M., 1961, *Free Radicals in Biological Systems* (New York: Academic Press).

Blois, M. S., Jr., Brown, H. W., and Maling, J. E., 1961, *Free Radicals in Biological Systems* (New York: Academic Press), p. 117.

Breit, G., and Rabi, I. I., 1931, *Phys. Rev.*, 38, 2082–3.

Castner, T. G., Jr., 1959, *Phys. Rev.*, 115, 1506–15.

Cohen, E. R., and Du Mond, J. W. M., 1965, *Rev. mod. Phys.*, 37, 537–94.

Davidson, N., *Statistical Mechanics* (New York: McGraw-Hill Book Company, Inc.).

Faulkner, E. A., 1962, *J. scient. Instrum.*, **39**, 135.
Feher, G., 1957, *Bell Syst. tech. J.*, **36**, 449–84.
Gambling, W. A., and Wilmshurst, T. H., 1963, *Phys. Lett.*, **5**, 228–9.
Hollocher, T. S., From, W. H., and Bromberg, N. S., 1964, *Physics Med. Biol.*, **9**, 65–72.
Hughes, D. G., and MacDonald, D. K. C., 1961, *Proc. phys. Soc.*, **78**, 75–80.
Ingram, D. J. E., 1958, *Free Radicals as Studied by Electron Spin Resonance* (London: Butterworth).
Jen, C. K., Foner, S. N., Cochran, E. L., and Bowers, V. A., 1958, *Phys. Rev.*, **112**, 1169–82.
Känzig, W., and Cohen, M. H., 1959, *Phys. Rev. Lett.*, **3**, 509–10.
Känzig, W., 1962, *J. Phys. Chem. Solids*, **23**, 479–99.
Kashiwagi, M., and Kurita, Y., 1966, *J. phys. Soc. Japan*, **21**, 558–9.
Klein, M. P., and Barton, G. W., Jr., 1963, *Rev. scient. Instrum.*, **34**, 754–9.
Kurita, Y., 1964, *J. chem. Phys.*, **41**, 3926–7.
Kurita, Y., and Kashiwagi, M., 1966, *J. chem. Phys.*, **44**, 1727–8.
Laboratory Practice, Special Number: Electron Spin Resonance, Nov. 1964.
Livingston, R., 1966, *Nucl. Sci. Ser. natn. Res. Coun.*, **43**, 3–16.
Livingston, R., and Zeldes, H., 1966, *J. chem. Phys.*, **44**, 1245–59.
McConnell, H. M., and Robertson, R. E., 1957, *J. phys. Chem.*, **61**, 1018.
Nafe, J. E., and Nelson, E. B., 1948, *Phys. Rev.*, **73**, 718–28.
Pake, G. E., 1962, *Paramagnetic Resonance* (New York: W. A. Benjamin Inc.).
Portis, A. M., 1953, *Phys. Rev.*, **91**, 1071–8.
Schonland, D. S., 1959, *Proc. phys. Soc.*, **73**, 788–92.
Segal, B. G., Kaplan, M., and Fraenkel, G. K., 1965, *J. chem. Phys.*, **43**, 4191–200.
Smith, R. C., and Wyard, S. J., 1961, *J. chem. Phys.*, **35**, 2254–5.
Sommerfield, C. M., 1957, *Phys. Rev.*, **107**, 328–9.
Stone, A. J., 1963a, *Molec. Phys.*, **6**, 509–15; 1963b, ibid., **7**, 311–6.
Teaney, D. T., Klein, M. P., and Portis, A. M., 1961, *Rev. scient. Instrum.*, **32**, 721–9.
Townes, C. H., 1960, *Phys. Rev. Lett.*, **5**, 428–30.
Ward, R. L., and Weissman, S. I., 1954, *J. Amer. chem. Soc.*, **76**, 3612.
Weissman, S. I., 1954, *J. chem. Phys.*, **22**, 1378–9.
Wilkinson, D. T., and Crane, H. R., 1963, *Phys. Rev.*, **130**, 852–63.
Wilmshurst, T. H., Gambling, W. A., and Ingram, D. J. E., 1962, *J. Electron. Control*, **13**, 339–60.
Wyard, S. J., 1962, *Proc. XIth Colloque Ampère*, 388–92; 1965, *Proc. phys. Soc.*, **86**, 587–93.
Zavoisky, E., 1945, *J. Phys. U.S.S.R.*, **9**, 211.

CHAPTER TWO

DOUBLE RESONANCE TECHNIQUES IN BIOLOGICAL APPLICATIONS OF MAGNETIC RESONANCE

J. M. Baker

The Clarendon Laboratory, Oxford, England

2.1 INTRODUCTION

In this section we shall discuss two closely related techniques, electron nuclear double resonance (ENDOR) (Feher, 1956) and nuclear magnetic resonance (NMR) which is enhanced by dynamic nuclear polarization (Overhauser, 1953; Jeffries, 1963). Both of these techniques involve simultaneous excitation of electron and nuclear magnetic resonance, and they are used in systems in which there are unpaired electrons which can interact with the nuclei which have a magnetic moment. Such an interaction between electron and nucleus gives rise to hyperfine structure. We shall give first a qualitative discussion of hyperfine structure before describing the experimental techniques and what can be learned from them.

2.2 HYPERFINE STRUCTURE

Hyperfine structure arises from the interaction of two magnetic moments, one belonging to the nucleus (μ_n) which has relatively small spatial distribution ($r \sim 10^{-12}$ cm), and one belonging to the electron (μ_e) which is distributed over the whole atom ($r \sim 10^{-8}$ cm). The energy of interaction between the two magnetic moments may be written down using standard electromagnetic theory if one divides the electron magnetic moment into small elements $d\mu_e$ occupying a small region of space. The interaction energy between the nucleus and one of these small elements is then integrated over the electron distribution.

$$W_I = \int \frac{\mu_n \cdot d\mu_e}{r^3} - \int \frac{3(\mu_n \cdot \mathbf{r})(\mathbf{r} \cdot d\mu_e)}{r^5}. \qquad (2.1)$$

It is often more helpful pictorially to use one of two other ways of looking at the interaction. First, one can think in terms of the magnetic field $\mathbf{H}_e$ set up at the nucleus by the unpaired electron, when the interaction energy is:

$$W_I = -\mu_n \cdot \mathbf{H}_e. \qquad (2.2)$$

Second, one can think in terms of a sort of average magnetic field $\mathbf{H}_n$ set up by the nucleus and experienced by the electron's magnetic moment, so that the interaction energy is:

$$W_I = -\mu_e \cdot \mathbf{H}_n. \qquad (2.3)$$

As these three expressions all describe the same interaction they are all equal.

Of these three descriptions the second is the most useful for discussing the differences between contributions from different types of electron wave function. Any wave function can be decomposed into contributions from s-electron wave functions, p-electron wave functions and so on; and one can also decompose $\mathbf{H}_e$ into the contributions from each type of wave function.

The s-electron wave function is spherically symmetric, and there is no orbital angular momentum for the spin to couple to; so that the spin and the magnetic moment are free to orient in any direction. The distribution of electron magnetic moment can be divided into uniformly magnetized spherical shells. The magnetic field at the center of a uniformly magnetized shell is zero, so the only contribution to H_e comes from the part of the wave function which is inside the nucleus. Because of the spherical symmetry and the freedom of the electron spin to orient in any direction, H_e always has the same magnitude and the hyperfine structure is isotropic.

p-Electrons have a small electron density at the nucleus, so that there is little contribution to H_e from the part of the wave function inside the nucleus; but they are not isotropically distributed in space, so there is a resultant magnetic field $H_e \sim \mu_e \langle r^{-3} \rangle$ where $\langle r^{-3} \rangle$ is the average value of r^{-3} taken over the electron wave function. Chemical combination, or the strong electrostatic crystal field effects in an ionic solid, often hold the p-orbits in definite orientations in a molecule or crystal, so that μ_e and hence H_e is a function of the direction of the applied magnetic field H_0. In this case, the hyperfine structure is anisotropic. In some kinds of molecular orbitals which have contributions from both s- and p-electrons, there is both an isotropic and an anisotropic component of the hyperfine structure.

In the ESR literature, the various contributions to the energy of the quantum states of the paramagnetic center are described by the spin-Hamiltonian (Pake, 1962a). In this spin-Hamiltonian, the hyperfine structure is described in terms of the quantum numbers S and I by a term

$$\mathscr{H} = A S \cdot I. \tag{2.4}$$

This is equivalent to equations (2.1)–(2.3), and $A = \mu_n H_e / J$. If the hyperfine structure is anisotropic, the spin-Hamiltonian becomes:

$$\mathscr{H} = A_z S_z I_z + A_x S_x I_x + A_y S_y I_y$$

where x, y, and z are principal directions in the molecule or crystal.

For most of the following, we shall continue to describe the hyperfine structure in terms of H_e. For most nuclei of paramagnetic ions, H_e is greater than the typical external fields H_0 (3 kOe for X-band) used for ESR. For nuclei of paramagnetic molecules or of the ligands of paramagnetic ions, H_e may be comparable to or less than H_0.

In the field H_e, the nuclear spin I is allowed $2I + 1$ orientations corresponding to the values of $\langle I_z \rangle = I, I - 1, I - 2, \ldots, -I$. Writing $\mu_n = g_n \beta I$ the interaction energy is:

$$-g_n \beta H_e \cdot I = -g_n \beta H_e \langle I_z \rangle. \tag{2.5}$$

Take as an example an electron with $S = \frac{1}{2}$ and a nucleus with $I = \frac{3}{2}$. In the external field $\mathbf{H}_0$ the electron has energy

$$-\boldsymbol{\mu}_e \cdot \mathbf{H}_0 = g\beta\mathbf{S} \cdot \mathbf{H}_0 = g\beta H_0 \langle S_z \rangle. \tag{2.6}$$

There is also a similar term for the energy of the nuclear magnetic moment in the external field

$$-\boldsymbol{\mu}_n \cdot \mathbf{H}_0 = -g_n\beta\mathbf{I} \cdot \mathbf{H}_0 = -g_n\beta H_0 \langle I_z \rangle \tag{2.7}$$

but this can often be neglected as being small compared with the other two terms. For $\langle S_z \rangle = +\frac{1}{2}$ there are four energy levels corresponding to the four values of $\langle I_z \rangle$ as shown in Fig. 2.1. There are also four levels for $\langle S_z \rangle = -\frac{1}{2}$ but their order is reversed as the inversion of the electron spin reverses the direction of H_e, and we have assumed that $H_e > H_0$. Electron paramagnetic resonance occurs with selection rules $\Delta S_z = \pm 1$, $\Delta I_z = 0$, so that there are four (in general, $2I + 1$) allowed transitions. It is the

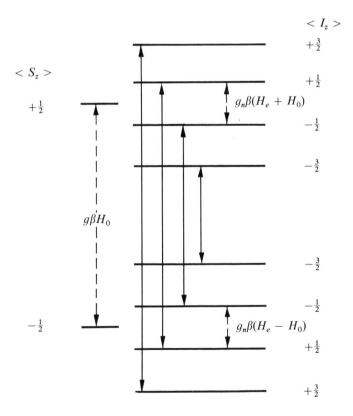

Fig. 2.1   Energy levels of a system with $S = \frac{1}{2}$, $I = \frac{3}{2}$ at constant H_0, showing the allowed ESR transitions.

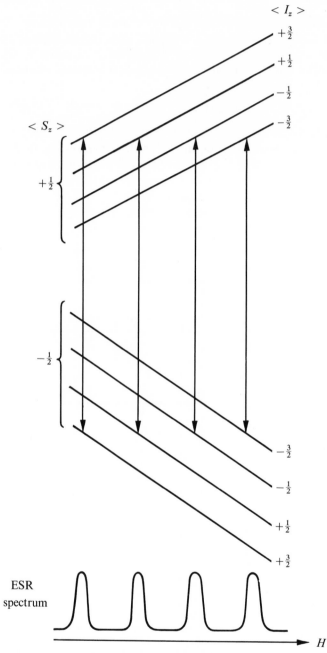

Fig. 2.2   Energy levels of a system with $S = \frac{1}{2}$, $I = \frac{3}{2}$ as a function of field H, and the allowed ESR transitions.

splitting up of the ESR line into $2I + 1$ components which is known as hyperfine structure. Although it is in principle possible to scan through an ESR spectrum as a function of frequency at constant external magnetic field H_0, it is usual to maintain a constant frequency and vary the magnetic field. In Fig. 2.2 we show the energy levels for the above example as a function of magnetic field H_0, and the four-line hyperfine structure one observes for a constant microwave frequency. The lines are, to a first approximation, equally spaced.

The splitting up of the ESR lines into $2I + 1$ components may be viewed in terms of the field H_n set up by the nucleus. The resonance condition for the ESR is

$$hv = g\beta H. \qquad (2.8)$$

But **H** is made up of two components, the applied field $\mathbf{H}_0$ and the field $\mathbf{H}_n$.†

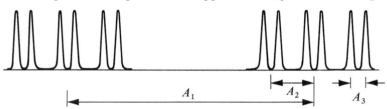

Fig. 2.3   Imaginary hyperfine structure for an electron interacting with three nuclei, two with $I = \frac{1}{2}$ and one with $I = 1$.

There are $2I + 1$ different values of H_n corresponding to the different values of $\langle I_z \rangle$, so that there are $2I + 1$ different values of H_0 for which equation (2.8) can be satisfied.

Often the electron is in an orbital where it interacts with several nuclei. For example, the unpaired electron in a molecule may interact with several of its nuclei because it moves in a molecular orbital on these nuclei (Staff of Varian Associates, 1960b); also in a paramagnetic salt the electrons of a paramagnetic ion usually interact with the several ligand nuclei (Griffith, *et al.*, 1953; Owen, 1955; Owen and Thornley, 1966). Each nucleus gives rise to its own hyperfine structure, the hyperfine components from one nucleus being split up by those from all of the others. In equation (2.8) $H = H_0 + \sum H_n$, the sum being taken over all nuclei. Figure 2.3 shows, for example, the hyperfine structure for interaction with three nuclei, of which numbers 1 and 3 have $I = \frac{1}{2}$ and number 2 has $I = 1$. In the figure we have labelled the hyperfine structure separations in terms of the spin-Hamiltonian parameter A which is usually used to describe the interaction in the ESR literature.

† Or more correctly its component in the direction of $\mathbf{H}_0$. As $H_0 >> H_n$, the component of the H_n perpendicular to H_0 makes little contribution to the magnitude of $\mathbf{H}_0 + \mathbf{H}_n$.

Sometimes, several of the nuclei with which an electron may interact are equivalent, e.g., the three protons in a CH_3 group. The proton has $I = \frac{1}{2}$ so the hyperfine structure comprises two lines. Figure 2.4(a) shows the hyperfine structure due to interaction with one of the protons only. The

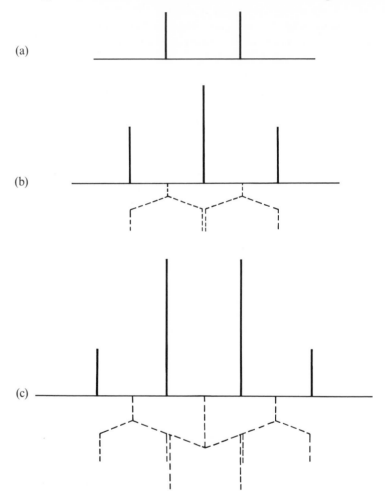

Fig. 2.4   Hyperfine structure for (a) one proton, (b) two equivalent protons, (c) three equivalent protons.

interaction with the second proton splits each of these components into a two-component hyperfine structure. As the line separation for each of the protons is the same, the two central lines are coincident, leading to the pattern shown in Fig. 2.4(b). Interaction with the third proton splits up each of the lines in Fig. 2.4(b) into two components.   The equality of the separations again causes coincidences leading to the pattern shown in Fig. 2.4(c).   This argument can be extended to derive the hyperfine structure pattern for any number n of equivalent protons.   The lines are always equally spaced by the hyperfine structure interval of an individual proton, and the intensities of the lines vary from one end of the pattern to the other as the binomial coefficients $_nC_r$, where r varies from 1 to n.

2.3   LINE WIDTH AND STRUCTURE

Even if the electron does not move in an orbital on neighboring nuclei, the dipolar fields enable it to interact with these nuclei.   More distant nuclei have smaller interactions, so the hyperfine line separation is smaller.   Also at greater distances there are more equivalent nuclei, so the hyperfine structure pattern contains more lines.   Eventually, at sufficient distance the hyperfine structure gets lost in the line width.   Sometimes even the structure from the nearest nuclei is lost in the line width.   ESR lines comprising a large number of unresolved hyperfine components are quite common and have been given the name 'inhomogeneous' (Portis, 1953).   It is worth noting that each component of the unresolved structure corresponds to the resonance of an electron in a different field H, and therefore arises from a different atom in the specimen.   If the ESR of one of these atoms were observable it would be a very much sharper line than the ESR line from all of the atoms.   Sometimes, because of other line broadening mechanisms, such as for example rapid spin-lattice relaxation, or rapid random rotation in liquids, the ESR lines from individual atoms are no narrower than the ESR line from all of the atoms.   In this case, the latter does not comprise a lot of narrow unresolved lines; this sort of line is called 'homogeneous' (Portis, 1953).

Often one would like to resolve the hyperfine structure which makes up an inhomogeneous line.   This cannot be done using conventional ESR for the obvious reason that the hyperfine components are not resolved.   However, it often can be done using ENDOR.

The ESR and ENDOR spectra of liquids and solids are rather different, and hence are better discussed separately.   In a single crystal, the paramagnetic ions are usually similarly oriented, so that any anisotropy of the hyperfine structure can be studied by varying the direction in which H_0 is applied.   In a polycrystalline solid, all orientations of H_0 with respect to the crystal axes are observed at once, so that one sees an averaged spectrum. The isotropic components give a spectrum similar to that in a single crystal, but the anisotropic components contribute to the line width.   For this reason, little ESR has been done in powders; the lines are usually too wide to give much information.   The situation in a liquid is similar to that in a powder in that the orientation of different molecules or paramagnetic complexes is random, but is different in that the molecules undergo random rotational Brownian motion.   If this motion is rapid enough, the ESR line becomes narrow (Pake, 1962b): the criterion for motional narrowing being that the correlation frequency of rotation v_c has to be greater than the anisotropic frequency broadening Δv, in which case the observed line width $\delta v \sim (\Delta v)^2/v_c$.   Hence the broadening effect of the anisotropic hyperfine structure is washed out and only the isotropic component of the hyperfine structure contributes to the line positions.

For these reasons, lines in liquids tend to be homogeneous while in most solids the lines are inhomogeneous.   This makes the discussion of ENDOR rather different for the two cases.

2.4   ENDOR IN SOLIDS

As ENDOR was first performed in solids, and most of the experiments so far performed have been in solids, we shall discuss them first.

We shall illustrate the technique, which was invented by Dr. G. Feher (1956), with a system with $S = \frac{1}{2}$ and $I = \frac{1}{2}$, whose energy levels and transitions are illustrated in Fig. 2.5.   ESR looks at transitions a and b, and if they are resolved A can be measured by finding ΔH.

One can also measure A by observing the transitions c and d for which $\Delta S_z = 0, \Delta I_z = \pm 1$.   These transitions constitute NMR in the field H_e† at frequency $v = g_n \beta H_e/h = \frac{1}{2}A/h$.   They are normally too weak to measure. The weakness does not arise from the difficulty of causing the transitions, but rather because the detection sensitivity is low, and because dilute material (10^{18} spins/ml) has to be used in order to obtain narrow lines. These transitions can be detected by a double resonance technique, which is the basis of ENDOR.

The strength of the ESR line a, for example, depends upon the relative populations of the levels 1 and 4.   If one excites either of the transitions c or d one disturbs the populations of either 1 or 4, and the size of the ESR signal changes.   To observe this effect, one maintains a steady magnetic field H_0 and a steady microwave frequency v_0, and one searches for the ENDOR by varying the frequency of a second r.f. field at the specimen until the ESR signal level changes.

The advantage of ENDOR over ESR in solids lies in the much smaller line width.   As one works at fixed frequency v_0 and fixed magnetic field H_0,

† Strictly, the effect of expression (2.7) should be included, so that transition c is in a field $H_e + H_0$ and transition d is in a field $H_e - H_0$, so that they occur at different frequencies, from which both the value of H_e and that of μ_n can be calculated.

the only atoms undergoing ESR are those which experience a total field H such that

$$h\nu_0 = g\beta H = g\beta(H_0 + \sum H_n) \tag{2.9}$$

where the sum is taken over all of the nuclei.   Only one of the unresolved hyperfine components is 'on resonance', and the others are unaffected,

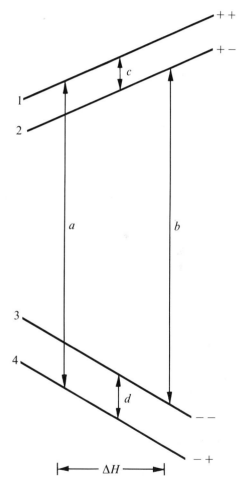

Fig. 2.5   Energy levels for a system with $S = \frac{1}{2}$, $I = \frac{1}{2}$. Levels have been labelled $++$, etc., the first sign being that of $\langle S_z \rangle$ and the second that of $\langle I_z \rangle$.

except by spin diffusion.† In some specimens this selection of one particular component, or 'spin packet' as it has been called by Portis (1953), can be demonstrated experimentally by 'burning a hole' in the ESR line. Saturation of an ESR line decreases its intensity, and when the microwave power is reduced to well below the saturation level the intensity recovers in a time of the order of the spin-lattice relaxation time T_1. Saturation of one hyperfine component of an inhomogeneous line decreases the size of that component without changing the size of the rest of the ESR line. If the whole ESR line is scanned within a time T_1 of saturating the one spin packet, one can observe the decreased intensity of that spin packet as shown in Fig. 2.6. The spin packet may be only a few kHz wide, compared with the width of the ESR line which is usually a few MHz or more. As only one

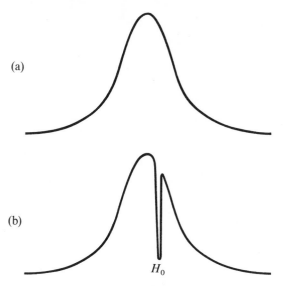

(a)

(b)

H_0

Fig. 2.6   (a) ESR line before saturation of the spin packet at H_0. (b) ESR line observed in a time less than T_1 after prolonged saturation of the spin packet at H_0.

† There are several ways in which the energy of orientation of a spin in the field H_0 can change. In addition to spin-lattice relaxation in which the energy of an electronic transition is radiated into the thermal energy of the lattice, there are more rapid spin-spin interactions in which the energy lost in one electronic transition is absorbed by a neighboring electron. This process goes on most rapidly when energy is conserved, so that both electrons have to have identical ESR frequencies for the energy emitted by one to be absorbed exactly by the other, i.e., they have to be in the same spin packet. A similar process which nearly conserves energy occurs more slowly when the spin-spin interaction is between spins in neighboring spin packets. The latter process allows the saturation of one spin packet to spread out slowly to the neighboring spin packets. This process is known as spin diffusion (Feher and Gere, 1959).

spin packet is saturated in an ENDOR experiment, the resultant lines have the width of the spin packet. Hence the resolution of an ENDOR experiment may be three orders of magnitude better than an ESR experiment.

In case this sounds too much of a panacea, it should be pointed out that the increased resolution is purchased at the expense of spectral complexity. Each neighboring nucleus gives its own spectrum. These can be recognized through differences in nuclear spin; the number of expected equivalent nuclei; the variation of the spectrum as a function of the direction of H_0; the size of the interaction, as this is expected to decrease with distance. However, to make a complete analysis of a complicated spectrum one has to have a good knowledge of the crystal or molecular structure.

A nice example of the application of this technique has been given by Feher (1956) for donor impurities in silicon crystals. The wave function of the additional unpaired electron spreads out a long way and interacts with many neighbors. Measurement of the Si^{29} ENDOR enabled the wave function to be mapped out to several lattice spacings from the donor nucleus.

It would presumably be information of this sort which would be of most value to the biological and medical fields. Some ENDOR work has been done on irradiated succinic acid (Cole, *et al.*, 1961). The measurement of H_e at nuclei which are neighbors of an unpaired electron can be interpreted in terms of admixtures of unpaired *s*- and *p*-electron wave functions on these nuclei, the isotropic part of the H_e giving the *s*-electron contribution and the anisotropic part the *p*-electron contribution. Such information for all of the neighboring nuclei enables one to build up a complete wave function of the unpaired electron. For example, it is known that the hyperfine structure due to one unpaired 1*s*-electron on a hydrogen nucleus is 506 Oe, so that a measured isotropic hyperfine structure of x oersted can be interpreted as a spin density of $(x/506)\%$ 1*s* character on the H nucleus. Any admixture of 2*s*- or higher *s*-electron wave functions invalidates this conclusion and needs more careful calculation.

2.5   ENDOR IN LIQUIDS

It is even more likely that information of the type discussed in the last paragraph would be valuable for free radicals in liquid specimens. Here, because of the motional narrowing, the ESR lines are homogeneous, and the ENDOR lines would have the same width as the ESR lines, typically 100 kHz. Only a few cases have so far been reported in the literature of ENDOR in a liquid (Hyde and Maki, 1964; Hyde, 1965).

The short electron spin-lattice relaxation times T_1 in liquids necessitate large r.f. magnetic fields to induce the nuclear transitions in a time short compared with T_1. Hence, for example, Hyde and Maki (1964) have used a pulse technique so that the r.f. field is switched on for a short time only and the heating associated with high c.w. r.f. power is reduced.

There are two main advantages which might be gained over ESR by using ENDOR in a liquid.

First, for an electron interacting with several nuclei the ENDOR spectrum is likely to be less complex than the ESR spectrum, hence ENDOR may be helpful when the ESR spectrum is difficult to elucidate. Each nucleus in the molecule gives rise to two ENDOR lines, one due to resonance at $H_0 + H_e$ and one at $H_0 - H_e$: these are equally disposed about the free NMR frequency in the field H_0, so that the nature of the nucleus is easily recognized. Suppose one had a molecule with five inequivalent protons. The ENDOR spectrum would comprise ten lines, five at greater and five at lesser frequencies than the free proton resonance. The ESR spectrum would comprise $2^5 = 32$ lines near $g = 2$ with much greater overlap and possibility of confusion. As the number of nuclei is increased the ESR spectrum rapidly becomes much more complex than the ENDOR spectrum. Also, in the ESR spectrum hyperfine structure lines due to different types of nuclei are superimposed, whereas the ENDOR spectra are at different frequencies because different nuclei have different NMR frequencies. Hence, although the line width is no less in the ENDOR spectrum the simpler spectrum might make interpretation easier.

The second possible advantage might be used when several molecular species have overlapping spectra, so that one observes a broad line without resolved structure. This is like the inhomogeneous lines in a solid so that ENDOR can still be performed on the various nuclei. A difficulty here would be that one could measure a variety of hyperfine coupling constants to various nuclei, but it would not be obvious which coupling constants belonged together in one radical. A triple resonance experiment might help to elucidate this. Simultaneous excitation of a second NMR in a radical already undergoing ENDOR would affect the ENDOR signal differently if the second nucleus were coupled to the same electron as the first nucleus. This is an alternative use for the double ENDOR experiment which has been used to measure the relative signs of the coupling constants (Cook and Whiffen, 1964).

2.6 NUCLEAR MAGNETIC RESONANCE

Similar, but slightly different information from that discovered by ENDOR is available from a study of NMR in diamagnetic species. The NMR suffers a chemical shift due to the diamagnetic circulation of paired electrons around the nucleus (Andrew, 1956; Staff of Varian Associates, 1960a). Also the NMR may be split up into a sort of hyperfine structure due to interactions

(J coupling) with another neighboring nucleus (Andrew, 1956). Such interactions are only large when they proceed through the intervening electrons, i.e., nucleus a interacts with an electron which in turn interacts with nucleus b, so that the size of the interaction is related to the nature of the electron wave function. Measurements of the chemical shift and splitting can, in principle, be interpreted in terms of models of the electronic structure and electronic states of the system, although at present such interpretations are rather phenomenological.

Most NMR work of this sort has been done on protons as $I = \frac{1}{2}$ and μ_n is large so that the signal is large (P and F satisfy the same conditions).

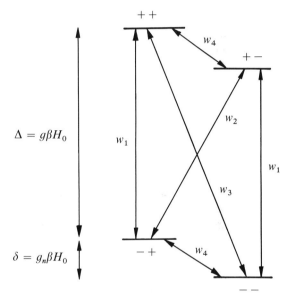

Fig. 2.7   Energy levels for a system with $S = \frac{1}{2}$, $I = \frac{1}{2}$ labelled as in Fig. 2.5. Here the coupling between unpaired electron and nucleus is assumed to be small.

To look for D, ^{13}C, or ^{15}N is much more difficult because of either low abundance or low μ_n. The NMR signal strength can often be enhanced by using a technique, which is closely related to ENDOR, so that the NMR signals are more easily observed.

The specimen must contain some paramagnetic impurities; e.g., paramagnetic ions may be dissolved or substituted in the specimen, or unpaired electrons may be produced by chemical action or irradiation. A concentration of $\sim 10^{19}$ paramagnetic centers per ml is desirable. These centers then interact through their dipolar fields with the nuclei. Figure 2.7 shows a schematic energy level diagram for one of the electron centers with $S = \frac{1}{2}$ coupled to a nucleus with $I = \frac{1}{2}$. The situation here is different from that envisaged in the discussion of ENDOR as the field H_e is considered to be small. Using ENDOR, one studies the nuclei which are close to a paramagnetic center, whereas here one studies nuclei which are distant from the paramagnetic centers so that most of the nuclei are sufficiently far away from the center for $H_0 >> H_e$. Expression (2.7) can no longer be neglected, in fact it is greater than (2.5). This not only affects the separation of the nuclear levels but also their order; compare with Fig. 2.5. In such a system the Boltzmann distribution is maintained over all of the levels by the spin-lattice relaxation which proceeds via transitions of the sort w_1, w_2, and w_3 in Fig. 2.7. The transitions w_1, in which the orientation of the nucleus does not change are the normal electron spin-lattice relaxations. The dipolar coupling between the nucleus and the electron makes the transitions w_2 and w_3 possible. Figure 2.8 shows the populations of the various levels in thermal equilibrium. The nuclear resonance frequency w_4 is the same for both

| | Boltzmann distribution | | Saturation of $+ - \leftrightarrow - +$ | |
	$\langle I_z \rangle = +\frac{1}{2}$	$\langle I_z \rangle = -\frac{1}{2}$	$\langle I_z \rangle = +\frac{1}{2}$	$\langle I_z \rangle = -\frac{1}{2}$
$++$	$\exp\left[-(\Delta + \delta)/kT\right]$		$\exp\left[-\Delta/kT\right]$	
$\underline{+ -}$		$\exp\left[-\Delta/kT\right]$		1
$- +$	$\exp\left[-\delta/kT\right]$		1	
$\underline{= \ --}$		1		$\exp\left[\Delta/kT\right]$
sum	$e^{-\delta/kT}(1+e^{-\Delta/kT})$	$(1+e^{-\Delta/kT})$	$(1+e^{-\Delta/kT})$	$e^{\Delta/kT}(1-e^{-\Delta/kT})$
difference between sums	$(1 + e^{-\Delta/kT})(1 - e^{-\delta/kT})$		$(1 + e^{-\Delta/kT})(1 - e^{-\Delta/kT})$	
	$\approx 2\dfrac{\delta}{kT}$		$\approx 2\dfrac{\Delta}{kT}$	

Fig. 2.8   Populations of energy states for Boltzmann distribution, and when the transition $+ - \leftrightarrow - +$ is saturated. The strength of the NMR signal is proportional to the difference between the total population of $\langle I_z \rangle = +\frac{1}{2}$ and $\langle I_z \rangle = -\frac{1}{2}$ states.

electron spin states so that the strength of the NMR signal depends upon the difference of the populations of the states with $\langle I_z \rangle = +\frac{1}{2}$ and those with $\langle I_z \rangle = -\frac{1}{2}$.

Although w_1 are the 'allowed' ESR transitions, the 'forbidden' transitions w_2 and w_3 can be induced because of the admixtures of states caused by the dipolar coupling between electron and nuclei. Suppose the transition w_2 were to be saturated by applying a lot of microwave power. This equalizes the populations of the states $++$ and $--$. The rapid relaxation for transitions w_1 maintains the Boltzmann distribution between the levels they connect, but the much slower relaxation for transitions w_2 and w_3 is dominated by the microwave saturation. Hence the populations of the various levels change upon saturation of w_2 to have the values given in the right-hand side of Fig. 2.8. The difference in populations of the states with $\langle I_z \rangle = +\frac{1}{2}$ and those with $\langle I_z \rangle = -\frac{1}{2}$ is now much greater; a polarization of the nuclei has been produced. This process is known as dynamic nuclear polarization, as the polarization only persists so long as the microwave transition is being saturated. As the NMR signal is proportional to the nuclear polarization, a much greater NMR signal is expected when the microwave power is on. As Δ is about three orders of magnitude greater than δ the enhancement of the NMR should theoretically be three orders of magnitude. In practice, the enhancements produced are smaller, often much smaller, because the relaxation processes across w_3 and those across w_4 both tend to reduce the nuclear polarization. In favorable materials enhancements of several hundred times have been observed.

2.7 EXPERIMENTAL DETAILS

The experimental arrangements for both ENDOR and dynamic nuclear polarization are similar. Both excite ESR and NMR simultaneously and so need to be a combination of microwave and r.f. resonance apparatus. The differences lie in the emphasis on what is to be measured. In ENDOR one is concerned to have a good ESR spectrometer into which is injected some r.f. power (Feher, 1959; Lambe, et al., 1961; Seidel, 1961; Baker and Williams, 1962; Holton and Blum, 1962; Cook, 1966); whereas in dynamic nuclear polarization it is the NMR spectrometer which has to be of good quality, but arranged so that the specimen can be bathed in a lot of microwave power (Richards and White, 1964; see also references in Jeffries, 1963).

A number of methods have been used to introduce the r.f. into a microwave cavity for ENDOR experiments; perhaps the simplest uses a single loop of wire so placed that it is always perpendicular to the microwave electric field. In this way, it does not lower the Q of the microwave cavity. The power requirements for ENDOR are usually fairly modest. The detection sensitivity is greatest if the ESR transition is about 50% saturated. For $T_1 > 10^{-6}$ sec the microwave power required is less than 50 mW, which is obtainable from most klystrons. For a solid sample, T_1 can always be made long enough by cooling the specimen. As this expedient is not available for liquid specimens there may be difficulties in performing ENDOR for short T_1. It is advantageous to drive the nuclear resonance as hard as possible, which requires the largest possible r.f. magnetic field at the sample. The best way to do this appears to be to pass a large current through the single loop coil. Many turn coils have been used but they have the compensating disadvantage that they tend to lower the Q of the microwave cavity. A tuned coil could be used but this has the disadvantage that it has to be tuned as well as the oscillator when searching for unknown lines. Because of these difficulties most workers have matched a single loop to the r.f. oscillator as well as possible. For work at low temperatures, r.f. powers of less than 1 watt have been adequate, but some work at room temperature, where the relaxation times are shorter, has required several watts (Seidel, 1961). Typically, the magnitude of the change in the ESR signal when ENDOR is performed is a few per cent, so there is little point in attempting to observe ENDOR on an ESR signal with a signal-to-noise ratio of less than 100.

For observing NMR enhanced by dynamic polarization, the important thing is to have a sensitive NMR spectrometer, so that one requires a multiturn coil with a good filling factor. The fact that the Q of the microwave cavity may be reduced by the coil is not so important as the reduction in Q can always be compensated for by using more microwave power. For these experiments, sometimes overmoded cavities have been used and sometimes no cavity at all. Another technique employs a helix as a microwave 'cavity'; in fact the same helix may carry microwave and r.f. current (Webb, 1962). Here, as for ENDOR the power required to saturate the ESR depends upon the spin-lattice relaxation time. The fact that it is a 'forbidden' line that one is trying to saturate does not necessarily mean that it is any more difficult than saturating the 'allowed' transition, because usually the relaxation time is longer for the forbidden transition which compensates for the fact that it is harder to induce.

2.8 CONCLUSION

The two techniques we have described give one detailed information either about the interaction of an unpaired electron with its neighboring nuclei (from ENDOR) or about the interaction of a nucleus with its diamagnetic surroundings and other nuclei through the medium of the surrounding electrons (from NMR). The interpretation of such measurements in terms of meaningful models of the electronic structure around the nuclei is a complex and incompletely understood problem. Most of the problems met in medical or biological applications will probably be more complex than the similar problems encountered in the physical and chemical applications of these techniques, and even these simpler problems are little understood in terms of a complete theory. All that can realistically be hoped for in biological and medical applications is some guidance in selecting from a number of different models, or qualitative indications of the differences between the electronic structure of different molecular species.

REFERENCES

Andrew, E. R., 1956, *Nuclear Magnetic Resonance* (Cambridge: University Press), Section 5.6.
Baker, J. M., and Williams, F. I. B., 1962, *Proc. R. Soc.* A, **267**, 283–94.
Cole, T., Heller, C., and Lambe, J., 1961, *J. chem. Phys.*, **34**, 1447–8.
Cook, R. J., 1966, *J. scient. Instrum.*, **43**, 548–53.
Cook, R. J., and Whiffen, D. H., 1964, *Proc. phys. Soc.*, **84**, 845–8.
Feher, G., 1956, *Phys. Rev.*, **103**, 834–5; 1959, *Phys. Rev.*, **114**, 1219–44.
Feher, G., and Gere, E. A., 1959, *Phys. Rev.*, **114**, 1245–56.
Griffith, J. H. E., Owen, J., and Ward, I. M., 1953, *Proc. R. Soc.* A, **219**, 526–42.
Holton, W. C., and Blum, H., 1962, *Phys. Rev.*, **125**, 89–103.
Hyde, J. S., 1965, *J. chem. Phys.*, **43**, 1806–18.
Hyde, J. S., and Maki, A. H., 1964, *J. chem. Phys.*, **40**, 3117–8.
Jeffries, C. D., 1963, *Dynamic Nuclear Orientation* (New York: Interscience).
Lambe, J., Laurance, N., McIrvine, E. C., and Terhune, R. W., 1961, *Phys. Rev.*, **122**, 1161–70.
Overhauser, A., 1953, *Phys. Rev.*, **92**, 411–5.
Owen, J., 1955, *Discuss. Faraday Soc.*, **19**, 127–34.
Owen, J., and Thornley, J. H. M., 1966, *Rep. Prog. Phys.*, **29**, 675–728.
Pake, G. E., 1962a, *Paramagnetic Resonance* (New York: Benjamin), Ch. 3; 1962b, ibid., Ch. 5.
Portis, A. M., 1953, *Phys. Rev.*, **91**, 1071–8.
Richards, R. E., and White, J. H., 1964, *Proc. R. Soc.* A, **279**, 474–80.
Seidel, H., 1961, *Z. Phys.*, **165**, 218–38.
Staff of Varian Associates, 1960a, *NMR and EPR Spectroscopy* (New York: Pergamon), Ch. 2; 1960b, ibid., Ch. 3.
Webb, R. H., 1962, *Rev. scient. Instrum.*, **33**, 732–7.

CHAPTER THREE

ELECTRON SPIN RESONANCE STUDIES OF RADIATION DAMAGE IN BIOLOGICAL MATERIALS

S. J. Wyard

Physics Department, Guy's Hospital Medical School, London, England

and J. B. Cook

Haileybury and Imperial Service College, Hertford, England (Previously of *Physics Department, Guy's Hospital Medical School*)

3.1   INTRODUCTION

The study of radiation damage in biological materials is a large subject with a history of many years, which is more familiar under the names of radiation chemistry and radiation biology.   (It is perhaps preferable to use the more neutral description of 'radiation effects' or 'changes induced by radiation', but we have used 'radiation damage' as being more familiar to physicists.) The procedure in these studies is to irradiate some material of biological interest, which may vary in complexity from pure water to a living animal, and investigate the effects, such as the production of new molecules in chemical samples, or alteration in behavior of a cell or animal in living samples.   Most chemical studies have been made with liquids, and the results are usually explained in terms of free radicals which are precursors of the stable products of the radiation.   Until very recently the free radicals were not observed.   In biological studies also, free radicals are usually thought to be involved in the process by which the energy absorbed from the radiation produces the observed effects, although, because of the greater complexity there is little understanding of the details of the process.   An introduction to these subjects will be found in *Mechanisms in Radiobiology*, edited by Errera and Forssberg (1961).

From the physics of the subject, it is known that the initial effect of ionizing radiation is to produce electrons and positive ions (or positive holes), and excited molecules; and from these species come the free radicals referred to above.   Something is known about the distribution in both time and space of these species; and how they vary for different types of radiations. (An introduction to this topic can also be found in *Mechanisms in Radiobiology*, referred to above.)   All these species contain unpaired electrons, and hence can be detected by ESR spectroscopy, provided of course that they last long enough, are present in sufficient concentration, and that the spectral line width is not too great.   Hence an obvious experiment would be to take any of the materials already studied in radiation chemistry or radiation biology, to irradiate it, and then from the ESR spectrum to identify the radical species produced and measure their yields.   One would also hope to measure the distribution in space of these species, to follow their reactions with each other and with other molecules in the sample, and to see how these effects were influenced by such factors as type of radiation, LET† of ionizing radiation, wavelength of ultraviolet radiation, total dose, dose-rate, temperature of the sample and presence in the sample of substances such as water or oxygen.   With chemical samples, one would be able to test the free radical theory, and supply quantitative data.   With biological samples, one could at least look for correlations between the radicals observed and the later biological effects.   However, there are several difficulties in the way of performing such an experiment.

† Linear energy transfer (LET) is the linear-rate of loss of energy (locally absorbed) by an ionizing particle traversing a material medium.

One difficulty arises from the fact that the majority of materials so far studied by radiation chemistry are liquids; likewise, most biological samples contain a good deal of water.   The radical species produced by radiation are generally very reactive, and often the reaction rate is limited only by diffusion (Matheson, 1964; Fricke and Thomas, 1964).   For this reason the spectrum must be recorded either during the irradiation or else very shortly afterwards; and the concentration of any radical species will be proportional to the product of the intensity of the radiation and the lifetime of the species. Because of the complexity of the experiment very few ESR studies of irradiated liquids have been undertaken.   Fessenden and Schuler (1960, 1963) report an important investigation of transient radicals in liquid hydrocarbons during irradiation by a beam of electrons.   The radicals could be identified from the spectra, which were well resolved with narrow lines.   The concentrations of the radicals were also determined from the spectra, and from these the rate constants for the disappearance of the radicals were calculated. Fessenden (1964) has also reported direct measurements of radical lifetimes in the msec range using ESR techniques.   Similar experiments with aqueous systems would be most interesting.   They would be more difficult, because of the dielectric loss of water, but would seem to be feasible using current techniques.   This point is further discussed in chapter 5.

Because of the difficulty of detecting short-lived radicals, most ESR studies have been made on irradiated solid samples.   It has been found that in many dry or frozen materials, some of the radical species produced by irradiation are 'trapped' or 'stabilized'.   (For a general discussion of this subject see *Formation and Trapping of Free Radicals*, edited by Bass and Broida (1960).)   With such samples, a sufficient concentration of radicals can be built up by prolonged irradiation, and the spectrum recorded at leisure.   In many materials of biological interest, radicals are trapped at room temperature; in other materials lower temperatures, down to that of liquid helium, have to be used.   It must be realized that this type of experiment is different from those described in the previous paragraph.   The radical species which are observed are those which, for some reason or other, happen to be trapped in the sample.   The energy absorbed from the radiation appears initially in the 'primary products', electrons, positive ions, and excited molecules.   There may then be a whole series of reactions between these products and the molecules of the sample, involving the production of new radical species and ending up with radical species which have been trapped along the way, stable molecular products, and heat.   The course of these reactions, and the radical species which are trapped, may be affected by parameters such as the temperature of the sample during irradiation; any subsequent heat treatment; presence of impurities such as water, dissolved gases, and especially 'radical scavengers', the state of the sample, e.g., single crystal, amorphous, glassy; external factors such as the application of a strong magnetic field.   Hence there may not be any simple correlation between ESR measurements of trapped radicals, and experiments in radiation chemistry and radiation biology which involve the same molecules.   At least, it would be rash to draw sweeping conclusions from a single ESR measurement.

In most of the early ESR studies of radiation damage, polycrystalline materials were irradiated at room temperature, and the spectra recorded. Gordy and his co-workers carried out a fairly extensive survey of this kind (Gordy, et al., 1955a, b; McCormick and Gordy, 1958; Shields and Gordy, 1958; Gordy and Shields, 1958; Gordy, 1959; Rexroad and Gordy, 1959). Materials studied include amino acids, peptides, polypeptides, proteins, nucleic acids and their constituents, fatty acids, enzymes, lipids, hormones, vitamins, carbohydrates, mitochondria, thyroid, parathyroid, and liver. These researches showed that irradiation of practically any dry biological material produces radical species which are stable for long periods at room temperature, and are easily detectable by ESR.   Although many interesting and suggestive facts came to light which have stimulated further research, these experiments did not produce much definite information, because anisotropic hyperfine coupling and anisotropic g-values gave rise to poorly resolved spectra; so that in most cases it was not possible to make a positive identification of the radical species produced.   There is a further difficulty that, since the g-values of radicals are mostly very close to the free spin value, spectra from different species will usually overlap.   Hence a complicated sample, containing a number of different molecules, may give an apparently simple spectrum, after irradiation, which is really the envelope of a number of spectra.

In recent years, ESR studies of irradiated biological materials have tended to follow a number of different lines.   One fruitful field has been the study of irradiated single crystals of the simpler biological molecules.   It turns out that the radicals produced are oriented in these crystals, and often give well resolved spectra from which a positive identification may be made. The emphasis has been on producing oriented radicals, identifying them, measuring the spectroscopic factors and interpreting these from the electronic wave functions of the radical.   In another type of study, mainly using polycrystalline samples, quantitative measurements are made of the yield of radicals; and this can always be done, whether or not the species can be identified.   The yield is an important parameter in any attempt to correlate ESR with other studies of radiation damage; it is obviously important to know whether the spectrum represents a major part of the damage, or some relatively unimportant part which happens to get trapped and shows up in the spectrum.   In other studies, one follows changes in the spectrum when low concentrations of impurities such as oxygen or 'protective agents' are introduced into the sample.   A recent development has been the irradiation of samples at a low temperature, and the observation of various changes in the spectrum as the sample is subsequently brought back to room temperature.   In the rest of this chapter, we will discuss many of these developments.†   We shall exclude proteins, materials containing only hydrogen and oxygen, and also the general subject of energy transfer, since these are discussed in detail in chapters 5 and 6.   We shall also exclude single crystal studies, which are discussed in chapter 4.

At this point it is interesting to calculate the radiation dose required to produce a detectable ESR spectrum.   We assume a spectrometer as described in chapter 1, operating at 9 GHz, with a sample volume of 0.1 ml and a material of unit density.   We assume an effective line width of 10 Oe, taking the line-splitting by hyperfine interaction into account, and a signal-to-noise ratio of 10 to 1 to give a reasonable spectrum.   Then we need 5×10^{14} spins per gram of sample.   A typical yield of ion pairs in a gas, or free radicals in a liquid, is 3 per 100 eV; and as a basis for calculation we assume the same yield of radicals produced and trapped in the sample. The radiation dose is usually measured in rads, where 1 rad equals 100 ergs absorbed per gram.   Hence the dose required is

$$D_{req.} = \frac{5 \times 10^{14}}{3} \times 100 \times \frac{1.6 \times 10^{-12}}{100} = 240 \text{ rads.} \qquad (3.1)$$

This dose is comparable to those used in animal experiments, so that we might say that an ESR spectrometer is as sensitive as a mouse in detecting radiation.   Actually, considerably larger doses are usually given, of the order of 1 Mrad.   This is partly because the factors are often less favorable than our calculations assume, and partly to obtain as good a signal-to-noise ratio as possible.   It should be checked that for smaller doses the spectrum is the same, and the number of radicals directly proportional to the dose; and that there is no reason to doubt that this holds true down to doses so small that no detectable spectrum is produced.

3.2   RADICAL YIELDS
3.2.1   GENERAL

In an investigation of radiation damage, the measurement of the number of radical species produced comes next in importance to the identification of the species.   With the ESR method it is much easier to measure a yield than

† Some of the topics of this chapter are discussed in considerable detail in 'Electron spin resonance and the effects of radiation on biological systems', *Nucl. Sci. natn. Res. Coun.*, U.S.A., 1966, **43**.

to identify a radical, since the number of unpaired electrons in the sample is directly proportional to the area under the absorption curve (chapter 1, equation (1.12)), and it is not necessary to use single crystals. Radical yields have been measured in a number of laboratories, and the values obtained have differed far more than one would expect from what appears to be a simple procedure. We therefore begin with a brief account of the technique, the errors involved, and the accuracy to be expected.

3.2.2 TECHNIQUE

It is possible, from the area under the absorption curve, to make an absolute determination of the number of spins in the sample. However, this involves determining a number of constants of the spectrometer which are not usually known; and, in practice, it is much simpler, as well as more accurate, to compare the sample with a standard containing a known number of spins. Provided the operating conditions, including sample temperature, are the same in each case, the ratio of the numbers of spins in the two samples will be the same as the ratio of the areas under their absorption curves. For the standard, a paramagnetic salt such as copper sulfate can be used, for which the number of spins may be determined by weighing; alternatively, a stable free radical such as α, α-diphenyl β-picryl hydrazyl (DPPH) or potassium disulfonate (Fremy's salt) can be used, for which the number of spins may be determined by chemical titration. Because of practical difficulties involved in the use of these absolute standards, we have found it very convenient to use a sample of powdered coal as a substandard. The sample used (supplied by Professor D. J. E. Ingram, and labelled D.13) contains 1.74×10^{19} spins/g, which is a convenient concentration because it is comparable with those of irradiated biological materials. The line width is 5 Oe between points of inflexion, which is also comparable with irradiated biological materials; and the spins are stable with the sample exposed to air at room temperature. The calibration has been checked a number of times in the past few years, by comparison with paramagnetic salts, with results agreeing to within $\pm 10\%$.

Most spectrometers employ high frequency magnetic modulation to obtain good sensitivity, and present the spectrum as the first derivative of the absorption curve. A double integration must therefore be performed to obtain the number of spins; and since this is very tedious when done by counting squares, methods have been described using electronic circuits (Randolph, 1960), a moment balance (Burgess, 1961; Köhnlein and Müller, 1962) and numerical analysis with a desk calculating machine (Wyard, 1965). It is worth pointing out that the integrated area is strictly proportional to the modulation amplitude of the magnetic field, even for modulation amplitudes several times the line width, which give a very distorted line shape (Randolph, 1960; Verdier, *et al.*, 1961). Hence, for samples with few spins, the modulation amplitude may be set at the value which gives the maximum signal. Another point to notice is that sizeable errors can be introduced by cutting off the tails of the derivative spectra too soon. If the tails are cut off when the amplitude has fallen to 2% of the maximum value, the error in area is 24% for a Lorentzian shape spectrum, but only 1% for a Gaussian shape. Hence, for accurate measurements, it may be necessary to record the tails at higher gain than the center part of the spectrum.

3.2.3   ERRORS

We now present a list of errors and corrections which arise in the measurement of yields. A discussion covering many of these points was given by Zimmer, *et al.* (1963).

A. *g-VALUE NOT EQUAL TO 2*

Equation (1.12) of chapter 1 assumes free spins. If $g \neq g_e$, the transition probability is altered, and so is the area under the absorption curve. Bleaney (1960) has derived formulae from which the magnitude of this effect can be calculated. For free radicals, whose g-value is very close to 2, the correction is likely to be negligible, but it could be appreciable for a paramagnetic salt used as an absolute standard. With copper sulfate, for example, the correction can be as much as 30%, depending on the orientation of the crystal.

B. H_1 *NOT CONSTANT*

Referring again to equation (1.12), we see that a determination of the number of spins from a comparison of areas under the absorption curves assumes that H_1 (the amplitude of the microwave magnetic field) is the same for both samples. There are a number of reasons why H_1 may differ.

(i) The sample is usually placed in the cavity where H_1 is at a maximum, since this position gives the largest signal. For an extended sample H_1 must vary throughout the sample. A correction could be calculated from the known variation of H_1 throughout the cavity, but since the amplitude of the magnetic modulation also varies, it is simpler to determine the correction experimentally using a 'point' sample.

(ii) The microwave magnetic field may be distorted by the presence of dielectric material in the cavity. This effect (sometimes called the 'lens effect') is particularly noticeable when the sample is placed in a quartz tube or quartz dewar.   Table 3.1 gives typical increases in signal size due to this effect for a 9 GHz spectrometer.   The sample itself may also distort the microwave magnetic field.   This error can be avoided by measuring a number of samples of different sizes and extrapolating back to zero.   As an indication of the magnitude of this effect, Singer and Kommandeur (1961) report that the signal from a small solid sample increased by a factor of 2 when it was moved from a position 1 mm above a drop of water in the cavity to a position inside the drop.

Table 3.1 *Errors due to the lens effect*

Material round sample	Increase in signal
3 mm O.D. quartz tube	× 1.15
4 mm O.D. quartz tube	× 1.25
Quartz dewar	× 1.8

(iii) A lossy sample will absorb microwave power, and reduce the effective Q of the cavity, thus reducing the signal size.   Köhnlein and Müller (1962) have described a double cavity in which the sample and standard can be measured at the same time, so that changes in Q are cancelled out. Singer (1959) has described an alternative method of correcting for changes in Q, in which a crystal of synthetic ruby mounted inside the cavity gives a monitor signal sufficiently displaced from $g = 2$ not to overlap the sample signal.

As Ehrenberg (1961) pointed out, these methods will not correct for the distortion of the microwave field by the sample; and this is best done by extrapolation to a sample of zero size.

C. *POWER SATURATION*

Equation (1.12) assumes that the sample is not saturated, whereas free radicals often saturate rather easily.   This fact was not appreciated in some early work, which led to an underestimation of the yield.   It is worth pointing out that saturation is determined by the value of H_1, and it follows from equations (1.44) and (1.46) that saturation sets in at much lower powers in a spectrometer operating at higher frequencies, as compared to the conventional 9 GHz spectrometer.   Lowering the temperature of the sample also makes saturation occur more easily.

Factors considered so far apply to the operation of the spectrometer. We now consider those that are directly related to the preparation and irradiation of the sample.

D. *SATURATION OF RADICAL CONCENTRATION*

It is clear that there must be a limit to the number of radicals which can be trapped in a given sample, and one would expect the yield curve (radical concentration plotted against radiation dose as in Fig. 3.1, for example) to level off eventually. For meaningful results, sufficient measurements of yield at different radiation doses must be made to ensure that the yield is being measured on the initial straight-line portion of the curve. Radical

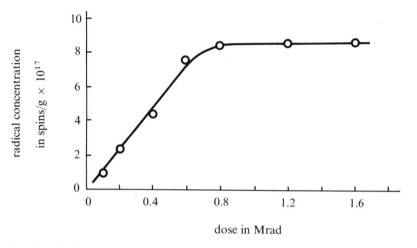

Fig. 3.1   Radical yield curve for a sample of DNA.

concentrations in most biological materials saturate at surprisingly low values, and ignorance of this led to an underestimation of the initial yield in some of the early measurements. The shape of the yield curve and the reasons for saturation will be discussed later.

E. *RADICAL DECAY*

In many materials, the number of trapped radicals decreases over a period of hours or days following the irradiation (Randolph, 1961; Ehrenberg, 1961; Müller, 1963). In such cases, it is necessary to follow the decay and to extrapolate back to zero time. It is often found that the decay is accelerated by the presence of moisture or oxygen, and especially of the two together. Hence it is becoming standard practice to dry materials thoroughly and then to seal them in an evacuated tube before irradiation, thus removing water and oxygen as far as possible.

F. *IRRADIATION PROCEDURES*

Most irradiations have been carried out with radiation of low LET (X- or γ-rays) at low intensities, and these may be taken as the standard conditions. A few measurements have been made with radiation of higher LET, and, as in radiation chemistry, it is found that the radical yield depends on the LET. For example, Müller, *et al.* (1963) found considerably lower yields, in most cases, in amino acids when using α-particles as compared to X- or γ-rays.

Since the trapped radicals seen by ESR are often the result of reactions between the primary products of the irradiation and the material of the sample, it would seem to be possible for the yield to depend on the intensity, because the concentration of short-lived species goes up with the intensity, and this could affect the reactions which take place. Hence one might find a difference with pulsed radiation (e.g., from a linear accelerator) even though the LET and average dose rate were the same as for γ-rays. Obviously, the intensity must be kept sufficiently low that the overall temperature of the sample does not rise appreciably. Rotblat and Simmons (1963b) have reported thermal effects when this precaution was not taken.

G. *SAMPLE PREPARATION*

It is well known in radiation chemistry, that small concentrations of 'scavengers' can have a big effect on the yield of molecular products, and a similar effect can be expected for the yields of trapped radical species measured by ESR. Evidence for this effect in proteins is presented in chapter 6.

The state of the material—i.e., single crystal, powder, glass, polymer —might also influence the yields. This does not seem to have been much investigated, although Wyard (unpublished) found no difference in radical yields in frozen samples of $H_2O_2-H_2O$ when these were irradiated either in the glassy or polycrystalline state. On the other hand, Henriksen (1966) did find some variation of yield with crystallite size for a number of organic molecules. The radical yield was greatest for freeze-dried material and decreased as the size of the crystallite increased. The largest variation in yield was 60%, for trypsin. It was suggested that this variation is due to radicals being trapped in imperfections, which are more common on the surface of a crystallite, and therefore more abundant in the smaller crystallites.

3.2.4 ACCURACY OF MEASUREMENT

In view of the large number of possible sources of error discussed in the previous sections, and also the fact that ESR spectrometers are not usually designed specifically for the purpose of measuring yields accurately, it is not surprising that values of published yields vary considerably.

Considering the spectrometer first, it is not unusual for the calibration to vary by 20–30% in the course of a day. The accuracy can of course be improved by repeated checks with a substandard, or by use of a double cavity or ruby monitor as described in section 3.2.3. Several workers have reported that a measurement on a given sample can be repeated to within 2–3% and claim accuracies of 10–20% for absolute determinations of the number of spins. Considering all the sources of error described in the previous section, it would seem that in favorable cases (g-value close to 2, adequate signal-to-noise ratio, dielectric loss not excessive) relative measurements, comparing one sample with another on the same spectroscope, should have errors not exceeding 10–20%; and absolute determinations of spin concentration should have errors not exceeding 30–40%. However, when a number of laboratories made measurements on the same sample, differences of a factor of 2 were common, and up to a factor of 3 in the worst cases (Köhnlein and Müller, et al., 1963), indicating that the difficulties of making accurate measurements are greater than is often supposed. The magnitude of these errors points to the fact that one should be cautious at drawing deductions from small differences in yields of radicals as determined by ESR.

When one compares radical yields for a given substance measured in different laboratories one often finds much bigger variations, up to factors of 10 or more in some cases (see, for example, Tables 3.2 and 3.4). Such variations cannot possibly be due to experimental errors in the ESR determination. They could be due to mistakes in a particular measurement, to use of inadequate techniques, to differences in the preparation of the sample, or to differences in the irradiation procedure.

3.2.5   RESULTS AND DISCUSSIONS

We shall not attempt to give a complete list of the yields which have been measured so far. Values will be found in the surveys by Zimmer and Müller (1965) and by Boag (1963). Many of these measurements are for amino acids. Values for proteins will be found in chapter 6, for hydrogen–oxygen systems in chapter 5, and for DNA and its constituents in this chapter, section 3.3.

Yields are generally expressed in terms of the G-value used in radiation chemistry, defined as the number of radical species formed by radiation per 100 eV of energy absorbed by the sample. For most of the materials studied, G-values of trapped radicals fall within the range 1–10. This is of the same order as the yield of ions in irradiated gases, and of molecular products in irradiated solutions. Yields are generally lower by approximately an order of magnitude in ring compounds and in unsaturated compounds.   Some measurements have been made for irradiations carried out at low temperatures (e.g., 77°K) and measured either at 77°K or at room temperature (Prydz and Henriksen, 1961; Henriksen, 1962a, 1962b; Henriksen, *et al.*, 1963; Müller and Köhnlein, 1964; Castelijn, *et al.*, 1964).   In many cases, yields are greater with low temperature irradiation; but in a few materials they are less, however.   It should be realized that the spectra are often different according to whether the sample is irradiated and measured at room temperature, irradiated and measured at low temperature, or irradiated at low temperature and measured at room temperature; so that the comparison is often between yields of different radical species.

It is possible for some radical species to be undetected by the ESR method, and this is likely if the line width is particularly large.   It should therefore be of interest to compare the ESR measurements with another method, such as measurement of magnetic susceptibility.   The sensitivity of this method is about 10^{14} spins at room temperature and 10^{16} spins at low temperature, which is quite adequate.

3.2.6 THE YIELD CURVE

The maximum number of radicals which can be trapped in organic solids averages around 10^{18} spins per gram, but varies considerably, from 2×10^{17} for adenine (Köhnlein and Müller, 1964) to 10^{20} for glycylglycine (Castelijn, *et al.*, 1964).   This means that radicals cannot be trapped closer together than about 100 Å in most substances; and the reason for this is not immediately clear.

It was discovered by Rotblat and Simmons (1963a) and also by Müller (1963) that for many substances the yield curve fits closely to an exponential function.[†]   Rotblat and Simmons pointed out that an exponential shape is obtained on the assumption that radiation destroys the radicals, as well as producing them, and they derived an equation

$$N = \frac{n}{\alpha} \left[1 - \exp \left(-\alpha D \right) \right] \qquad (3.2)$$

where n is the initial yield, and α the rate of recombination.   The saturation yield $N_{max} = n/\alpha$.   Since N_{max} is usually smaller than the number of molecules in the sample by a factor of 10^3—10^4, this explanation would imply some transference of energy absorbed by the sample to the radicals.   This might be by a migration of short-lived radical species, or by a local heating effect which allowed radicals previously trapped to recombine.   Simmons

[†] This is by no means a universal rule.   In frozen hydrogen peroxide solutions, for example, the concentration of radicals rises to a maximum at 200 Mrad and then decreases again at still higher doses.

(1965) has shown that hydrogen is a product of irradiated glycine, which gives some support to the suggestion that in this case the shape of the yield curve is due to a back reaction between atomic hydrogen, produced by the radiation, and the trapped radicals.   The point might be settled by measuring the yield of hydrogen, which was not done in this case, unfortunately.

3.3   RADIATION DAMAGE IN DNA AND ITS CONSTITUENTS
3.3.1   INTRODUCTION

Radiobiologists have long been intrigued by the sensitivity of living cells to radiation damage.   Thus a dose of 1000 rad, which would cause very little change in a chemical system, will destroy the viability of 1 in 5 *Eschericia coli* cells.   In recent years, the conviction has been growing that 'radiation damages a vital macromolecule; that vital macromolecule is DNA; this damage sets in train a series of biochemical events which lead to the visible effects, cell death, chromosome abnormalities, mutation and so on . . .' (Stacey, 1963).   Molecular biology has shown that DNA performs two vital functions, synthesis of RNA for the normal functioning of the cell and synthesis of new DNA when the cell divides.   (An excellent introduction to molecular biology has been written by Watson (1965).)   Zimmermann, *et al.* (1964) showed that the ability of DNA to synthesize RNA *in vitro* is reduced by 30% by a dose of 1000 rad.   Additional support for the identification of DNA as the main site of radiation damage in the cell is given by a simple numerical calculation.

Consider a sample containing among other things n molecules of average molecular weight M_n, giving a total weight of nM_n/N_0 gram, where N_0 is Avogadro's number.   Let irradiation produce a yield of G 'damage sites' per 100 eV absorbed by these molecules.   Then a dose of r rads to the sample produces $1.04 \times 10^{-12} nM_nGr$ damage sites.   Supposing now that each damage site results in the molecule breaking into two fragments, then since each break adds one fragment the effect of b breaks is to reduce the average molecular weight from M_n to $M_n' = nM_n/(n + b)$.   Hence

$$\frac{1}{M_n'} = \frac{1}{M_n} + 1.04 \times 10^{-12}Gr. \tag{3.3}$$

Equation (3.3) has been verified for chemical polymers (Alexander, *et al.*, 1954) where irradiation under suitable conditions causes a decrease in the molecular weight (an effect known as 'degradation').   A plot of the reciprocal of the molecular weight against the radiation dose gives a straight line, and from the slope of the line the value of G can be calculated.   It is found that a typical value is $G = 3$, much the same as the yield of ion pairs in a gas, of radical species in solution, and of radicals in organic solids.   The dose required to halve the molecular weight is $10^{12}/GM_n$ rads; expressed in the terminology of radiation biology this is the D_{37} dose, i.e., the dose for which $1/e$ or 37% of the molecules are undamaged.   The molecular weights of chemical polymers are of the order of 3×10^5, so a typical D_{37} dose will be 10^6 rads, and very much larger than typical values in radiation biology.

Early estimates of the molecular weight of DNA were of the order of 10^6.   This would give a D_{37} of 3×10^5 rad for inactivation of DNA and would raise serious difficulties for the idea that destruction of a cell is due to damage in its DNA.   However, it is now realized that the early molecular weights were far too low because of breakage occurring during the preparation of DNA.   From an autoradiograph by Cairns (1963) the molecular weight of DNA in *E. coli* is calculated as about 2×10^9.   Assuming a typical G value of 3, this gives a D_{37} of 170 rads.

A direct measurement of breakage in DNA has recently been made by McGrath and Williams (1966).   Using a very gentle method of preparation they were able to extract pieces of single stranded DNA from *E. coli* with an average molecular weight of 2.2×10^8.   Irradiation reduced the average molecular weight and a plot of the reciprocal molecular weight against dose gave a straight line, agreeing with equation (3.3).   A dose of 20 krad halved the average molecular weight, corresponding to a G-value of 0.23.   Thus the dose required to halve the average molecular weight of each strand of the intact DNA in the cell would be 3.3 krad.   Comparison with the D_{37} for killing cells is complicated by the fact that most strains of bacteria have a mechanism for repairing damaged DNA.   However, the strain of *E. coli* B_{s-1} apparently does not, and for this strain D_{37} is about 3 krad, in very nice agreement.

The importance of DNA in the life of the cell, and probably also in radiobiology, has naturally stimulated several ESR studies of radiation damage in DNA.   The experiment of McGrath and Williams demonstrated the likelihood that radiation kills cells (at least bacteria) by breaking DNA. It is difficult to see how damage to any of the other cell constituents (e.g., RNA, enzymes) could be effective at the doses required for killing, because the molecular weight is much too small; also there are many identical molecules in the cell and, if a few are destroyed, the cell could soon make new ones to repair the damage.   The only other substance of sufficiently high molecular weight is the cell membrane, regarded as a single molecule. It is conceivable that radiation could kill a cell by punching a hole in the membrane, in a manner similar to the way in which lysozyme is believed to act (Johnson and Phillips, 1965).   However, there has been no ESR work on cell membranes and so this idea will not be pursued here.

Before discussing ESR of DNA it should be emphasized that, in every case, the samples have been either dry or frozen, so the results may not be very relevant to what happens in a living cell.   Also, because of the complexity of the DNA molecule, one would expect a number of radicals with overlapping spectra, making identification of any of them very difficult.   It will be seen that in this respect ESR spectroscopy has been surprisingly successful.   It remains to be shown what connection, if any, the radiation damage studied by ESR has with the biological effects of radiation.   For the sake of readers who are unfamiliar with the subject we will give next a brief description of the DNA molecule.

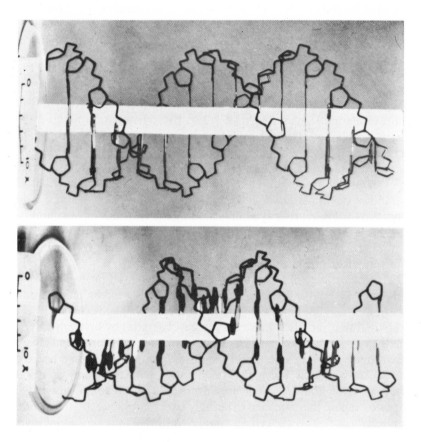

Fig. 3.2   Photographs of a rough scale model of the structure of DNA. The pairs of bases are represented by metal plates; the white plates represent the area between the bases in which the hydrogen bonding takes place. The fiber axis is represented by a Perspex rod. (After Crick and Watson, 1954, and reproduced by permission of the Royal Society.)

The structure of the DNA molecule is generally accepted to consist of a very long double helix (Watson and Crick, 1953; Wilkins, *et al.*, 1953; Franklin and Gosling, 1953; Crick and Watson, 1954; Marvin, *et al.*, 1958) as shown in Figs. 3.2 and 3.3.   Each helical coil is made up of alternate sugar (2-deoxy-*D*-ribose) and phosphate groups.   A side group consisting of either a purine or a pyrimidine base is attached to each sugar.   Two purines, adenine and guanine, and two pyrimidines, cytosine and thymine, are commonly present.   The two coils are joined together by hydrogen bonds between a purine base on one coil and a pyrimidine base on the other.

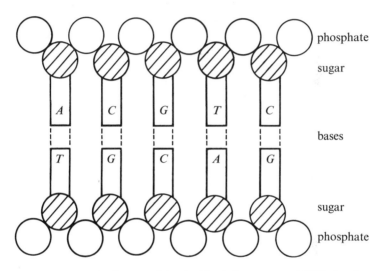

Fig. 3.3   Schematic diagram of the double chain structure of DNA showing how the two chains are joined by hydrogen bonds between the base pairs.

Adenine always bonds with thymine, and guanine with cytosine, accounting for the observed molar equivalence of adenine and thymine, and of guanine and cytosine.   The base ratio $(A + T)/(G + C)$ does vary with the source of the DNA.   Extreme values of the ratio for bacteria are 0.39 and 2.7 (Ki Yong Lee, *et al.*, 1956); values for T_2 bacteriophage and for calf thymus are 1.92 and 1.25 respectively (Lehman, *et al.*, 1958); and the ratio is close to 1.25 for all preparations of DNA commonly used.

The structure of the DNA molecule is based on X-ray diffraction photographs taken from fibers in which the molecules are oriented approximately parallel to the fiber axis.   Three forms have been found for DNA fibers, designated A, B, and C.   At high relative humidities the paracrystalline B form occurs, in which the water content may vary from 40 to several hundred % of the dry weight.   Form B is also observed in intact biological systems.   As the relative humidity is lowered there is a continuous and reversible transition to one of the other two forms.   The crystalline form A, found when the sodium salt of DNA is used, occurs at 75% relative humidity and contains about 30% of water by weight.   Form C is found when the lithium salt is used, and occurs at 44% relative humidity.   Dry specimens give very disordered X-ray patterns, indicating an irregular structure.   The bases have a planar structure and are arranged in pairs in the centre of the molecule, between the two helices.   In form B, the plane of the bases is approximately perpendicular to the fiber axis; the transition to form A is accomplished by a tilting of the planes of the bases, producing a decrease in the length of the fiber.   The bases are also slightly tilted in form C.   The combination of a base and sugar is called a nucleoside; the combination of base, sugar, and phosphate is called a nucleotide.   All these constituents of DNA are available for study separately.   The molecular weights of the nucleotides are about 300, while the molecular weight of fibrous DNA in prepared samples in the solid state is of the order of 10^7.

With this background, we shall proceed to the consideration of radiation damage in DNA.   The results obtained so far are somewhat conflicting and confusing, partly because of the complexity of the DNA molecule and partly because of the difficulty of obtaining highly purified samples.   This difficulty led to earlier reports of intense paramagnetic resonances in unirradiated DNA (Blumenfeld, 1959).   These resonances were found to be due to metallic ions, especially iron (Walsh, et al., 1961).   The resonance from iron was much larger than was expected from its concentration because the iron was partly present in a ferromagnetic form so that the normal Boltzmann statistics (see chapter 1, section 1.2.2) were not obeyed.   Blois, et al. (1963) showed that, if DNA was prepared and purified with sufficient care, no paramagnetic resonance could be detected.

3.3.2   RADICAL YIELDS IN IRRADIATED DNA

Early investigators reported low yields from DNA irradiated and measured at room temperature (Shen-Pei-Gen, et al., 1959) with G-values of 0.05 (Shields and Gordy, 1959), 0.0002 and 0.0009 (Dorlet, et al., 1962).   These low values were due either to the presence of moisture in the sample, or to the use of a single high radiation dose (7 Mrad or more).   It was reported by Shields and Gordy (1959), and has been since confirmed by several investigators, that the ESR signals in DNA are stable for several days under vacuum or in dry air, but decay rapidly in moist air.   Müller (1962) showed that the concentration of radicals in DNA, irradiated at room temperature, levels off at a comparatively low radiation dose, with a D_{37} equal to 205 krad (D_{37} is the reciprocal of the coefficient α in equation (3.2)).   Consequently, in the more recent measurements moisture has been carefully excluded, and the dose has been kept sufficiently low to ensure a correct value of the initial yield.   Values obtained are given in Table 3.2.

Table 3.2   *Recent values for radical yields in DNA irradiated at room temperature*

Authors	Source of DNA	G-value
Müller (1962)	Calf thymus	0.6
Müller (1963)	*E. coli*	3.3–12.5; av. 6.7
Henriksen (1963)	Not stated	5.7
Ehrenberg, *et al.* (1963)	Calf thymus	0.4
van de Vorst (1964)	Herring sperm	0.3
van de Vorst and Villée (1964)	Salmon sperm	0.6
van de Vorst, *et al.* (1965)	Chicken erythrocytes	
	mol. wt. 6×10^6	1.0
	mol. wt. 2.7×10^5	1.6[a]
Ormerod (1965)	Salmon sperm	2.0

[a] Same sample as previous one, after degradation by ultrasonics.

There is a difference of a factor of more than 40 between the smallest and the largest values of Table 3.2, which is considerably more than can be attributed to the experimental errors discussed in section 3.2.3.   In order to see whether the yield depends on the source or the method of preparation of DNA, the present authors compared yields under identical conditions for a number of samples.   The samples were dried, sealed in evacuated tubes, irradiated, and measured at room temperature.   The yield curves were determined by measurements at several doses between 0.1 and 1.5 Mrad, and were similar in shape to those given by Müller (1963).   Values of initial yields are given in Table 3.3 (Cook and Wyard, 1966c).

Table 3.3   *Comparison of yields in different samples of DNA irradiated at room temperature*

Supplier	Source	G-value
King's College, London	Salmon sperm	2.0
King's College, London	Calf thymus	1.4
L. Light and Co. Ltd.	Salmon sperm	0.8
L. Light and Co. Ltd.	Herring sperm	1.5
L. Light and Co. Ltd.	Calf thymus	1.4
British Drug Houses Ltd.	Calf thymus	0.8

The variation in Table 3.3 is a factor of 2.5, which can reasonably be ascribed to experimental errors plus differences in method of purification, resulting in differing concentrations of impurities, particularly protein and metallic ions, differing water contents, and possibly differing molecular weights.

It is of interest to compare yields in DNA with yields in its constituent parts. Table 3.4 summarizes the results for irradiation at room temperature of the bases, nucleosides, nucleotides, and the sugar. Some early results (Shen-Pei-Gen, et al., 1959; van de Vorst and Williams-Dorlet, 1963) have been omitted because the radiation doses used were greater than the radical saturation dose.

Table 3.4   *Radical yields (G-values) in constituents of DNA irradiated at room temperature*

Constituent		Müller (1964)	Henriksen (1963)	Cook and Wyard (1966b)	Ormerod (1965)
Cytosine	base	0.4	0.4	0.1	
	nucleoside	1.0			
	nucleotide	5			
Thymine	base	0.1	<0.1	0.1	0.4
	nucleoside	0.4		0.4	0.33
	nucleotide	2		2	
Adenine	base	0.1	0.1	0.04	
	nucleoside	1.4			
	nucleotide	2			
Guanine	base	0.8	0.1	0.05	
	nucleoside	0.9			
	nucleotide	3			
Sugar		4			

The discrepancies between the G-values obtained by different workers, given in Table 3.4, are larger than would be expected for relatively simple molecules. Nevertheless, one can be reasonably sure on two points, first, that radical yields for room temperature irradiation increase with the size of the molecule, from base through nucleoside to nucleotide, and second, that the yield in DNA is not very different from the yield in the nucleotides. Further, the spread of the values in Tables 3.2, 3.3, and 3.4 suggests that one should be cautious about accepting conclusions based on small differences in yields. The low D_{37} values found in DNA and the correspondingly low saturation values for radical concentration led to the early speculation that one DNA molecule can contain only one radical (*Radiation Effects in Physics, Chemistry and Biology*, 1963, p. 213). However, later estimates (Müller, 1963) gave up to 100 for the maximum number of radicals per DNA molecule. Furthermore, the D_{37} values and radical saturation values are also low in the bases, nucleosides, and nucleotides, with D_{37} lying between

0.3 and 7 Mrad (Müller, 1964; Müller and Köhnlein, 1964; Köhnlein and Müller, 1964). It is likely that radical saturation in DNA and its constituents is due neither to the existence of a limited number of radical traps nor to the delocalization of the unpaired electron over the macromolecule, as has been suggested in the literature, but to a mechanism of the kind suggested by Rotblat and Simmons (1963a) whereby an equilibrium is reached between the rate at which radicals are produced by one process, and the rate at which they are destroyed by another process.

Radical yields have also been determined in DNA and its constituents following irradiation at low temperature although fewer measurements have been made than at room temperature. (The radicals produced at low temperature are not the same as at room temperature; this point will be discussed in the next section but for the moment we only concern ourselves with the yields.) An early paper by Alexander, *et al.* (1961) gave $G = 0.3$ for irradiation at 77°K while more recently Lett, *et al.* (1964) and Ormerod (1965) gave $G = 1.3$ for the same conditions. Van de Vorst, *et al.* (1965) irradiated DNA at 100°K and recorded the number of radicals at 150°K; they found $G = 1.8$ for the native product with a molecular weight of 1.9×10^6, but $G = 2.4$ if the DNA was first degraded to a molecular weight

Table 3.5 *Radical yields (G-values) in constituents of DNA irradiated and measured at low temperature (77 or 100°K), and after warming up to room temperature*

Constituent		(1)	(2)	(3)	(4)	(5)
tosine	base		$0.8 \rightarrow 0.3$	$0.7 \rightarrow 0.2$		
	nucleoside		$1.0 \rightarrow 0.4$			
	nucleotide	$0.3 \rightarrow 0.4$				
ymine	base		$1.5 \rightarrow 0.7$	$0.1 \rightarrow\, <0.1$		$0.47 \rightarrow 0.20$
	nucleoside		$0.4 \rightarrow 0.4$			$0.17 \rightarrow 0.085$
	nucleotide	$0.4 \rightarrow 0.3$				
lenine	base		$0.14 \rightarrow 0.03$	$0.3 \rightarrow 0.1$	0.1	
	nucleoside		$1.0 \rightarrow 0.5$		0.2	
	nucleotide	$0.2 \rightarrow 0.17$			0.4	
					(1.3 for poly A)	
lanine	base		$1.3 \rightarrow 0.3$	$0.6 \rightarrow 0.1$		
	nucleoside		$1.8 \rightarrow 0.4$			
	nucleotide	$0.3 \rightarrow 0.15$				
gar			$2.0 \rightarrow 1.0$			

Notes (*a*) Authors are: (*1*), Alexander, *et al.*, 1961 (yields were measured after a dose of 10 rad, which may be too high); (*2*), Köhnlein and Müller, 1964; Müller and Köhnlein, 1964; (*3*), nriksen, 1963; (*4*), Singh and Charlesby, 1965; (*5*), Ormerod, 1965.

(*b*) $0.3 \rightarrow 0.4$ means that the *G*-value was 0.3 for irradiation and measurement at 77°K, and e number of radicals increased in the ratio 0.4 to 0.3 as the sample was brought up to room tempera- re; and similarly for the other samples.

of 4.1 × 10^5 by ultrasonification.   Henriksen (1963) gave $G = 3.0$ at 77°K. Patten and Gordy (1964) report a G of the order of unity for irradiation of dry DNA at 4.2°K.   Several authors have noted that D_{37} values are higher at 77°K than at room temperature.

Thus the low temperature yields, although showing a fair amount of spread, are not very different from yields at room temperature.   Ormerod (1965) has compared yields for the same sample of DNA irradiated at 77°K and room temperature, obtaining G-values of 1.3 and 2.0 respectively.   On the other hand, when a sample irradiated at 77°K was brought to room temperature, the number of radicals decreased by nearly 40%, from $G = 1.3$ to $G = 0.8$.   Cook and Wyard (1966a) found a decrease of only 15% in a similar experiment but the difference between this and Ormerod's value could be due to experimental errors.   Müller (1963) reported that the radical yield after irradiating at 77°K and warming up to 300°K was the same as after irradiation at 300°K.

Low temperature yields in the constituents of DNA are given in Table 3.5, together with the yield after warming up to room temperature. There is the usual variation between different workers; but there are two general tendencies, firstly an increase in yield going from the smaller to the larger molecule, and secondly a decrease in yield on warming up.

3.3.3   IDENTIFICATION OF RADICALS IN IRRADIATED DNA

Because of the complexity of the DNA molecule one would expect irradiation to produce a number of radicals with overlapping spectra, and in a polycrystalline sample with anisotropy present, a lack of resolution and difficulty in identifying any radicals.   For these reasons, Elliott and Wyard have commenced a study of oriented DNA, using fibers similar to those used in the X-ray diffraction studies.   In these fibers the axes of the helices are all approximately parallel, so that each repeating component has the same orientation with respect to the fiber axis.   Consequently, when the fiber is aligned to be parallel to the magnetic field, there should be no anisotropy in the ESR spectrum, which should therefore be sharp and well resolved.   For other orientations of the fibers there should be anisotropy and a smearing out of any hyperfine structure in the spectrum.   Preliminary results (Elliott and Wyard, 1965) have confirmed these predictions to some extent, since in the parallel position a narrow symmetrical spectrum was obtained which changed to a broader asymmetrical spectrum as the fibers were rotated to the perpendicular position.   However, it was not possible to relate these spectra to that from the same sample of DNA irradiated in a polycrystalline form.

Before discussing polycrystalline DNA we will first consider radicals identified in the constituents of DNA, since these should be a guide to the production of radicals in the complete molecule.   At the time of writing, only two of the constituents have been studied as single crystals, cytosine monohydrate by Cook, *et al.* (1967) and thymidine by Pruden, *et al.* (1965). In both cases, the investigations were carried out at room temperature.   The results for cytosine monohydrate are discussed in detail in chapter 4; we summarize here by stating that three radicals were detected of which two were identified.   One of these was formed by subtraction of a hydrogen atom, the other by rupture of a double bond and the addition of a hydrogen atom.

In the case of thymidine, two radicals were identified, although the assignment of one, produced in lower concentration, was not unambiguous.

(A)   (B)   (C)

Structure (*A*) is that of thymidine, X being the sugar which does not appreciably affect the ESR spectrum.   Structure (*B*) is the radical produced in higher concentration, and is formed by rupture of a double bond with the addition of a hydrogen atom.   The unpaired electron has an appreciable interaction with only five β-protons.   Hence the anisotropies in the couplings are small, and the spectra show little change as the crystal is rotated in the magnetic field (see section 4.4.2 of chapter 4).   The ESR spectrum for structure (*B*) consists of eight lines, equally spaced, with relative intensities 1:3:5:7:7:5:3:1.   It is deduced that the methyl group is rotating freely, thus giving a quartet with lines of relative intensity 1:3:3:1, since the three protons are equivalent.   The other two protons with which the unpaired electron interacts are also found to be equivalent, giving a 1:2:1 pattern. Normally, this would result in a 12-line spectrum with relative intensities 1:3:3:1:2:6:6:2:1:3:3:1.   However, it so happens that in this radical the coupling to the methylene (CH_2) hydrogens, 40.5 Oe, is nearly twice that to the methyl (CH_3) hydrogens, 20.5 Oe; and the resultant overlapping gives the 8-line spectrum instead.   Structure (*C*) is probably the radical produced in lower concentration, and would be formed by the removal of a hydrogen atom.   The unpaired electron interacts with two equivalent α-hydrogen atoms giving a 1:2:1 triplet with an isotropic coupling of 23 Oe.

Several authors have published spectra from the constituents of DNA in a polycrystalline form, the most complete sets being those of Shields and Gordy (1959) and of Köhnlein and Müller (Müller and Köhnlein (1964); Müller (1964); Köhnlein and Müller (1964)). From these spectra it is only possible to guess at the radicals present. However, it is notable that in thymine, thymidine, and thymidine monophosphate the spectra include a group of eight well-resolved lines with a spacing of about 20 Oe, similar to the spectrum from the radical of structure (B). The good resolution obtained from these radicals in polycrystalline samples is rather a special case, due to the free rotation of the methyl group and also to the fact that the hyperfine splitting is due to β-protons for which the anisotropy is small.

Returning now to DNA, the earliest papers reported a single line spectrum (Shields and Gordy, 1959; Shen-Pei-Gen, et al., 1959; Boag and Müller, 1959). Some structure was reported by Dorlet, et al. (1962) and also by Müller (1963), but in neither case was there any attempt to identify the radicals. The first identification of a radical in irradiated DNA came from Ehrenberg, et al. (1963) and from Salovey, et al. (1963); both groups obtained an 8-line spectrum superimposed on another spectrum. A strong resemblance was noted between this spectrum and the 8-line spectra from polycrystalline samples of thymine and thymidine. Since 1963, the 8-line spectrum in DNA has been observed by a number of workers, and is generally attributed to an unpaired electron localized on the thymine base, the radical having the structure (B). Cook and Wyard (1966c) have pointed out that the relative intensities of the eight lines in DNA differ slightly from those in thymidine; but this may be due to small differences in the coupling constants for the two molecules, or to an underlying unresolved spectrum in DNA. Figure 3.4 shows a particularly well resolved 8-line spectrum in DNA due to Cook and Wyard (1966c).

Because of conflicting reports in the literature about the existence of the 8-line spectrum in DNA, the present authors irradiated a number of different samples under similar conditions. The samples were used without further purification, and were irradiated in vacuo at room temperature. With one exception, all the samples gave a well resolved 8-line spectrum. The percentages of radicals giving the 8-line spectrum were estimated from the spectra, and are given in Table 3.6.

On visual inspection, sample 4, whose ESR spectrum consisted of a single line, appeared powdery rather than fibrous and, when examined by the method of Marmur and Doty (1962), showed no hyperchromic effect, indicating that the sample did not contain double stranded DNA. Thus, in our experience, in all genuine DNA samples irradiated in vacuo at room temperature, about 50% of radicals are located on the thymine base.

However, it is still not clear under exactly what conditions the 8-line

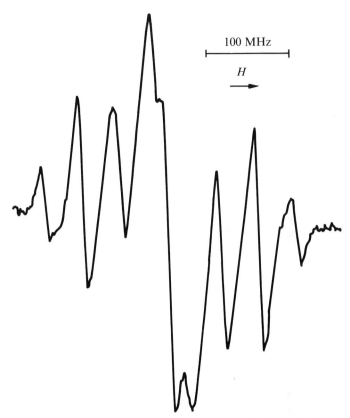

Fig. 3.4   Derivative spectrum of DNA sample number 1 irradiated and
recorded at 300°K.

spectrum is produced, and the conditions seem to be quite critical.   We have
already mentioned that a DNA sample which gave a good 8-line spectrum in
the polycrystalline form failed to give any hyperfine structure when the

Table 3.6   *Production of 8-line spectrum in DNA*

Sample number	Suppliers	Source	G-value for all radicals	Percentage of radicals giving 8-line spectrum
1	King's College, London	Salmon sperm	2.0	50
2	King's College, London	Calf thymus	1.4	50
3	L. Light and Co. Ltd.	Salmon sperm	0.8	50
4	L. Light and Co. Ltd.	Herring sperm	1.5	0
5	L. Light and Co. Ltd.	Calf thymus	1.4	40
6	British Drug Houses Ltd.	Calf thymus	0.8	50

molecules were oriented in fibers.   Gordy, *et al.* (1965) did not obtain any significant 8-line spectrum in several commercial samples irradiated *in vacuo* at room temperature, although a few samples did show weak thymidine-like signals after heavy irradiation.   These signals were appreciably enhanced when the irradiation was carried out in an atmosphere of hydrogen gas.   It will be recalled that the main radical in irradiated thymidine is formed by the addition of a hydrogen atom.   It is not clear where the hydrogen atom comes from in any of the cases when the 8-line spectrum is produced in a molecule containing the thymine base, but it is clear that in DNA the hydrogen atom can come from hydrogen gas if this is adsorbed in the sample.   It was initially noted by Ehrenberg, *et al.* (1963) that the 8-line spectrum in DNA was the first to disappear when moist air was admitted to the sample.   Cook and Wyard (1966a) found that, when irradiated DNA is heated to temperatures between 50 and 80°C, the 8-line spectrum is again the first to disappear.   This suggests that the radical on the thymine base is less stable than other radicals formed in DNA, and that unless the conditions are just right it is either not formed at all, or else it is destroyed as quickly as it is formed, so that no observable concentration is built up.   The maximum reported yield for this radical is a G-value of 1 (sample 1 of Table 3.6).   If all the energy for the production of these radicals comes from the thymine nucleotide, the corresponding G-value is 3.5.   This value is not so high as to necessitate an explanation in terms of energy transfer either across the hydrogen bonds (i.e., from the adenine nucleotides) or along the helices of the DNA molecule, especially as the G-values in general increase with the size of the molecule (Table 3.4).   It seems more likely, as will be discussed later, that the chemical bonds affect the radical yields indirectly by changing the stability of the radicals formed.   van de Vorst and Richir (1965) report that if DNA is degraded by ultrasonification to a molecular weight of 2.7 or 4.1×10^5, irradiated at 100°K and warmed to room temperature, a spectrum with a strong 8-line component is formed.

It is possible that, because of its good resolution and possibility of identification, overmuch attention has been paid to the 8-line spectrum in irradiated DNA.   Although other radicals are produced, generally in greater concentration, it has not been possible to identify them.   However, Gordy, *et al.* (1965) have suggested that the spectrum obtained by Dorlet, *et al.* (1962) (at very low yield) is due to the addition of a hydrogen atom to the guanine ring.   van de Vorst and Villée (1964) found a resemblance between a spectrum from DNA irradiated at 100°K and warmed to 300°K and the superposition of spectra from guanine and cytosine.   In a later paper van de Vorst and Krsmanovic-Simic (1966) show that there is a close resemblance between the spectrum of DNA irradiated *in vacuo* at room temperature and the spectrum from a mechanical mixture of the four bases in certain proportions, irradiated under similar conditions. With polycrystalline samples, however, the experimental evidence is too inconclusive to be certain about such assignments.

So far, we have considered irradiation of DNA at room temperature. Alexander, *et al.* (1961) reported a change in the spectrum of DNA, irradiated at 77°K, on warming to room temperature. Similar observations were made by Shields and Gordy (1959) and by Müller (1963). Salovey, *et al.* (1963) found an increase in the relative strength of the 8-line spectrum on warming to room temperature for samples irradiated at ∼200°K. Ormerod (1965) also observed an increase in the concentration of the thymine radical as DNA irradiated at 77°K was warmed to room temperature, from 6 to 15% of the total number of radicals present. Cook (1965) obtained a similar result, but with different numerical values, the percentage of the thymine radical increasing from a negligible amount at 77°K to 50% at room temperature. Both authors reported that irradiation at room temperature produces the same spectrum as irradiation at 77°K and warming to room temperature. Cook and Wyard (1966a) also observed three distinct changes in the spectrum as the sample was warmed from 77°K after irradiation at that temperature. These occurred at 100, 210 (where the 8-line spectrum mainly appeared), and 260°K. Furthermore, the single line obtained at 77°K differed both in width and g-value from the single line obtained at room temperature after the 8-line spectrum had been removed by annealing to 80°C. Ormerod (1965) suggested that at least part of the DNA spectrum at 77°K consists of the spectrum of trapped electrons. This suggestion is based partly on the fact that the ESR spectrum of hydrogen atoms is not observed in DNA after irradiation at 77°K, and partly on the fact that the addition to DNA of electron scavengers reduces or completely suppresses the yield of thymine radicals on warming. The suggested reactions are

$$T + e^- \rightarrow T^- \tag{3.4}$$

at 77°K, followed by either

$$T^- + RH \rightarrow T\dot{H} + R^- \tag{3.5a}$$

or

$$T^- + RH^+ \rightarrow T\dot{H} + \dot{R} \tag{3.5b}$$

on warming, where T represents the thymine ring, $T\dot{H}$ the thymine radical and RH some other part of the DNA molecule.

Irradiation of the constituents of DNA at low temperature produces similar results, in that the spectrum is generally different but becomes identical with the room temperature spectrum on warming to room temperature. In particular, Cook and Wyard (1966a) found that irradiation of thymidine at 77°K gave a well resolved 8-line spectrum the same as at room temperature, but that thymine and thymidine monophosphate gave single lines at 77°K. On warming, the 8-line spectrum appeared at 120°K in thymine, and 160°K in thymidine monophosphate. Thus, if we accept Ormerod's suggestion, reaction (3.5) occurs at 77°K in thymidine, at 120°K in thymine, at 160°K in thymidine monophosphate, and at 210°K in DNA. Hence the temperature at which the reaction occurs is greatly altered by the part of the molecule which has no measurable effect on the shape of the ESR spectrum.

3.3.4   OTHER ESR STUDIES ON DNA

In this section, we briefly discuss other ESR measurements on DNA which are relevant to those already discussed. These are of two kinds, first, experiments in which radicals are produced by means other than ionizing radiation—specifically by ultraviolet radiation or by bombardment with hydrogen atoms—and second, experiments using ionizing radiation where the effect of various additive substances is investigated.

From the point of view adopted in this chapter, the interest in producing radicals by other means is in the assistance it gives to understanding the effects of ionizing radiation. Caution is necessary here, because even if the ESR spectrum shows that the same radical is trapped following some alternative procedure, the initial species produced and the subsequent physical and chemical events may be very different. Platzman (1962) has pointed out and given reasons for the very large differences between the primary products of ionizing radiation and those of conventional u.v., which includes wavelengths down to about 2000 Å only.

The interest in adding various substances to biological materials before irradiation came originally from a search for substances which would protect living organisms against the injurious effects of ionizing radiation. Although this search has not been very successful, such experiments are also of interest for the light they throw on mechanisms of 'energy transfer', i.e., the physical and chemical processes by which some of the energy initially absorbed at one point in the sample eventually appears in a different form elsewhere.

Eisinger and Shulman (1963) discovered that the 8-line spectrum in DNA is also produced by u.v. radiation. The mechanism of production is different than with ionizing radiation, since in both DNA and thymine the 8-line spectrum appears at 77°K. Other radicals are also produced by u.v.; in the case of DNA, the additional spectrum is a broad line. A thorough investigation into the production of the thymine radical in DNA by u.v. radiation has been carried out by Pershan, et al. (1964, 1965).

The results for u.v. irradiation of DNA may be summarized as follows.

(1) For the 8-line spectrum, the coupling for the methyl protons is 20.8 $\pm$ 0.3 Oe, and for the methylene protons 37.7 Oe.   These values may be compared with 20.5 $\pm$ 0.5 and 40.5 $\pm$ 0.5 for a single crystal of thymidine (Pruden, *et al.*, 1965) and with values ranging from 20.0 to 21.3 and from 34.5 to 37.5 for polycrystalline samples of thymine, thymidine, thymidilic acid, and DNA (Ormerod, 1965).   It is quite conceivable that small differences exist in the coupling for the same proton in different molecules.   On the other hand, the separation between the peaks in a spectrum from a poly-crystalline sample is unlikely to give the coupling exactly.

(2) If DNA is moistened (by equilibriating in air at relative humidity $\sim 100\%$) before u.v. irradiation and measurement at 77°K, the proportion of the 8-line spectrum is greatly increased.   In moistened samples, the 8-line spectrum is stable at 195°K, but not at room temperature.

(3) Denaturation of the DNA by heating before irradiation has no significant effect on the ESR spectrum.

(4) Different samples of DNA (both from different suppliers and from different sources) give different, but reproducible, spectra with varying proportions of the 8-line spectrum.   In these experiments, the proportion of the 8-line spectrum varies from 10 to 80%, with 50% as a typical value for moist calf thymus DNA.   By subtracting a theoretical 8-line spectrum from the observed spectra, five other spectra are obtained under differing conditions.   These have not been identified, but one is similar to the spectrum observed in polycrystalline cytidine.

(5) The quantum efficiency for production of the thymine radical is about 5×10^{-4}, with some variation for u.v. intensity and for sample temperature.   At saturation, about 5% of thymine molecules are converted to radicals.

(6) The presence in the DNA of paramagnetic ions, in the proportion of 1 ion to 10 phosphate groups, reduces the yield of thymine radicals by a factor between 2 and 6.

Nucleic acids and their constituents have been bombarded by low velocity hydrogen and deuterium atoms by Herak and Gordy (1965, 1966a, 1966b), by Heller and Cole (1965) and by Holmes, *et al.* (1966).   Although the samples are in the form of a powder, the resolution of the spectra is good, partly because the proton couplings in the radicals are nearly isotropic and partly because in many cases only a single radical is produced.   Herak and Gordy found H-addition radicals in all the bases, nucleotides, and nucleo-sides, and in RNA, after bombardment at either 300 or 77°K; but found no evidence of H-addition radicals in DNA.   Heller and Cole obtained a very well resolved spectrum for thymine from which they deduced that the coupling for the methyl protons is 20.5 Oe, as in thymidine, but that the couplings to the methylene protons are unequal at 34.3 and 40.3 Oe, unlike thymidine. This supports the suggestion of Cook and Wyard (1966c) that the coupling constants for the thymine radical may vary slightly depending on the molecule in which it is formed. Holmes, *et al.* (1966) had the sample in the ESR cavity during bombardment, and were thus able to show that in some cases an initial spectrum changes after further bombardment. There is no doubt that bombardment by hydrogen and deuterium atoms is a useful technique, both for producing well resolved spectra, and also, since hydrogen atoms are important intermediates in radiation damage, in elucidating the secondary reactions following ionizing radiation.

Lett, *et al.* (1964) studied DNA extracted from bacteria grown in media containing 5-bromodeoxyuridine. In this DNA, 49% of the thymine is replaced by 5-bromouracil (BU). The BU-containing DNA was irradiated with γ-rays at 77°K *in vacuo*, giving a single ESR line with a G-value of 1.7. On warming to room temperature, the spectrum changes slightly, but there is no sign of the 8-line spectrum. The suggested interpretation of this result is that bromouracil scavenges hydrogen atoms more efficiently than thymine.

Ormerod (1965) studied the effect of adding either iodoacetamide or cystamine to sperm heads. Sperm heads consist of 65% DNA and 35% protein, and when irradiated at 77°K give a normal low temperature DNA spectrum. On warming to room temperature a marked 8-line spectrum appears. In samples of sperm heads with 5% additive, irradiation at 77°K gives a normal DNA spectrum plus spectra characteristic of the additive, iodoacetamide or cystamine. On warming to room temperature, however, the 8-line spectrum appears in reduced yield with cystamine, and is completely absent with iodoacetamide. The suggested interpretation is that the additive scavenges electrons produced by the radiation and suppresses the formation of the precursor of the thymine radical.

3.4   ESR OF IRRADIATED TISSUES AND ORGANISMS

3.4.1   INTRODUCTION

With the more complicated biological systems, usually containing a large number of different kinds of molecules randomly oriented, one would expect a broad ESR spectrum after irradiation, this being an envelope of a large number of spectra from the individual radicals. The only information to be obtained would be the radical yield; and the interest would lie in trying to correlate the yield with the conditions of irradiation, and with other forms of biological damage. Somewhat surprisingly, however, certain radicals are preferentially stabilized in a number of biological tissues, so that characteristic patterns often appear in the spectra. In some cases, where the molecules are naturally oriented, it has even been possible to identify the radicals.   In other cases where the radicals cannot be identified, it may still be possible to recognize in the ESR spectrum a number of different 'signals' or 'resonances', characterized by different g-values and line widths, and to correlate these separately with other forms of radiation damage.

Considerable caution is needed when interpreting the ESR spectra of irradiated tissues, since ESR spectra in these materials may be due to a variety of causes besides irradiation, and even for different radicals the spectra may be indistinguishable because of the poor resolution.   Thus spectra may be due to paramagnetic ions or to radicals produced by enzymatic processes.   Melanins are very widely distributed in biological tissues and give a strong ESR signal (see chapter 7 for a full discussion).   Strong ESR signals have been observed in a number of unirradiated freeze-dried tissues (Miyagawa, *et al.*, 1958) and in freeze-dried bacteria (Lion, *et al.*, 1961; Dimmick, *et al.*, 1961).   The intensity of the signal is dependent on the oxygen tension in all cases although the form of the dependence varies. Ulbert (1962) showed that mechanical damage to keratins (hoof, fingernail, feather, etc.) produces ESR spectra very similar to those produced by X-irradiation, but of greater intensity and better resolution.   He points out the possibility of many ESR spectra of biological objects being artefacts caused by mechanical damage during the treatment of the samples.   Burke, *et al.* (1962) found that certain oxidizing agents produce free radicals in wool and silk with spectra similar to those produced by ionizing radiation.   Even the application of water alone produced small quantities of radicals in wool under the experimental procedure which was employed.

In order to stabilize the radicals produced by radiation, it is necessary first either to freeze the sample or else to dry it (as was explained in section 3.1), unless one is working with a material which has a low water content in its natural state.   This forms a convenient way of classifying the samples and we shall follow it in the following sections.

3.4.2   FROZEN SAMPLES

Very little has been done with frozen samples, but Smaller and Avery (1959) have published an interesting study on yeast.   Suspensions of yeast in water were quickly frozen to $77°K$ and irradiated and examined at that temperature. To some samples a small quantity of β-mercaptoethylamine, a radiation protective agent, was added shortly before freezing.   It was possible to distinguish three components in the ESR spectrum, one due to water, one due to yeast, and one due to β-mercaptoethylamine.   The separation of the components was assisted by using heavy water, and by varying the microwave power level at which the spectra were recorded.   It was found that the presence of β-mercaptoethylamine reduced the yield of free radicals coming from the yeast, without affecting those from water.   When the sample was annealed at 125°K for 1 min the water signal disappeared, but the other signals were not affected.

3.4.3   FREEZE-DRIED SAMPLES

Again, little work has been done with freeze-dried (lyophilized) tissues and organisms.   Gordy (1959) has reported on resonances in irradiated liver, thyroid, parathyroid, and mitochondria; and Lion, *et al.* (1961) give spectra for irradiated bacteria.   Although there was a certain amount of structure in some of the spectra, none of the radicals were identified, and the interest of the experiments came from changes in the spectra when the samples were treated by heat, by oxygen, or by radiation protective agents.   A point of interest with the bacteria is that they are not destroyed by freeze-drying, provided they are stored in a vacuum.   Hence it is possible to compare the ESR spectrum with loss of viability due to subsequent treatment.

3.4.4   NATURALLY DRY SAMPLES

There are a number of biological tissues and organisms for which the water content in the natural state is sufficiently low that some radicals produced by irradiation are stabilized at room temperature.   There is an obvious attraction in working with such materials, in that there is no need for freezing or drying which may alter the properties of the material in some unknown way.

The materials fall mainly into two groups: first, tissues such as hair, feathers, silk, which are composed mainly of proteins, and second, embryonic tissue such as spores or seeds in the resting state.   The second group are of much greater interest to the radiobiologist, because they contain a high proportion of nucleic acid, and also because they are viable, so that the ESR spectra may be compared directly with other biological damage.   However, the first group has been more rewarding to the spectroscopist.

A. NATIVE PROTEINS

The first materials of this kind to be investigated were the celebrated toe-nail of Professor Gordy and the hair from the tail of a black horse (Gordy, 1955). Both these samples gave ESR spectra with the same beautiful structure, and Gordy and his co-workers extended the list to include feathers, hide, horn, wool, fish scale, bone, and silk (Gordy, *et al.*, 1955a; Gordy and Shields, 1958, 1960).   Cow tail hairs have also been studied by Pohlit, *et al.* (1961); feather quills by Rajewsky and Redhardt (1962); and bones by Swartz (1965). We will confine ourselves to a brief summary of these experiments, because radiation damage in proteins is discussed in some detail in chapter 6.

Gordy and co-workers found that most native proteins irradiated at room temperature give an ESR spectrum which is either like that from hair, or else like that from silk, or is a combination of both these types of spectra. The hair-like spectrum, which occurs in all keratin proteins, and is similar also to spectra from polycrystalline cystine or cysteine, is characterized by asymmetry and a g-value considerably higher than the usual value for free radicals.   By comparison with the spectra from single crystals of sulfur-containing organic compounds (see section 4.4.6 of chapter 4) it was established that the unpaired spin density in the hair-like spectrum is concentrated mainly on the sulfur.

Silk contains no sulfur, and its ESR spectrum after irradiation at room temperature consists of a well resolved symmetrical doublet.   A similar doublet is obtained from glycylglycine.   In an elegant experiment which

$$
\begin{array}{c}
\overset{\displaystyle H}{\underset{\displaystyle |}{}} \qquad \overset{\displaystyle O}{\underset{\displaystyle \|}{}} \\
\ldots \diagdown N \diagdown \underset{\underset{\displaystyle H}{\displaystyle |}}{\dot{C}} \diagup C \diagdown \ldots
\end{array}
$$

utilized the natural orientation of the molecules in silk fibers and in feather quills, Gordy and Shields (1960) deduced the principal g-values and coupling constants and showed that the radical is formed in the polypeptide backbone; and is as shown in the diagram.   It was also possible from the ESR spectra to obtain information about the orientation of certain groups and bonds in the native proteins, and thus to supplement other methods of structure determination.

In the case of bone, Gordy and Shields (1958) found a marked oxygen effect, in that three days' exposure to oxygen converted a doublet spectrum, similar to that found in silk, to an asymmetrical singlet, believed to be due to a peroxide radical.   It was considered that a similar effect might occur in many other proteins, but is especially marked in bone because of its porous nature.   The effect of oxygen on the hair-like spectrum was simply to destroy it, but it was not discovered how this came about.

Pohlit, *et al.* (1961) and Rajewsky and Redhardt (1962) investigated the influence of moisture content and of temperature on the ESR spectra of irradiated hairs and feather quills, and also measured radical yields.   They found evidence of additional resonances besides the cystine-like resonance noted by Gordy and co-workers, but found that these other resonances were less stable.   From measurements of yield they concluded that energy transfer processes related to a special protein structure do not play an essential part in the production of cystine-like radicals.

Swartz (1965) irradiated rat femurs under a variety of conditions, including low temperature, immersed in saline, after extraction of organic material by ethylenediamine, as well as in the living animal. In every case ESR spectra were obtained. From the *in vivo* irradiations, spectra were observed with doses as low as 750 rads, and the limit was set not by the sensitivity of the spectrometer but by the presence of an ESR spectrum in unirradiated bones.

B. *SPORES, SEEDS, ETC.*

There have been several papers on seeds, starting with Zimmer, *et al.* (1957), who made a preliminary investigation using barley embryos. Irradiation of dry embryos gave an ESR spectrum consisting of a single line, 11 Oe wide, at $g = 2.004$. The only information which could be obtained from the spectrum was the number of radicals present; however, only relative measurements of radical concentration were made. Irradiations were made in both air and nitrogen, in each case with a relative humidity of 30%, and the yield was somewhat higher in air than in nitrogen. There was a noticeable decay of the radicals during the first few hours after irradiation, but a portion of the radicals appeared to be more stable. A small ESR signal was present in unirradiated embryos.

In order to obtain more accurate and meaningful values of the radical yield, Ehrenberg and Ehrenberg (1958) worked with seeds of *Agrostis stolonifera*, which are sufficiently small for whole seeds to be used. Particular attention was paid to errors due to dielectric losses from the water content of the seeds, and to decay of radicals during the irradiation. It was found that after correcting for these errors the initial radical yield was independent of the water content for the range studied (which was from 3 to 10%, due to storing the seeds in air with from 0 to 30% relative humidity). However, the decay pattern varied with the water content in that the proportion of semi-stable radicals (those remaining after several days) was smaller in the wetter seeds.

A cautious attempt was made to associate the semi-stable radical fraction with the radiosensitivity of the seeds. The radiosensitivity measured by inhibition of growth also varies with water content and is in fact at a minimum for a water content of about 12%, corresponding to the bound water. It was suggested that water may protect the seeds by allowing a certain proportion of radicals to recombine, so that when the seeds are germinated there are fewer radicals to do damage. An experiment by Sparrman, *et al.* (1959) in which dry seeds were stored in an atmosphere of nitric oxide after irradiation in nitrogen gave support to this suggestion. It was found that the radical concentration decayed fairly rapidly, due to reaction with the nitric oxide.   In another set of experiments, it was found that for seeds irradiated and stored in nitric oxide the radiosensitivity was low and independent of water content up to 12%.   Apparently, if the nitric oxide removes the radicals causing some of the radiation damage, the presence of water has no additional effect.   For water contents above 12%, the radiosensitivity increases again, both in air and in nitric oxide.   However, no ESR measurements were made at the higher water contents, presumably because the radical decay is too rapid.

Conger and Randolph (1959) measured the production and decay of radicals in seeds and embryos of barley and wheat, with different water contents, and in the presence of air, oxygen, or nitrogen.   For most of the experiments, wheat germ, ground into a powder, was used.   The results obtained were very similar to those of Ehrenberg and Ehrenberg (1958), although the width of the ESR absorption line was rather larger.   It was tentatively concluded that most of the radicals observed came from the protein and nucleic acid content of the seeds.   A G-value of 0.2 was obtained for dry wheat germ (water content 1.5%) irradiated in air at room temperature.   However, this value is probably an under-estimate for the initial yield, since no correction was made for decay of radicals during irradiation, which lasted several hours.

In a later paper, Conger (1961) found several correlations between radical decay and reduction in growth when barley seeds were stored in various gases, at various temperatures and with various water contents, between irradiation and germination.   This suggested that radicals stored in the seeds after irradiation could either react and disappear harmlessly, or could react with certain molecules in the seeds to disappear and produce biological damage which showed up when the seed was germinated.

The formation and decay of radiation-produced radicals in seeds of greater water content (up to 72%) has been studied by Cook (1963).   He was able to do this by the use of a specially designed spectrometer operating at 300 MHz, at which frequency the presence of water in the sample has a much smaller effect on the operation of the spectrometer, and in which spectra could be recorded during irradiation at a dose rate of 1.2 Mrads/hr.   White mustard seeds were used, and in all cases the spectra were single lines of width 13.5 Oe.   For seeds of normal water content ($\sim 8\%$) the initial radical yield was $G = 0.6$; for wetter seeds the G-value was lower as measured, i.e., without correcting for radical decay.   If seeds of normal water content were moistened at the end of irradiation, it was found that the rate of decay increased with amount of water taken up.   With 72% water the number of radicals fell to a half in about 10 min; presumably some of this time is taken by the water penetrating the seed.

Klingmüller, et al. (1959) irradiated parts of Vicia faba.   Radiation produced radicals in all parts of dry seeds (water content 4–5%) but none that could be detected in seeds stored normally (water content 10–12%). The radicals probably decayed too quickly for detection under the experimental conditions used in the latter case.

Experiments carried out on spores (Powers, *et al.*, 1960; Powers, *et al.*, 1961; Powers, 1961) were similar in many ways to those on seeds and, on the whole, with similar results. There are, however, some interesting differences. Dry spores of *Bacillus megaterium* were irradiated under a variety of conditions, exposed to various post-irradiation treatments, and then the ESR spectrum was compared with the biological damage. The criterion of biological damage was failure of the irradiated spore to form a visible colony on incubation in a culture medium. Somewhat surprisingly the ESR spectra showed a certain hyperfine structure, which varied with the conditions of the experiment. Irradiation at 77°K gave a 3-line spectrum which changed into a 5-line spectrum on warming the spores to room temperature in the absence of air. This spectrum was further modified by storage for 24 hr at room temperature, by heating to 100°C for 10 min and by exposure to nitric oxide or oxygen. Irradiation of deuterated spores, obtained by growing *B. megaterium* for several generations in a medium in which the water was replaced by D_2O, gave ESR spectra with a single narrow line (8 Oe), showing that the hyperfine structure was due to replaceable protons. It was not possible to identify any of the radicals produced and, although it would have been possible to measure radical concentrations, this was not done. However, there did appear to be a close correlation between the amount of biological damage and the ESR spectra for many of the variables studied, although not for all.

Randolph (1961) has reported briefly on *Tradescantia* pollen. The G-value was 0.5, the spectrum had at least two components which decayed at different rates, and the decay was very dependent on atmospheric moisture. No attempt was made to correlate the spectrum with biological damage.

The last two materials to be discussed in this section are bacteriophage (Zimmer and Müller, 1965) and sperm heads (Alexander, *et al.*, 1961; Ormerod and Alexander, 1963; Ormerod, 1965). These materials are of considerable interest because they consist mainly of nucleic acid and associated protein, which are likely sites for the initiation of radiation damage in cells; and also because they can retain their biological integrity in a dry state —i.e., the ability to infect bacteria or to fertilize eggs. Zimmer and Müller (1965) found pronounced variability in spectra, dose curves, and yields in irradiated bacteriophage even in seemingly identical experiments. They also obtained some very high G-values (from 2 to 16). They discussed the difficulty of comparing ESR data with other radiobiological experiments, citing the apparent discrepancy between dose-yield curves for radicals and dose-irradiation curves for biological damage.   The experiments on sperm heads we have already discussed in section 3.3.4.

C. ANTS

A preliminary report on ESR in living ants has recently been published by Krebs and Benson (1965).   This was mainly concerned with spectra from unirradiated ants; but it was mentioned that irradiation produces a relatively narrow line close to $g = 2$, without hyperfine structure, and that this spectrum slowly decayed following irradiation.

3.5 CONCLUSIONS AND FUTURE PROSPECTS

It is evident from the preceding sections that there is some disagreement about the results of ESR measurements of radiation damage in biological materials, a certain amount of confusion about the interpretation of these results, and considerable uncertainty concerning the relationship of these results with other biological experiments.   This is not surprising in a new subject, and usually occurs when a new physical technique is applied to materials as complex and variable as biological tissues.   No doubt, the work of identifying the radicals will continue, for which the most powerful method is the use of single crystals, to be discussed in chapter 4.   The steps by which these radicals are produced from the primary products of the radiation will also be further elucidated; and it seems likely that the explanation will be in terms of existing physical and chemical processes, without the necessity of invoking any special properties for proteins, nucleic acids, and living tissues.

However, there are two fundamental drawbacks to the ESR methods so far discussed.   The first is that observation is restricted to those species which for some reason or other become trapped in the material under the experimental conditions used.   The second is that it is very difficult to use wet samples.

The first drawback can be overcome to some extent by the use of low temperatures.   By irradiating the sample and recording the spectrum at the temperature of liquid nitrogen, or better still at the temperature of liquid helium, one would hope to get nearer to the primary products.   Then, by following changes in the spectrum as the sample is warmed up to room temperature, one hopes to follow the subsequent physical and chemical processes. A start has already been made on these lines, in experiments described in this and other chapters, and it has been shown that usually, but not always, a different spectrum is obtained with irradiation at a low temperature than at room temperature.   The low temperature spectrum, however, will not necessarily be that of the primary products, partly because some movement and chemical reactions take place even at 4.2°K, and partly because of the local heating effect of radiation, so that even though the bulk of the sample is at 4.2°K, small volumes surrounding points where radiation is absorbed may temporarily be raised to considerably higher temperatures. (For references on this point see Smith and Wyard, 1961; Norman and Spiegler, 1962; Seitz and Kohler, 1956.)   As an example (discussed in more detail in chapter 5), consider the ESR spectrum of irradiated frozen solutions of H_2O_2 in H_2O.   The primary products will be electrons, positive ions, and excited molecules from ionizing radiation, or OH radicals from u.v. radiation.   None of these species appears in the spectra, even when irradiation is carried out at 4.2°K; the spectra are mainly due to HO_2 radicals with either type of radiation.

The drawback about not being able to use wet samples is that, although the primary products of radiation may be the same in wet and dry samples (apart from the products from the extra water in the wet samples), the subsequent reactions may be very different in the two cases, due to the much greater mobility in wet samples.   A good example of this comes from the work on seeds, discussed in section 3.4.4.B, where increasing the water content up to the normal amount of bound water decreases radiosensitivity, but beyond this point increases it again; and the effect of nitric oxide is also reversed beyond the same point.   Although there is not a sharp boundary, we may say that dry seeds are in a solid state in which the primary products of radiation take part in one set of reactions while wetter seeds are in a semi-liquid state in which the primary products take part in another set of reactions.   ESR experiments to date have been concerned almost exclusively with the solid state.

Both the drawbacks referred to might be overcome by a combination of ESR spectroscopy with pulse radiolysis, and it is possibly in this direction that the biggest advances will now be made.

There still remains an important question concerning the biological significance of the work described in this chapter.   Assuming, as now seems likely, that the main cause of death of a cell following irradiation is breakage of a DNA molecule, what connection is there between this and the radicals observed by ESR?   To this question there is at present no answer.

ACKNOWLEDGEMENTS

This work forms part of the research program of the Physics Department, Guy's Hospital Medical School, London, and was supported by the British Empire Cancer Campaign.   We are grateful to Professor C. B. Allsopp for his interest and support and to Dr. J. P. Elliott for many helpful discussions.

REFERENCES

Alexander, P., Charlesby, A., and Ross, M., 1954, *Proc. R. Soc.* A, **223**, 392–404.

Alexander, P., Lett, J. T., and Ormerod, M. G., 1961, *Biochim. biophys. Acta*, **51**, 207–9.

Bass, A. M., and Broida, H. P., 1960, editors, *Formation and Trapping of Free Radicals* (New York and London: Academic Press).

Bleaney, B., 1960, *Proc. phys. Soc.*, **75**, 621–3.

Blois, M. S., Jr., Maling, J. E., and Taskovich, L. T., 1963, *Biophysics Laboratory Report* (U.S.A.: Stanford University).

Blumenfeld, L. A., 1959, *Biofizika*, **4**, 515–20.

Boag, J. W., 1963, in *Radiation Effects in Physics, Chemistry and Biology* (Amsterdam: North-Holland Publ. Co.), p. 194.

Boag, J. W., and Müller, A., 1959, *Nature*, Lond., **183**, 831–2.

Burgess, V. R., 1961, *J. scient. Instrum.*, **38**, 98–9.

Burke, M., Kenny, P., and Nicholls, C. H., 1962, *Nature*, Lond., **196**, 667–8.

Cairns, J., 1963, *J. molec. Biol.*, **6**, 208–13.

Castelijn, G., Depireux, J., and Müller, A., 1964, *Int. J. Radiat. Biol.*, **8**, 157–64.

Conger, A. D., 1961, *J. cell. comp. Physiol.*, **58**, 27–32.

Conger, A. D., and Randolph, M. L., 1959, *Radiat. Res.*, **11**, 54–66.

Cook, J. B., 1965, Ph.D. Thesis, University of London.

Cook, J. B., Elliott, J. P., and Wyard, S. J., 1967, *Molec. Phys.*, **13**, 49–64.

Cook, J. B., and Wyard, S. J., 1966a, *Nature*, Lond., **210**, 526–7; 1966b, *Int. J. Radiat. Biol.*, **11**, 225–7; 1966c, ibid., **11**, 357–65.

Cook, R. F., 1963, *Int. J. Radiat. Biol.*, **7**, 497–504.

Crick, F. H. C., and Watson, J. D., 1954, *Proc. R. Soc.* A, **223**, 80–96.

Dimmick, R. L., Heckly, R. J., and Hollis, D. P., 1961, *Nature*, Lond., **192**, 776–7.

Dorlet, C., van de Vorst, A., and Bertinchamps, A. J., 1962, *Nature*, Lond., **194**, 767.

Ehrenberg, A., 1961, in *Free Radicals in Biological Systems* (New York and London: Academic Press), pp. 337–50.

Ehrenberg, A., and Ehrenberg, L., 1958, *Ark. Fys.*, **14**, 133–41.

Ehrenberg, A., Ehrenberg, L., and Löfroth, G., 1963, *Nature*, Lond., **200**, 376–7.

Eisinger, J., and Shulman, R. G., 1963, *Proc. natl. Acad. Sci. U.S.A.*, **50**, 694–6.

Elliot, J. P., and Wyard, S. J., 1965, *Nature*, Lond., **208**, 483–5.

Errera, E., and Forssberg, A., 1961, editors, *Mechanisms in Radiobiology* (New York and London: Academic Press).

Fessenden, R. W., 1964, *J. phys. Chem.*, Ithaca, **68**, 1508–15.

Fessenden, R. W., and Schuler, R. H., 1960, *J. chem. Phys.*, **33**, 935–6; 1963, ibid., **39**, 2147–95.

Franklin, R. E., and Gosling, R. G., 1953, *Nature*, Lond., **171**, 740–1.

Fricke, H., and Thomas, J. K., 1964, *Radiat. Res. Suppl.*, **4**, 35–53.

Gordy, W., 1955, *Discuss. Faraday Soc.*, **19**, 182–3; 1959, *Radiat. Res. Suppl.*, **1**, 491–510.

Gordy, W., Ard, W. B., and Shields, H., 1955a, *Proc. natl. Acad. Sci. U.S.A.*, **41**, 983–96; 1955b, **41**, 996–1004.

Gordy, W., Pruden, B., and Snipes, W., 1965, *Proc. natl. Acad. Sci. U.S.A.*, **53**, 751–6.

Gordy, W., and Shields, H., 1958, *Radiat. Res.*, **9**, 611–25; 1960, *Proc. natl. Acad. Sci. U.S.A.*, **46**, 1124–36.

Heller, H. C., and Cole, T., 1965, *Proc. natl. Acad. Sci. U.S.A.*, **54**, 1486–90.

Henriksen, T., 1962a, *J. chem. Phys.*, **36**, 1258–62; 1962b, ibid., **37**, 2189–95; 1963, *Electron Spin Resonance Studies on the Formation and Properties of Free Radicals in Irradiated Sulfur-containing Substances*, Norsk Hydro's Institute for Cancer Research, Oslo, Norway; 1966, *Acta chem. scand.*, **20**, 2898–900.

Henriksen, T., Sanner, T., and Pihl, A., 1963, *Radiat. Res.*, **18**, 147–62.

Herak, J. N., and Gordy, W., 1965, *Proc. natl. Acad. Sci. U.S.A.*, **54**, 1287–92; 1966a, ibid., **55**, 1373–78; 1966b, ibid., **56**, 7–11.

Holmes, D. E., Myers, L. S., Jr., and Ingalls, R. B., 1966, *Nature*, Lond., **209**, 1017–8.

Johnson, L. N., and Phillips, D. C., 1965, *Nature*, Lond., **206**, 761–3.

Ki Yong Lee, Wahl, R., and Barbu, E., 1956, *Annls. Inst. Pasteur*, Paris, **91**, 212–24.

Klingmüller, W., Lane, G. R., Saxena, M. C., and Ingram, D. J. E., 1959, *Nature*, Lond., **184**, 464–5.

Köhnlein, W., and Müller, A., 1962, *Physics Med. Biol.*, **6**, 599–604; 1964, *Int. J. Radiat. Biol.*, **8**, 141–55.

Köhnlein, W. and Müller, A., Henriksen, T., Ehrenberg, A., Ehrenberg, L. and Löfroth, G., ten Bosch, J. J. and Braams, R., Redhardt, A., and Randolph, L., 1963, in *Radiation Effects in Physics, Chemistry and Biology* (Amsterdam: North-Holland Publ. Co.), p. 194.

Krebs, A. T., and Benson, B. W., 1965, *Nature*, Lond., **207**, 1412–13.

Lehman, I. R., Zimmerman, S. B., Adler, J., Bessman, M. J., Sims, E. S., and Kornberg, A., 1958, *Proc. natl. Acad. Sci. U.S.A.*, **44**, 1191–6.

Lett, J. T., Parkins, G., Alexander, P., and Ormerod, M. G., 1964, *Nature*, Lond., **203**, 593–6.

Lion, M. B., Kirby-Smith, J. S., and Randolph, M. L., 1961, *Nature*, Lond., **192**, 34–6.

McCormick, G., and Gordy, W., 1958, *J. Phys. Chem.*, Ithaca, **62**, 783–9.
McGrath, R. A., and Williams, R. W., 1966, *Nature*, Lond., **212**, 534–5.
Marmur, J., and Doty, P., 1962, *J. molec. Biol.*, **5**, 109–18.
Marvin, D. A., Spencer, M., Wilkins, M. H. F., and Hamilton, L. D., 1958, *Nature*, Lond., **182**, 387–8.
Matheson, M. S., 1964, *Radiat. Res. Suppl.*, **4**, 1–23.
Miyagawa, I., Gordy, W., Watabe, N., and Wilbur, K. M., 1958, *Proc. natl. Acad. Sci. U.S.A.*, **44**, 613–7.
Müller, A., 1962, *Int. J. Radiat. Biol.*, **5**, 199–200; 1963, ibid., **6**, 137–42; 1964, ibid., **8**, 131–40.
Müller, A., and Köhnlein, W., 1964, *Int. J. Radiat. Biol.*, **8**, 121–30.
Müller, A., Schambra, P. E., and Pietsch, E., 1963, *Int. J. Radiat. Biol.*, **7**, 587–99.
Norman, A., and Spiegler, P., 1962, *J. appl. Phys.*, **32**, 2658.
Ormerod, M. G., 1965, *Int. J. Radiat. Biol.*, **9**, 291–300.
Ormerod, M. G., and Alexander, P., 1963, *Radiat. Res.*, **18**, 495–509.
Patten, R. A., and Gordy, W., 1964, *Nature*, Lond., **201**, 361–3.
Pershan, P. S., Shulman, R. G., Wyluda, B. J., and Eisinger, J., 1964, *Physics*, **1**, 163–82; 1965, *Science*, N.Y., **148**, 378–80.
Platzman, R. L., 1962, *Vortex*, **23**.
Pohlit, H., Rajewsky, B., and Redhardt, A., 1961, in *Free Radicals in Biological Systems* (New York and London: Academic Press), pp. 367–72.
Powers, E. L., 1961, *J. cell. comp. Physiol.*, **58**, 13–25.
Powers, E. L., Ehret, C. F., and Smaller, B., 1961, in *Free Radicals in Biological Systems* (New York and London: Academic Press), pp. 351–66.
Powers, E. L., Webb, R. B., and Ehret, C. F., 1960, *Radiat. Res. Suppl.*, **2**, 94–121.
Pruden, B., Snipes, W., and Gordy, W., 1965, *Proc. natl. Acad. Sci. U.S.A.*, **53**, 917–24.
Prydz, S., and Henriksen, T., 1961, *Acta chem. scand.*, **15**, 791–802.
Radiation Effects in Physics, Chemistry and Biology, 1963, Ed. M. Ebert and A. Howard (Amsterdam: North-Holland Publ. Co.).
Rajewsky, B., and Redhardt, A., 1962, *Nature*, Lond., **193**, 365–6.
Randolph, M. L., 1960, *Rev. scient. Instrum.*, **31**, 949–52; 1961, in *Free Radicals in Biological Systems* (New York and London: Academic Press), pp. 249–61.
Rexroad, H. N., and Gordy, W., 1959, *Proc. natl. Acad. Sci. U.S.A.*, **45**, 256–269.
Rotblat, J., and Simmons, J. A., 1963a, *Physics Med. Biol.*, **7**, 489–97; 1963b, ibid., **7**, 499–504.
Salovey, R., Shulman, R. G., and Walsh, W. M., Jr., 1963, *J. chem. Phys.*, **39**, 839–40.

Seitz, F., and Kohler, J. S., 1956, *Solid State Phys.*, **2**, 307–448.

Shen-Pei-Gen, Blumenfeld, L. A., Kalmanson, A. E., and Pasynski, A. G., 1959, *Biofizika*, **4**, 263–74.

Shields, H., and Gordy, W., 1958, *J. phys. Chem.*, Ithaca, **62**, 789–98; 1959, *Proc. natl. Acad. Sci. U.S.A.*, **45**, 269–81.

Simmons, J. A., 1965, *Nature*, Lond., **205**, 697.

Singer, L. S., 1959, *J. appl. Phys.*, **30**, 1463–4.

Singer, L. S., and Kommandeur, J., 1961, *J. chem. Phys.*, **34**, 133–40.

Singh, B. B., and Charlesby, A., 1965, *Int. J. Radiat. Biol.*, **9**, 157–64.

Smaller, B., and Avery, E. C., 1959, *Nature*, Lond., **183**, 539–40.

Smith, R. C., and Wyard, S. J., 1961, *Nature*, Lond., **191**, 897–8.

Sparrman, B., Ehrenberg, L., and Ehrenberg, A., 1959, *Acta chem. scand.*, **13**, 199–200.

Stacey, K. A., 1963, *Radiation Effects in Physics, Chemistry and Biology*, (Amsterdam: North-Holland Publ. Co.), p. 96.

Swartz, H. M., 1965, *Radiat. Res.*, **24**, 579–86.

Ulbert, K., 1962, *Nature*, Lond., **195**, 175.

Verdier, P. H., Whipple, E. B., and Schomaker, V., 1961, *J. chem. Phys.*, **1**, 118–19.

van de Vorst, A., 1964, *Int. J. Radiat. Biol.*, **8**, 111–20.

van de Vorst, A., and Krsmanovic-Simic, D., 1966, *C. R. hebd. Séanc. Acad. Sci. Paris*, **262**, 2288–90.

van de Vorst, A., and Richir, M., 1965, *C.R. hebd. Séanc. Acad. Sci. Paris*, **260**, 6458–61.

van de Vorst, A., and Villeé, F., 1964, *C.R. hebd. Séanc. Acad. Sci., Paris*, **259**, 928–31.

van de Vorst, A., Villée, F., and Duchesne, J., 1965, *Int. J. Radiat. Biol.*, **9**, 269–75.

van de Vorst, A., and Williams-Dorlet, C., 1963, *C.R. hebd. Séanc. Acad. Sci., Paris*, **257**, 2183–6.

Walsh, W. M., Jr., Shulman, R. G., and Heidenreich, R. D., 1961, *Nature*, Lond., **192**, 1041–3.

Watson, J. D., 1965, *Molecular Biology of the Gene* (New York: W. A. Benjamin Inc.).

Watson, J. D., and Crick, F. H. C., 1953, *Nature*, Lond., **171**, 737–8.

Wilkins, M. F. H., Stokes, A. R., and Wilson, H. R., 1953, *Nature*, Lond., **171**, 738–40.

Wyard, S. J., 1965, *J. scient. Instrum.*, **42**, 769–70.

Zimmer, K. G., Ehrenberg, L., and Ehrenberg, A., 1957, *Strahlentherapie*, **103**, 3–15.

Zimmer, K. G., Köhlein, W., Hotz, G., and Müller, A., 1963, *Strahlentherapie*, **120**, 161–90.

Zimmer, K. G., and Müller, A., 1965, in *Current Topics in Radiation Research* (Amsterdam: North-Holland Publ. Co.).

Zimmermann, F., Kröger, H., Hagen, U., and Keck, K., 1964, *Biochim. biophys. Acta*, **87**, 160–2.

CHAPTER FOUR

ELECTRON SPIN RESONANCE OF RADIATION DAMAGE IN ORGANIC SINGLE CRYSTALS

J. B. Cook

Haileybury and Imperial Service College, Hertford, England (Previously of *Physics Department, Guy's Hospital Medical School*)

and S. J. Wyard

Physics Department, Guy's Hospital Medical School, London, England

4.1 INTRODUCTION

Paramagnetic resonance was first observed by Zavoisky in 1945, and in the following years the method was used to investigate extensively the magnetic properties of the salts of transition elements. This work has been reviewed by Bleaney and Stevens (1953), by Bowers and Owen (1955) and by Orton (1959). Most of the experiments were made with single crystals, since it was quickly realized that with single crystals more accurate measurements could be made and more information obtained than from measurements with powders.

The first electron spin resonance (ESR) study of radiation damage in materials of biological interest used powders (Gordy, *et al.*, 1955) but this was quickly followed by reports of orientation effects in single crystals of glycine (Uebersfield and Erb, 1956) and alanine (van Roggen, *et al.*, 1956). The first detailed results were given by Ghosh and Whiffen (1958, 1959) who also studied glycine. Papers on dimethylglyoxime (Miyagawa and Gordy, 1959) and malonic acid (McConnell, *et al.*, 1960) soon followed and confirmed that it was possible to investigate radicals produced by irradiating single crystals, in a similar way to that which had been used to study paramagnetic ions. The early papers indicated that the radiation-produced radicals were highly oriented. The spectra were very different from those which had been obtained from polycrystalline samples, showing many more, and much narrower lines. When the crystal was rotated in the magnetic field, there were quite large changes in the spectrum. As an example of such changes, spectra from an irradiated crystal of L-hydroxyproline are given in Fig. 4.1, the crystal having been rotated through only 15° between the two recordings.

When studying radicals in organic single crystals, one difficulty is that the species produced by irradiation have first to be identified. In practice, certain bonds are preferentially ruptured, but the energy absorbed from the radiation is generally sufficient to break any of the bonds in a molecule and so even a simple molecule could produce a number of radical fragments. These could then react to produce further species, and so it is not possible to say in advance what will be found in an irradiated crystal. The analysis of the spectra is often involved and, in consequence, there are many radicals which have not been identified. A useful review on this subject has recently been written by Morton (1964a).

In this chapter, a summary of the relevant theory will be given and then a detailed description of the experimental procedure and method of interpreting the spectra. This will be followed by a review of previous ESR studies of radiation damage in irradiated organic single crystals which demonstrates the types of interaction which are generally observed. We have included a number of tables of *g*-values and hyperfine splittings of radicals classified according to the type of interaction. We would also refer readers to the exhaustive tables prepared by Fischer (1965) which include data from all publications on ESR spectroscopy of free radicals up to March 1964. Finally, as an example of the technique, our interpretation of the spectra from an irradiated crystal of cytosine will be described.

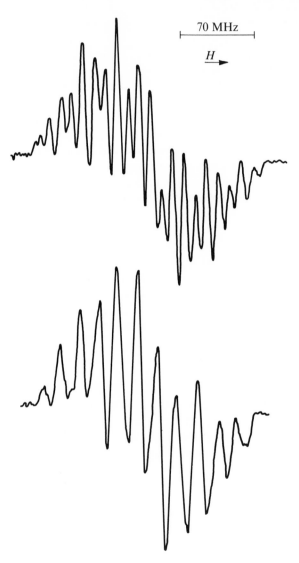

70 MHz

H

Fig. 4.1   Derivative spectra from an irradiated single crystal of L-hydroxyproline. The crystal was rotated through 15° between the two recordings.

4.2   THEORY

The detailed theory of electron spin resonance spectroscopy has been covered in the first chapter.   In single crystal work, the most interesting information arises from changes in shape of the spectrum as the crystal is rotated in the magnetic field.   Therefore, in this section, only the origin of hyperfine interaction and its interpretation in terms of a spin-Hamiltonian will be discussed.

4.2.1   ORIGIN OF HYPERFINE INTERACTION

If the orbital of an unpaired electron embraces an atom which has a nucleus with a magnetic moment and spin, there will be an interaction between this nucleus and the electron, resulting in a small splitting of the energy levels of the electron.   In the particular case of interaction with a single proton, the magnetic moment and spin of the proton will be lined up either parallel or antiparallel to the applied field and electron spin.   The proton itself has a spin $I = \frac{1}{2}$, and therefore only the two possible orientations, with components along the field of $\pm\frac{1}{2}$, are allowed.   For the general case of a nucleus with spin I, there would be $(2I + 1)$ possible orientations.   The magnetic moment of the proton will produce a small additional field at the electron and, according to whether the proton is quantized with its spin parallel or antiparallel to the field, this will add to, or subtract from, the effect of the external field. Hence the electron experiences a magnetic field which is either slightly greater, or slightly less than the applied field.   As the protons are approximately equally distributed between the two orientations, each of the electronic levels will be split into two.   When radiation of the resonant frequency is applied, the electron spins will change orientation, but in general the nuclear spins will remain unchanged during the electronic transition. Exceptions to this rule will be discussed in section 4.4.7.   Thus, transitions will only occur between levels which have the same quantized component of nuclear spin, and they are therefore governed by the selection rules $\Delta M_s = \pm 1$, $\Delta M_I = 0$.   Hence, there are two absorption lines whose separation is termed the hyperfine splitting and gives a direct measure of the interaction between the proton and the unpaired electron.   It follows that for the general case of a nuclear spin I, the spectrum will consist of $(2I + 1)$ equally spaced components.

Most hyperfine splittings are anisotropic, that is, their magnitude depends on the angle between the applied field and the orbital of the unpaired electron.   Hence, as an irradiated single crystal is rotated in the magnetic field, the spectrum changes, often very rapidly, as shown in Fig. 4.1.   If a particular hyperfine splitting can be measured at many crystal orientations, the isotropic and anisotropic components of the splitting can be determined and these often yield precise information of the site of the radiation damage and also of the orbital of the unpaired electron. The existence of hyperfine structure is therefore the chief diagnostic tool for studying free radicals by electron spin resonance techniques. Hyperfine splittings are usually measured in oersted but for theoretical reasons are often quoted in MHz, the conversion factor being 2.8025 MHz = 1 Oe, as mentioned in equation (1.4) of chapter 1.

4.2.2 THE SPIN-HAMILTONIAN

The energy of interaction between a nucleus and an unpaired electron in a magnetic field H is usually expressed as a 'Hamiltonian'. Whiffen (1961) has considered, in some detail, the Hamiltonian appropriate to organic single crystal studies, and so only its simplest form will be discussed here. The Hamiltonian may be written:

$$\mathscr{H} = -\beta\mathbf{S} \cdot g \cdot \mathbf{H} + \mathbf{S} \cdot A \cdot \mathbf{I} \qquad (4.1)$$

where β is the Bohr magneton, S is the electron spin operator, g is the tensor of the spectroscopic splitting factor, A is the hyperfine interaction tensor, and I is the nuclear spin operator.

The first term represents the direct coupling of the electron with the magnetic field. If the orbital angular momentum of the unpaired electron were completely quenched, then the tensor for g would be isotropic and equal to the free spin value of -2.0023. The sign of the g-value will be discussed in section 4.4.6. In fact, the orbital angular momentum is not completely quenched and small deviations in g-value are observed. However, with the exception of some sulfur-containing compounds, the g-values measured for free radicals trapped in organic single crystals depart from the free spin value by ± 0.01 or less. As this deviation is direction dependent, g is a symmetrical tensor with off-diagonal elements of this order. The second term represents the hyperfine interaction between the electron spin S and the nuclear spin I, described by the second-rank tensor A. In so far as g is nearly isotropic, the hyperfine tensor A will be a symmetrical 3×3 matrix which can be diagonalized and resolved into isotropic and anisotropic components. A term involving direct interaction between the nucleus and the magnetic field has been neglected since its primary effect is to relax the selection rule $\Delta M_I = 0$. Terms representing direct coupling between nuclei are also neglected as such couplings are negligible in the solid state.

In single crystal studies, it is the interaction between the electron spin S and the nuclear spin I which gives the spectroscopist the most interesting information through the hyperfine structure of the spectrum. The energy of this hyperfine interaction is expressed by the second term of equation (4.1).

The isotropic and anisotropic parts of the interaction can be separated by rewriting this term in the form of an effective Hamiltonian $\mathscr{H}'$ (Abragam and Pryce, 1951).

$$\mathscr{H}' = (\tfrac{8}{3}\pi g\beta\gamma)\psi^2(0)\mathbf{S} \cdot \mathbf{I} - g\beta\gamma[(\mathbf{S} \cdot \mathbf{I})r^{-3} - 3(\mathbf{S} \cdot \mathbf{r})(\mathbf{I} \cdot \mathbf{r})r^{-5}] \quad (4.2)$$

where γ is the gyromagnetic ratio for the nucleus and r is the mean distance between the unpaired electron and the nucleus. The eigenvalues of $\mathscr{H}'$ are the principal values of A, and the isotropic and anisotropic components of this tensor correlate with the first and second terms, respectively, of the last equation.

4.2.3 ISOTROPIC HYPERFINE INTERACTION

The first term in equation (4.2) gives rise to a hyperfine splitting only if there is a finite probability of finding the unpaired electron at the interacting nucleus, as indicated by the factor $\psi^2(0)$. For this reason, the isotropic interaction is usually called the 'contact' or Fermi interaction (Fermi, 1930). Thus only electrons in s-atomic orbitals will experience isotropic interactions. Likewise only σ-molecular orbitals have a finite electron density at the nucleus, although in the case of π-orbitals a special mechanism, configurational interaction, operates to modify this provision. It is possible to estimate the s-character of the orbital by comparing the experimentally determined isotropic hyperfine interaction with a parameter calculated from known wave functions, assuming the unpaired electron to be wholly in the s-orbital of the nucleus concerned. For example, a splitting of 1420 MHz is expected for an unpaired electron occupying the s-orbital of a hydrogen atom. A splitting of this order has been observed for hydrogen atoms formed in γ-irradiated frozen inorganic acids (Livingston, et al., 1955).

It has been mentioned that configurational interaction accounts for observed isotropic hyperfine interaction when the simple theory predicts zero electron density at the nucleus. This is the name given to the fact that it is possible for excited electron configurations with finite densities at the nucleus to be mixed with the ground state configuration. As a result, the electron density takes on a small amount of the distribution corresponding to the excited state. Such an excited state has unpaired electrons in the s-orbitals and hence the possibility of producing a large isotropic hyperfine splitting. Proton splittings, for example, are intrinsically large, 1420 MHz for a $1s$-electron, and so very little admixture is needed to explain observed splittings.

There are, however, two important cases not explained by the theory of configurational interaction. First, some observed splittings are much larger than the theory allows unless account is taken of a 'negative spin density' (Weissman, 1956; McConnell and Chesnut, 1958) on certain atoms. Spin polarization of bonds causes the unpaired spin density to perturb the paired electrons and effectively produce a partial unpairing, giving rise to a secondary spin density of opposite sign to that of the original electron. The algebraic sum of the spin densities for the whole molecule remains unity as there is a corresponding increase in the positive spin density of the original electron. The configurational interaction theory is still valid, but the effective spin density is now the sum of the moduli of the spin densities, which can easily exceed unity.

The second case arises because it has been observed experimentally that protons of methyl groups attached to the ring system of aromatic radicals produce hyperfine splittings of the same order as those attached directly to the ring (Venkataraman and Fraenkel, 1955). Methyl carbon atoms are sp^3 hybridized, and configurational interaction cannot explain the finite spin density at the protons required for such a splitting. However, the theory of hyperconjugation shows that, if consideration is given to the spatial arrangement of the three proton $1s$-orbitals, a linear combination of these orbitals can be taken with the same symmetry relative to the aromatic plane as the π-orbital containing the unpaired electron. The 'pseudo π-orbital' of the protons can then interact directly with the π-orbitals of the ring system, producing a splitting which depends on all three protons.

4.2.4 ANISOTROPIC HYPERFINE INTERACTION

The second term in equation (4.2) imparts to the effective Hamiltonian an anisotropic or direction-dependent character. It is frequently termed the dipolar hyperfine interaction and comes from the classical interaction between two magnetic dipoles. The anisotropic hyperfine energy is given by the expression (Frosch and Foley, 1952; Zeldes, et al., 1960):

$$g\beta\gamma M_I M_S \left\langle \frac{1 - 3\cos^2\alpha}{r^3} \right\rangle_{AV} (1 - 3\cos^2\theta) \tag{4.3}$$

where r is the distance from the nucleus to the unpaired electron, α is the angle between this line and a principal axis of the tensor, and θ the angle between the magnetic field and the same principal axis. For an interacting nucleus at the centre of a spherically symmetric electronic orbital, that is an s-orbital, the element of solid angle corresponding to $d\alpha$ is $2 \sin \alpha \, d\alpha$ and the effective magnetic field at the electron is proportional to the product $r^{-3}(1 - 3\cos^2\alpha)(2\sin\alpha \, d\alpha)$ integrated over all α. This is zero, and therefore the unpaired electron must have p- or d-character for there to be any anisotropic hyperfine interaction. It is possible to estimate the p-character of the orbital of an unpaired electron by comparing the observed anisotropic hyperfine splitting with a parameter obtained from known wave functions. Thus, s-atomic orbitals give isotropic splittings and p-atomic orbitals give anisotropic hyperfine splittings. In the case of a π-electron radical, the unpaired electron usually occupies a predominantly carbon $2p$-orbital perpendicular to the plan trigonal skeleton of the radical. The simple theory anticipates that only p-orbitals and therefore anisotropic interactions are involved, whereas in practice isotropic splittings are also observed. Configurational interaction and negative spin density through spin polarization in the bonding orbital are used to explain these observed isotropic splittings.

4.2.5   ADVANTAGES OF SINGLE CRYSTAL STUDIES

It has been shown that the hyperfine structure observed in the ESR spectra of organic free radicals can yield precise information of the structure of the radicals and the distribution of the odd electron. Many measurements have been made on systems in solution, for which state the anisotropic part of the coupling is averaged to zero by the comparatively fast tumbling of the radicals. Hence, the resulting spectra can only be interpreted in terms of their isotropic interactions. In the case of radicals trapped in amorphous or polycrystalline solids, the summation over all orientations of the anisotropic term results in a broadening of the individual lines, so that hyperfine structure may be blurred out and the spectra have false simplicity. This is particularly so when there are large anisotropic interactions and hence the interpretation of such spectra may not be very meaningful.

In order to obtain the couplings in a radical as a tensor, and thus derive the maximum amount of information, it is necessary for the radicals to be trapped at specific orientations. This condition is fulfilled for the radicals trapped in irradiated single crystals where both the anisotropic and isotropic couplings can often be evaluated. If there are large anisotropic interactions, the spectra are usually complex and their interpretation correspondingly involved. However, the single crystal studies are potentially rewarding in terms of the additional information on the nature of the radical that can be deduced from the observed anisotropic interactions.

4.3   EXPERIMENTAL TECHNIQUES AND INTERPRETATION OF SPECTRA

4.3.1   EXPERIMENTAL TECHNIQUES

The experimenter will wish to investigate the effects of radiation on a particular molecule or chemical grouping within a molecule. It is then necessary to find a compound containing the molecule or chemical grouping which can be readily crystallized. The minimum dimensions of the crystals should be about 2 mm and they should preferably have well developed faces. It is also preferable to choose crystals whose structure has been worked out, since without this it is difficult to interpret the spectra.

Crystals are usually grown from solution, most commonly aqueous solution, and the only apparatus needed is a constant temperature bath thermostatted to, say, $\pm 0.05°C$. Three simple methods have been used in our laboratory for growing single crystals: (a) slow cooling of a solution, (b) slow evaporation of the solvent from a solution held at a constant temperature, and (c) growth of a seed crystal in a supersaturated solution within a temperature range for which spontaneous nucleation does not occur. Methods (a) and (b) have been suitable for producing seed crystals, and method (c) the best for growing the larger crystals needed in ESR.

The crystals are usually irradiated with X- or γ-rays, but other radiations have been used. Care should be taken to ensure that the dose rate is low enough to avoid undue heating of the specimens during irradiation. The exact dose is usually unimportant as it is only necessary to produce sufficient free radicals to give a spectrum whose intensity is well above the spectrometer noise level. Doses from 1 to 10 Mrads are generally sufficient for this purpose. However, in the case of some unsaturated compounds with a low radical yield, much higher doses have been used.

In section 4.2.2 it was stated that when an unpaired electron couples to a nucleus with spin $I \geq \frac{1}{2}$, the resultant splitting observed in the electron spin resonance spectrum is direction-dependent, and hence needs a coupling tensor for complete expression. The elements of this tensor are inferred from measurements of the variation in the splitting while the crystal is rotated about three selected orthogonal axes. These axes are chosen with respect to external features for a crystal of the triclinic system, but will usually be the three crystallographic axes for an orthorhombic crystal, and two of the crystallographic axes together with the third member of an orthogonal set for a monoclinic crystal.

There are many ways of mounting the irradiated single crystal. However, the simplest method suitable for room temperature observations is to mount it on a quartz or teflon rod with a non-magnetic grease such as anhydrous lanoline. This mounting rod is attached to the head of an optical goniometer and the position of one selected axis adjusted so that it is parallel to the rod axis. The crystal is rotated about this axis, according to a right-handed system, and spectra, which will repeat themselves after a rotation of $180°$, are recorded at frequent intervals. A similar procedure is adopted for rotations about the other two axes of the orthogonal set. Rather than rotating the crystal in the magnetic field, the magnet could be rotated about the crystal. However, in this case, if high frequency modulation is used, care should be taken to ensure that it rotates with the main magnetic field so that the two are parallel at all orientations.

4.3.2 DETERMINATION OF THE ELEMENTS FOR A COUPLING TENSOR

It is the square of the coupling tensor which can generally be determined from the experimental observations and the elements of the actual coupling tensor are obtained from this. Assuming that a splitting can be followed for most spectra, it is measured directly and its square plotted against the orientation of the crystal in the magnetic field. There will be three graphs, one for each plane of observation. The splitting is required to be a smooth function of the crystal orientation and this function has to be fitted to the experimental points in order to determine the elements of the coupling tensor. If the square of an actual tensor is defined as:

$$A = \begin{pmatrix} A_{11} & A_{12} & A_{13} \\ A_{21} & A_{22} & A_{23} \\ A_{31} & A_{32} & A_{33} \end{pmatrix} \tag{4.4}$$

for a symmetric tensor:

$$A_{ij} = A_{ji}, \quad i, j = 1, 2, 3. \tag{4.5}$$

The squares of the splittings along the three selected orthogonal axes give the diagonal elements of this tensor. The off-diagonal elements are obtained from the phase and amplitude of the experimental splitting curves. These three curves are defined by the equations:

$$(S_{\theta_1})^2 = A_{33} \sin^2\theta + 2A_{32} \sin\theta \cos\theta + A_{22} \cos^2\theta \tag{4.6}$$

$$(S_{\theta_2})^2 = A_{11} \sin^2\theta + 2A_{13} \sin\theta \cos\theta + A_{33} \cos^2\theta \tag{4.7}$$

$$(S_{\theta_3})^2 = A_{22} \sin^2\theta + 2A_{21} \sin\theta \cos\theta + A_{11} \cos^2\theta \tag{4.8}$$

where θ is the angle between an axis of rotation and the magnetic field according to a right-handed axial system, and S_{θ_x}, $x = 1, 2, 3$, is the measured splitting at this angle during rotation about axis x. The off-diagonal elements of the tensor will be positive if the splitting curve has its maximum in the first quadrant, and negative if it falls in the second quadrant of rotation. The most accurate way of fitting the curve is to apply a least squares method to a large number of experimentally determined splittings at different angles of rotation. However, various quicker methods have been described (Weil and Anderson, 1958; Schonland, 1959).

The rotation axes are chosen for convenience and are therefore arbitrary with respect to interatomic directions in the free radicals. This feature is removed by diagonalizing the coupling tensor, that is, choosing a new set of orthogonal axes which makes all the off-diagonal elements zero.

The three roots λ_1, λ_2, λ_3 of the secular equation,

$$\det (A - \lambda I) = 0 \qquad (4.9)$$

where I is the unit matrix, are the squares of the principal values of the actual coupling tensor. The direction cosines of the principal axes satisfy

$$\sum_{j=1}^{3} A_{ij} l_{kj} = \lambda_k l_{ki}, \qquad i = 1, 2, 3 \qquad (4.10)$$

where the l_{kj}, $j = 1, 2, 3$, are the direction cosines corresponding to the roots λ_k, $k = 1, 2, 3$, of equation (4.9). Once the principal values of the actual coupling tensor and the direction cosines of its principal axes have been determined, the elements of the actual tensor are obtained by applying the usual algebraic processes. Many standard textbooks (for example, Atkin, 1956) discuss the algebra of the subject, and in section 4.5.2 of this chapter the working for the α-hydrogen coupling tensor is given in some detail to illustrate the method.

4.3.3   DETERMINATION OF THE ELEMENTS FOR A g-TENSOR

In addition to hyperfine interactions, the g-value is also direction dependent and hence needs a tensor for complete expression. The g-values are measured by comparing the position of the center of each radical spectrum with that of a standard such as α, α-diphenyl, β-picryl hydrazyl (DPPH). The DPPH is very finely ground in order to avoid asymmetry of the line in respect to its own anisotropic g-value (Weidner and Whitmer, 1953), and a smear put on the crystal so that the superimposed spectra are recorded. If the differences between the centers of the pattern are measured in frequency units, the g-values are calculated from:

$$g = \left(1 + \frac{\Delta v}{v}\right) g_D \qquad (4.11)$$

where $g = g$-value of the radical, $g_D = g$-value of DPPH, $\Delta v =$ frequency difference between the centers, and $v =$ frequency of measurement. The sign convention for this equation is that shifts to lower fields than DPPH are positive. Holden, $et\ al.$ (1950) have determined the g-value of DPPH as 2.0036 ± 0.0002. The squares of the measured g-values are plotted on three curves defined by equations similar to those for hyperfine interactions, that is:

$$(g_{\theta_1})^2 = g_{33} \sin^2\theta + g_{32} \sin\theta \cos\theta + g_{22} \cos^2\theta \qquad (4.12)$$

$$(g_{\theta_2})^2 = g_{11} \sin^2\theta + g_{13} \sin\theta \cos\theta + g_{33} \cos^2\theta \qquad (4.13)$$

$$(g_{\theta_3})^2 = g_{22} \sin^2\theta + g_{21} \sin\theta \cos\theta + g_{11} \cos^2\theta. \qquad (4.14)$$

Hence, using a method similar to that already described, the g-tensor can be evaluated.

4.3.4   SITE SPLITTING

The above discussion has assumed that the spectra arise from only one radical site with coupling to only one nucleus.   In practice, the spectra are often complex and it is not easy to link the absorption lines with various interactions.   The presence of chemically similar species in magnetically distinguishable positions produces site splittings, that is, every absorption line appears as a multiplet, one line for each of the sites.   Although in most cases only two non-equivalent radical sites are observed, this frequently complicates the spectra.   The space group of a crystal symbolizes the elements of symmetry present within the unit cell (Phillips, 1946) and these indicate at which crystal orientations site splitting is to be expected when each unit cell contains more than one molecule.

Whether or not two paramagnetic molecules situated in the same lattice are magnetically equivalent depends on their symmetry relations.   If they are related by a center of symmetry they are entirely equivalent.   For a diad rotation operation they are equivalent only if the magnetic field is directed along or perpendicular to the diad axis.   This can be understood by the following considerations.   If an unpaired electron 'sees' a magnetic dipole at a point P_1 (α, β, γ) in the crystal x, y, z system, the symmetry operations of the space group dictate the corresponding dipole coordinates of the other molecules comprising the unit cell.   Translation through a center of symmetry would give P_2 $(-\alpha, -\beta, -\gamma)$ and rotation about a diad y-axis would give P_3 $(-\alpha, \beta, -\gamma)$.   These sets of coordinates define vectors and the site splitting of the spectra is determined by the equivalence or otherwise of these angles θ_i, $i = 1, 2, 3$ between the vectors and the applied field.   If the applied field H has coordinates (H_x, H_y, H_z), these angles are obtained from the moduli of the relevant scalar products.   Thus:

$$\theta_1 = |\alpha H_x + \beta H_y + \gamma H_z| \tag{4.15}$$

$$\theta_2 = |-\alpha H_x - \beta H_y - \gamma H_z| \tag{4.16}$$

$$\theta_3 = |-\alpha H_x + \beta H_y - \gamma H_z|. \tag{4.17}$$

The sign effects can be removed by taking squares.   Hence:

$$\theta_1^2 = \alpha^2 H_x^2 + \beta^2 H_y^2 + \gamma^2 H_z^2 + 2\alpha\beta H_x H_y + 2\beta\gamma H_y H_z + 2\gamma\alpha H_z H_x \tag{4.18}$$

$$\theta_2^2 = \alpha^2 H_x^2 + \beta^2 H_y^2 + \gamma^2 H_z^2 + 2\alpha\beta H_x H_y + 2\beta\gamma H_y H_z + 2\gamma\alpha H_z H_x \tag{4.19}$$

$$\theta_3^2 = \alpha^2 H_x^2 + \beta^2 H_y^2 + \gamma^2 H_z^2 - 2\alpha\beta H_x H_y - 2\beta\gamma H_y H_z + 2\gamma\alpha H_z H_x. \tag{4.20}$$

Thus, as $\theta_1{}^2 = \theta_2{}^2$ for any position of the field, two molecules related by a center of symmetry will always be magnetically equivalent. However, $\theta_1{}^2 = \theta_3{}^2$ only when $H_y = 0$ or $H_x = H_z = 0$. Thus two molecules related by the symmetry operations of any diad axis are only magnetically equivalent when the field is parallel or perpendicular to this axis. It follows that the sites will have opposite signs in all off-diagonal elements of the coupling tensor for an orthorhombic crystal, and in the two off-diagonal elements obtained from observations in the planes containing the diad axis for a monoclinic crystal. When more than one off-diagonal element has sign duality, the relative signs are determined by comparing the spectra at some skew orientation with those predicted as a result of different relative signs in the off-diagonal elements.

The simplest spectra are generally recorded when the magnetic field is parallel to a crystallographic axis as site splitting does not occur, and these orientations are investigated first. If the spectra are extremely complicated and the absorption lines cannot be linked, then a useful procedure is to measure all possible splittings and plot them on a polar diagram. The presence of parallel curves in such a diagram often assists in the identification of various interactions.

4.3.5   SEPARATION OF OVERLAPPING HYPERFINE STRUCTURES

The main complication in ESR spectra is usually the fact that irradiation often produces more than one radical species. The g-values of organic free radicals rarely differ by more than 1% and hyperfine structures from two species are therefore generally overlapping. The presence of more than one radical is indicated if the spectra contain lines with different widths and also if the spectra recorded with the magnetic field parallel to a crystallographic axis lack a center of symmetry. There are various techniques for distinguishing between spectral lines arising from different radical species.

A. *ANNEALING*

If a crystal is aged at room temperature, then one radical may decay faster than others. Such a process can generally be accelerated by annealing, that is, the crystal is warmed and then cooled to room temperature. Immediately after irradiation, the spectra from a single crystal of malonic acid (McConnell, *et al.*, 1960; Horsfield, *et al.*, 1961b) contained up to 14 absorption lines. After storage at room temperature for two months or warming to 60°C for several hours, only a doublet remained.

B. *POWER SATURATION*

When microwave power saturation occurs, the amplitudes of absorption lines arising from two radicals are unlikely to increase at the same rate. Hence, simply by increasing the microwave power in the resonance cavity, it is often possible to differentiate between overlapping hyperfine structures.

C. *MEASUREMENTS AT TWO FREQUENCIES*

Although the *g*-values of two organic radicals may be only slightly different, the distance between the centers of the individual spectra will vary with the recording frequency. Thus, measurements on *X*-band (9 GHz) and *Q*-band (36 GHz) spectrometers will give different spectra, the relative shift of overlapping hyperfine structures often being as large as 20 MHz.

D. *ISOTOPIC SUBSTITUTION*

The nuclear spins and magnetic moments of isotopes are rarely the same. Isotopic substitution has therefore been used to confirm whether or not an observed interaction is with a given nucleus. In principle, provided the chemistry is not too difficult, any isotope could be employed but so far only deuterium, C^{13} and N^{15} have been used in single crystal studies. The results obtained with such substitutions will be discussed in later sections.

E. *LOW TEMPERATURE IRRADIATION*

Irradiation at 77°K and warming to room temperature before observation does not necessarily produce the same radicals as irradiation at 300°K. Although such a technique has not been used very much in single crystal studies, it is possible that low temperature irradiation could assist in the interpretation of complex spectra obtained after room temperature irradiation. It is in this field of low temperature irradiation and observation before and after warming to room temperature that the most recent advances have been made in studying radiation damage in organic single crystals by ESR techniques. A good example is the ESR study of single crystals of a number of malonic acids, irradiated at 77°K and examined at 77°K and also after annealing to 195°K and 300°K (Tamura, *et al.*, 1966b).

Having recorded the spectra and obtained the coupling tensors for the various interactions, it is now necessary to interpret these in terms of the orbital of the unpaired electron in the free radical. This process is best illustrated by a review of previous ESR studies of radiation damage in organic single crystals.

4.4   REVIEW OF PREVIOUS STUDIES

A considerable literature has accumulated on the subject of the ESR spectra of organic single crystals damaged by radiation.   The work has obviously centered on those substances from which single crystals can readily be grown, and most of the biologically significant compounds have been either saturated dicarboxylic acids and their salts, amino acids, or unsaturated acids. The radicals have generally been produced by ionizing radiations and almost all the irradiations and examinations have been made at room temperature. In some cases (Akasaka, *et al.*, 1964; Box and Freund, 1964; Box, *et al.*, 1965) different radicals have been trapped after irradiation and examination at the temperature of liquid nitrogen, and subsequent warm-up has not always yielded the same radicals as are produced by room temperature irradiation.   By far the most frequently observed damage has been the breaking of a C—H bond to give a π-electron radical centered on the carbon atom.   The hybridization is changed from tetrahedral sp^3 to planar sp^2 and the unpaired electron occupies what is predominantly a carbon $2p$-orbital directed perpendicular to the plane trigonal skeleton of the radical.   However, there are cases in which C—N, C—C, N—H, C—F, and S—S bonds have been ruptured by the radiation.

The hyperfine splitting of an ESR spectrum arises from the interaction of the magnetic moment of the unpaired electron with the magnetic moments of neighboring nuclei.   The types of interaction which have been observed in organic radicals will be treated individually and then consideration given to other phenomena detected in some spectra.   Finally, a section will be devoted to unsaturated compounds where additive rather than subtractive damage has sometimes been observed.

4.4.1   HYPERFINE INTERACTION WITH α-HYDROGEN ATOMS

An α-hydrogen atom is one which is directly attached to the free radical atom in a π-electron system.   The central atom is generally carbon, but in organic radicals it can be nitrogen.   As the proton has spin $I = \frac{1}{2}$, the spectrum consists of two lines whose separation shows a characteristic variation as the crystal is rotated about three mutually perpendicular axes in the magnetic field.   This variation is expressed in the form of a coupling tensor. The isotropic component of the diagonalized tensor is attributed to spin polarization of the Ċ—H bond and, in consequence, a small negative spin density appears at the proton.   This negative sign cannot be determined from the spectra but is inferred from the theory (McConnell and Chesnut, 1958; McConnell and Strathdee, 1959).   The isotropic proton hyperfine coupling $\mathscr{A}_H$, is proportional to the spin density on the central atom, ρ, according to the equation of McConnell and Chesnut (1958):

$$\mathscr{A}_H = Q\rho \qquad (4.21)$$

where Q is a 'constant' approximately equal to -64 MHz. For example, if a hydrogen atom has an isotropic hyperfine splitting of -51 MHz, then $\rho \sim 0.8$. The unpaired spin density at the hydrogen atom can also be calculated. An unpaired electron in the $1s$-orbital of a hydrogen atom would produce a splitting of 1420 MHz and so a splitting of 64 MHz indicates a spin density of -0.045 on the proton.

A large number of radicals containing α-hydrogen interactions have been identified and a comprehensive list is presented in Table 4.1. It is clear that the isotropic coupling is remarkably constant considering the varying nature of the substituents. Couplings less than the expected value show that not all the unpaired electron spin density is concentrated on the central atom, but is delocalized on other atoms.

Several nitrogen-centered radicals have also been studied and isotropic couplings of -64 MHz for the radical $H\dot{N}(SO_3^-)$ in potassium sulfamate (Rowlands, 1962), -64 MHz for $H_2{}^+\dot{N}(SO_3^-)$ in sulfamic acid (Rowlands and Whiffen, 1962) and -65 MHz for $H\dot{N}^+\langle$ in diammonium hydrogen phosphate (Morton, 1963) seem to indicate slightly higher values than for carbon-centered radicals. However, the evidence is not yet conclusive owing to insufficient examples.

In addition to this isotropic interaction, Table 4.1 shows that α-hydrogen atoms trapped in π-electron radical systems exhibit a characteristic anisotropic interaction. This is due to the dipole-dipole interaction between electron and proton. Ghosh and Whiffen (1959) have considered a planar $H\dot{C}R_1R_2$ fragment for which symmetry requires that the three principal directions of the tensor be parallel to the $\dot{C}$—H bond, perpendicular to the radical plane and the mutually perpendicular direction in the plane of the radical. For a stationary electron the interaction between its magnetic moment, μ_e, and the magnetic moment of a proton μ_p, considering both as point dipoles aligned in a field, is:

$$\mu_e\mu_p\left(\frac{1 - 3\cos^2\theta}{r^3}\right) \qquad (4.22)$$

where r is the distance between the electron and proton and θ the angle between the applied field and the line joining the electron and proton. However, as the electron is not stationary, this expression has to be averaged over the p-orbital. The interaction will be zero when $(1 - 3\cos^2\theta)$ is zero and this defines a nodal surface, a cone of half-angle $\cos^{-1}(\frac{1}{3})$. In Fig. 4.2(a), the field H_0 is parallel to the $\dot{C}$—H bond and the orbital is almost entirely within the cone. Thus the $\dot{C}$—H direction corresponds to the most positive

Table 4.1 *Hyperfine interaction (in MHz) with α-hydrogen atoms*

Host crystal	Radical	Hyperfine interaction			References
		Isotropic	Anisotropic		
Malonic acid	$H\dot{C}$—$(CO_2H)_2$	-59	$+32$ -1	-31	Cole, *et al.*, 1959; McConnell, *et al.*, 1960; Horsfield, *et al.*, 1961b
Malonic acid	$H_2\dot{C}$—CO_2H	$\{\begin{matrix}-59\\-63\end{matrix}$	$\begin{matrix}+29 & +4\\+26 & +4\end{matrix}$	$\begin{matrix}-32\\-29\end{matrix}$	Horsfield, Morton, and Whiffen, 1961b and 1961d; McConnell and Giuliano, 1961
Succinic acid	HO_2C—CH_2—$\dot{C}H$—CO_2H	-60	$+30$ $+1$	-32	Heller and McConnell, 1960; Pooley and Whiffen, 1961a
Glutaric acid	HO_2C—$(CH_2)_2$—$\dot{C}H$—CO_2H	$\{\begin{matrix}-56\\-51\end{matrix}$	$\begin{matrix}+30 & +3\\+28 & -1\end{matrix}$	$\begin{matrix}-32\\-28\end{matrix}$	Horsfield, Morton, and Whiffen, 1961a
Adipic acid	HO_2C—$(CH_2)_3$—$\dot{C}H$—CO_2H	-57	$+29$ $+7$	-37	Morton and Horsfield, 1961b
Potassium hydrogen malonate	^-OOC—$\dot{C}H$—COO^-	-57	$+30$ -1	-28	Lin and McDowell, 1961b
Hexamethylenedi-ammonium adipate	^-OOC—$(CH_2)_3$—$\dot{C}H$—COO^-	-55	$+30$ $+4$	-34	Kashiwagi and Kurita, 1963
Glycollic acid	$HO\dot{C}H$—CO_2H	-57	$+27$ $+2$	-29	Atherton and Whiffen, 1960a
Potassium glycollate	$HO\dot{C}H$—COO^-	-51	$+28$ $+1$	-29	Atherton and Whiffen, 1960b
Lithium glycollate anhydrous	$HO\dot{C}H$—COO^-	-54	$+27$ $+3$	-31	Pooley and Whiffen, 1961b
Lithium glycollate monohydrate	$HO\dot{C}H$—COO^-	-50	$+27$ $+3$	-29	Pooley and Whiffen, 1961b
Diglycollic acid	HO_2C—CH_2—O—$\dot{C}H$—CO_2H	-49	$+24$ $+3$	-27	Kurita, 1962
Thiodiglycollic acid	HO_2C—CH_2—S—$\dot{C}H$—CO_2H	-43	$+21$ -2	-23	Kurita and Gordy, 1961b
Glycine	H_3N—$\dot{C}H$—CO_2^-	-62	$+35$ -4	-30	Ghosh and Whiffen, 1959; Whiffen, 1961: Morton, 1964b

Compound	Structural formula					Reference
Glycylglycine	$H_3N^+—CH_2—CO—NH—CH—CO_2$	-51	$+27$	$+4$	-32	Lin and McDowell, 1961a
Glycylglycine hydrochloride	$H_3N(Cl)—CH_2—CO—NH—\dot{C}H—CO_2H$	-53	$+23$	-5	-18	Box, et al., 1963
N-Acetylglycine	$H_3C—CO—NH—\dot{C}H—CO_2H$	-51	$+23$	$+3$	-25	Miyagawa, et al., 1960
N-Carbamyl glycine	$H_2N—CO—CO—NH—\dot{C}H—CO_2H$	-54	$+26$	-8	-18	Rao and Katayama, 1962
α-Alanine	$H_3C—\dot{C}H—CO_2H$	-55	$+30$	$+5$	-34	Miyagawa and Gordy, 1960; Morton and Horsfield, 1961a; Miyagawa and Itoh, 1962
DL-Aspartic acid hydrochloride	$HO_2C—CH_2—\dot{C}H—CO_2H·HCl$	-63	$+24$	$+3$	-27	Rowlands, 1961; Jaseja and Anderson, 1962b
Urea oxalate	$HO_2C—H\dot{C}OH$	-47	$+24$	$+3$	-27	Rao and Gordy, 1961a
Methylurea	$H_2\dot{C}—NH—OCNH_2$	-60	$+32$	-2	-30	Jaseja and Anderson, 1961
Ethylurea	$H_3\dot{C}—\dot{C}H—NH—OCNH_2$	-51	$+23$	-8	-16	Jaseja and Anderson, 1961
Malonamide	$H\dot{C}(CONH_2)_2$	-59	$+30$	0	-30	Rexroad, et al., 1965
Fumaric acid	$HO_2C—RCH—\dot{C}H—CO_2H$	-60	$+27$	$+3$	-30	Cook, Rowlands, and Whiffen, 1963a
Maleic acid	$HO_2C—CH_2—\dot{C}H—CO_2H$	-57	$+29$	$+2$	-30	Cook, Elliott, and Wyard, 1967a
Potassium methoxy-acetate	$H_3C—O—\dot{C}H—CO_2^-$	-50	$+33$	-2	-32	Horsfield and Morton, 1962
Monofluoroacetamide	$F\dot{C}H—CO—NH_2$	-63	$+32$	0	-33	Cook, Rowlands, and Whiffen, 1962 and 1963b
Potassium methane disulfonate	$H\dot{C}(SO_3)_2^{2-}$	-60	$+32$	$+3$	-35	Horsfield, Morton, Rowlands, and Whiffen, 1962
Diketopiperazine	$OC—\dot{C}H—NH—CO—CH_2—NH$	-50	$+22$	$+3$	-25	Miyagawa, 1961; Lin and McDowell, 1963
ε-Caprolactam	$HN—\dot{C}H—(CH_2)_4—CO$	-57	$+28$	$+6$	-34	Kashiwagi and Kurita, 1964
Creatinine	$HNC—NH—CO—\dot{C}H—NCH_3$	-50	$+18$	0	-18	Ueda, 1964
Cytosine	$OC—NH—\dot{C}H—CH_2—C(NH_2)=N$	-55	$+19$	$+5$	-24	Cook, Elliott, and Wyard, 1967b

interaction.   In Fig. 4.2(b), where H_0 is in the radical plane but perpendicular to the Ċ—H bond, the orbital lies in the negative region and corresponds to the most negative interaction.   Finally, in Fig. 4.2(c) where H_0 is parallel to the p-orbital, the cone intersects the region of high electron density and the

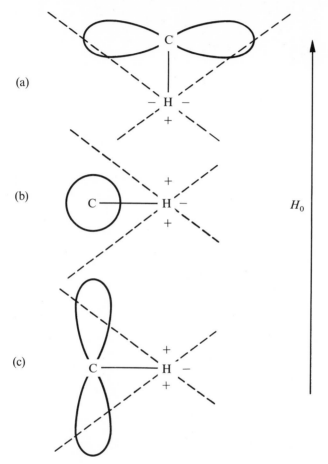

Fig. 4.2   Origin of anisotropic hyperfine interaction with α-hydrogen atoms. (a) H_0 parallel to C—H_α bond, (b) H_0 in radical plane perpendicular to C—H_α bond, (c) H_0 perpendicular to radical plane.

corresponding coupling will be numerically small.   The theoretical considerations of McConnell and Strathdee (1959) have shown that with an unpaired spin density of unity on the central atom, the anisotropic components of the principal values of the tensor should be $+43$ MHz along the direction of the $\dot{C}$—H bond, -5 MHz in a direction perpendicular to the radical plane, and -39 MHz in a direction mutually perpendicular to the other two. Table 4.1 indicates that the anisotropic interactions have remarkably constant values for α-protons which have been identified and the characteristic tensor is now regarded as being diagnostic of an α-hydrogen atom in a π-electron radical.

It is sometimes possible to infer radical geometry from the coupling tensor. For example, there are two α-protons in the $H_2\dot{C}$—(CO_2H) radical found in irradiated malonic acid (Horsfield, Morton, and Whiffen, 1961b) and the $H\dot{C}H$ angle has been calculated from the tensors to be $116 \pm 5°$. Furthermore, the molecular plane in fumaric acid (Cook, Rowlands, and Whiffen, 1963a) has been determined from spectral observations when no detailed crystal structure was available. In general, the directions of the principal values of the coupling tensor coincide with a radical orientation which is close to that of the parent molecule in the undamaged crystal.

4.4.2 HYPERFINE INTERACTION WITH β-HYDROGEN ATOMS

A β-hydrogen atom is one which is two bonds from the free radical atom, the most common form being $\rangle\dot{C}$—C—H_β with carbon as both the central and intermediate atom. Thus a β-hydrogen is much further from the orbital of the unpaired electron than an α-hydrogen and, as the dipole–dipole interaction is proportional to r^{-3}, little anisotropy is expected (Derbyshire, 1962). This is borne out by experiment where the principal values of the anisotropic tensor rarely exceed 10% of the isotropic coupling. The isotropic coupling arises from hyperconjugation between the $2p_z$-orbital of the free radical carbon and the π-electron system containing the β-hydrogen orbital. Observed values of isotropic β-proton couplings have varied from less than 10 MHz (Rao and Gordy, 1962; Whiffen, 1962) to over 120 MHz (Horsfield, Morton, and Whiffen, 1961a). The magnitude of the coupling is very dependent on the radical geometry, being small when the β-proton is in the nodal plane of the free radical atom's $2p$-orbital and large if it is far from this plane. Theoretical studies (McLachlan, 1958; Lykos, 1960) have shown that the isotropic coupling is positive and probably given by (Stone and Maki, 1962):

$$B_1 + B_2 \cos^2\theta \qquad (4.23)$$

where B_1 and B_2 are constants such that $B_1 < < B_2$ and θ is the angle between the C_β—H_β bond and the p-orbital direction projected perpendicular to the $\dot{C}_\alpha$—C_β bond. A value of B_1 less than 10 MHz has been evaluated from work with α-alanine at liquid nitrogen temperatures (Horsfield, Morton, and Whiffen, 1961c). The value of B_2 is 130 ± 10 MHz.

Table 4.2 shows various β-proton couplings which have been observed

Table 4.2 *Hyperfine interaction (in MHz) with β-hydrogen atoms*

Host crystal	Radical	Hyperfine Interaction				References
		Isotropic	Anisotropic			
Succinic acid	$HO_2C—CH_2—\dot{C}H—CO_2H$	$\begin{cases}+100 \\ +80\end{cases}$	+8 −1 −7 +9 −1 −8			Heller and McConnell, 1960; Pooley and Whiffen, 1961a
Succinic acid	$HO_2C—(CH_2)_2—\dot{C}(OH)O^-$	+78 +24 $\left.\begin{array}{c}+122 \\ +47\end{array}\right\}$	+6 −3 −3 +11 −2 −8			Box, *et al.* 1965
Glutaric acid	$HO_2C—(CH_2)_2—\dot{C}H—CO_2H$	+107				Horsfield, Morton, and Whiffen, 1961a
Adipic acid	$HO_2C—(CH_2)_3—\dot{C}H—CO_2H$	+33 +112 +74				Morton and Horsfield, 1961b
Ethyl malonic acid	$H_3C—CH_2—\dot{C}—(CO_2H)_2$	$\begin{cases}+70 \\ +57\end{cases}$	+5 +1 −6 +5 −1 −4			Rowlands and Whiffen, 1961
Valine	$(H_3C)_2—\dot{C}—HC(NH_3{}^+)—CO_2{}^-$	+8				Whiffen, 1962
DL-Isovaline	$H_3C—CH_2—\dot{C}(CO_2H)—CH_3$	$\begin{cases}+109 \\ +26\end{cases}$				Jaseja and Anderson, 1962a
Deuterated DL-serine	$(DO)_2\dot{C}—HCND_2—CH_2—OD$	+118	+5 −3 −3			Rao and Gordy, 1961b

Compound	Structure					Reference
N-Acetyl methionine	H_3C—CO—NH—HC(CO_2H)—$(CH_2)_2$—$\dot{S}$	+27				Cipollini and Gordy, 1962
L-Cystine dihydrochloride	HO_2C—H_2NCH—CH_2—$\dot{S}$	+25				Kurita and Gordy, 1961a
DL-Aspartic acid hydrochloride	HO_2C—CH_2—$\dot{C}H$—CO_2H·HCl	+116 +68				Rowlands, 1961; Jaseja and Anderson, 1962b
Acetyl L-glutamic acid	H_3C—CO—NH—HC(CO_2H)—CH_2—$\dot{C}H$—CO_2H	+98 +70				Katayama, 1962a
Deuterated DL-tartaric acid	DO_2C—$DO\dot{C}$—DOCH—CO_2D	+6	+10	-3	-7	Rao and Gordy, 1962
Fumaric acid	HO_2C—RCH—$\dot{C}H$—CO_2H	+56	+8	-4	-5	Cook, Rowlands, and Whiffen, 1963a
Maleic acid	HO_2C—CH_2—$\dot{C}H$—CO_2H	+81	+6	-2	-3	Cook, Elliott, and Wyard, 1967a
Itaconic acid	H_3C—$\dot{C}(CO_2H)$—CH_2—CO_2H	+47	+6	-2	-5	Fujimoto, 1963
Diketopiperazine	OC—$\dot{C}H$—NH—CO—CH_2—NH	+25				Miyagawa, 1961; Lin and McDowell, 1963
Thymidine	OC—NR—CH_2—$\dot{C}(CH_3)$—CO—NH	+114				Pruden, et al., 1965
Cytosine	OC—NH—$\dot{C}H$—CH_2—$C(NH_2)$=N	+104				Cook, Elliot, and Wyard, 1967b

and the magnitudes of their anisotropic hyperfine interactions where they have been computed. Most of the observed compounds contain methylene groups and so have two β-protons. The couplings to methylene protons are rarely the same, showing that chemical equivalence does not infer geometric equivalence. Kashiwagi and Kurita (1963) have demonstrated that, when irradiated crystals of hexamethylenediammonium adipate are cooled, there is a decrease in coupling to the β-protons.

As the fragment $\overset{\cdot}{C}H_3$ is too reactive to be trapped in the lattice of a single crystal, coupling to methyl protons has only been observed in radicals of the type $\overset{\cdot}{C}$—CH_3 and $\overset{\cdot}{N}$—CH_3. This is a special case of β-hydrogen coupling and, in consequence, the anisotropies are expected to be small. Geometric equivalence of the protons will occur if the methyl group is rotating freely, or at least 'tunnelling' at the temperature of observation. This is so at room temperature where the frequency of rotation is at least 1 GHz. The equivalence of the hydrogens results in a spectrum of four equally spaced lines with intensity ratio 1:3:3:1, and the small anisotropies mean that even polycrystalline samples give well resolved spectra. Table 4.3 lists methyl couplings which have been observed at room temperature. It is clear that the coupling to each proton is in the region 50–80 MHz and calculations using these values confirm that $B_2 = 130 \pm 10$ MHz.

Horsfield, Morton, and Whiffen (1961c) cooled an irradiated crystal of α-alanine to 77°K and observed that the spectra were very different from those recorded at 300°K. The methyl group was rotating at less than 10 MHz and the three protons became inequivalent. The average isotropic coupling was still 70 MHz but the individual couplings, instead of being equal, were 120, 76, and 14 MHz. The methyl group had taken up a skew position with respect to the —$\overset{|}{\underset{|}{C}}$—$\overset{\cdot}{C}$—$H_\alpha$ plane of the radical. Between 100 and 200°K there had been a gradual change in the spectrum (Miyagawa and Itoh, 1962; Horsfield, Morton, and Whiffen, 1962) and more recent detailed work by Delbousquet (1964) has shown that free rotation only occurs above 190°K. The temperature at which free rotation ceases varies from radical to radical and Heller (1962) observed that at 4°K the methyl group in the radical H_3C—$\overset{\cdot}{C}$—$(CO_2H)_2$ formed by irradiating methyl malonic acid was still nearly rotating freely. Two methyl groups are present in the radical $(H_3C)_2$—$\overset{\cdot}{C}$—CO_2H in α-amino isobutyric acid, and work by Morton (1964c) has indicated that at 40°K the protons of one group are inequivalent while those of the other methyl group are still rotating freely. At 4°K both groups have ceased to rotate freely. An apparent anomaly in the coupling to β-hydrogen atoms in irradiated ethyl malonic acid (Rowlands and Whiffen, 1961) and in irradiated n-propyl malonic acid (Tsvetkov, et al., 1964) has been removed by a low temperature examination of the ESR spectra (Tamura, et al., 1966a). The appearance of the spectra at room

Table 4.3 *Hyperfine interaction (in MHz) with methyl groups*

Host crystal	Radical	Hyperfine interaction				References
		Isotropic	Anisotropic			
Methyl malonic acid	H_3C—$\dot{C}$—$(CO_2H)_2$	$+71$	$+5$	-2	-2	Heller, 1962
Glycine	H_3N^+—$\dot{C}H$—CO_2^-	$+53$	$+11$	-3	-8	Ghosh and Whiffen, 1959; Whiffen, 1961; Morton, 1964b
α-Alanine	H_3C—$\dot{C}H$—CO_2H	$+70$	$+6$	-3	-3	Miyagawa and Gordy, 1960; Morton and Horsfield, 1961a; Miyagawa and Itoh, 1962
Acetyl DL-alanine	H_3C—CO—NH—$\dot{C}(CH_3)$—CO_2H	$+53$				Katayama, 1962b
Chloroacetyl DL-alanine	H_2CCl—CO—NH—$\dot{C}(CH_3)$—CO_2H	$+60$				Katayama, 1962b
α-Amino isobutyric acid	$(H_3C)_2$—$\dot{C}$—CO_2H	$+66$	$+4$	-1	-3	Horsfield, Morton, and Whiffen, 1961e
DL-Isovaline	H_3C—CH_2—$\dot{C}(CO_2H)$—CH_3	$+65$				Jaseja and Anderson, 1962a
Ethylurea	H_3C—$\dot{C}H$—NH—$OCNH_2$	$+64$				Jaseja and Anderson, 1961
Itaconic acid	H_3C—$\dot{C}(CO_2H)$—CH_2—CO_2H	$+67$	$+2$	0	-2	Fujimoto, 1963
Betaine hydrochloride	$(CH_3)_3$—$\dot{N}^+$	$+78$				Schoffa, 1964a and 1964b
Thymidine	OC—NR—CH_2—$\dot{C}(CH_3)$—CO—NH	$+57$				Pruden, et al., 1965

temperature was shown to be due to molecular motion, which was frozen out at 77°K.

A β-hydrogen also occurs with oxygen as the intermediate atom in a radical of the form $\rangle\dot{C}$—OH. In general, the hydrogen is in, or near, the nodal plane of the unpaired electron's orbital and thus only a small isotropic interaction is observed. There has been some doubt about the sign of the isotropic coupling, but on both theoretical (Derbyshire, 1962) and experimental (Henn and Whiffen, 1964) grounds it is now assumed to be negative. Some delocalization of the unpaired electron density in the π-system, from the carbon onto the hydroxyl oxygen, would give a small negative spin density at a hydrogen atom in, or near, the nodal plane of the unpaired electron's orbital. In the case of anhydrous lithium glycollate (Pooley and Whiffen, 1961b), the hydroxyl group is twisted from the plane of the radical and direct spin polarization produces a positive spin density at the proton, giving a fairly large positive coupling. A hydroxyl hydrogen is generally nearer the free radical carbon than the β-hydrogen in a $\rangle\dot{C}$—C—H_β fragment. Hence, the dipole–dipole interaction will be greater and the resulting anisotropies larger.

Finally, β-hydrogen atoms are found in a radical of the form $\rangle\dot{C}$—N—H_β, with nitrogen as the intermediate atom. The β-proton interacts with the unpaired electron in a similar manner to a β-proton with carbon as the intermediate atom. However, the splitting from the nitrogen is often of the same order of magnitude as the splitting from the β-proton and this confuses the spectrum, making quantitative measurements difficult.

4.4.3 HYPERFINE INTERACTION WITH γ-HYDROGEN ATOMS

A γ-hydrogen atom is one which is three bonds from the free radical atom and would be found in a radical such as $\rangle\dot{C}$—C—C—H_γ. Attempts to observe γ-proton couplings in the radical (HO_2C)—CH_2—CH_2—$\dot{C}H$—(CO_2H) formed by irradiating glutaric acid (Horsfield, Morton, and Whiffen, 1961a) and the radical (HO_2C)—CH_2—CH_2—CH_2—$\dot{C}H$—(CO_2H) found in irradiated adipic acid (Morton and Horsfield, 1961b) were unsuccessful, and it was concluded that the coupling was less than the line width of about 9 MHz. However, with oxygen as one of the intermediate atoms, some of the unpaired electron spin density is delocalized from the $2p$-orbital of the free radical carbon and up to 25% may appear on the adjacent atom. This has led to γ-proton couplings being detected in the radicals (HO_2C)—CH_2—O—$\dot{C}H$—(CO_2H) in diglycolic acid (Kurita, 1962) and H_3C—O—$\dot{C}H$—CO_2^- in potassium methoxy-acetate (Horsfield and Morton, 1962). The isotropic splittings were 12 and 6 MHz respectively. A similar effect is observed with sulfur as one of the intermediate atoms and an isotropic γ-proton coupling of 15 MHz was found by Kurita and Gordy (1961b) for the radical (HO_2C)—CH_2—S—$\dot{C}H$—(CO_2H) in irradiated thiodiglycollic acid.

4.4.4 HYPERFINE INTERACTION WITH THE NITROGEN NUCLEUS

An unpaired electron centered on a nitrogen atom as a result of radiation damage is mainly localized in the $2p$-orbital of this nucleus. The N^{14} nucleus has spin $I = 1$ and therefore the interaction between its magnetic moment and the magnetic moment of an unpaired electron will result in an ESR spectrum of three equal lines with even spacing. Table 4.4 lists the isotropic and anisotropic components of the hyperfine interactions for some N^{14} centered π-electron radicals. Theoretical treatments (McLachlan, et al., 1960; Fraenkel, 1962) indicate that the isotropic interaction will be positive. The s-character of the unpaired electron's orbital can be determined from the magnitude of the isotropic interaction, a splitting of 1540 MHz being observed if the electron occupies only an s-orbital. For example, an isotropic coupling of 45 MHz indicates 3% s-character.

Theoretically, the anisotropic hyperfine interaction should be of the form (Frosch and Foley, 1952; Zeldes, et al., 1960):

$$B_0(3\cos^2\theta - 1)\rho \qquad (4.24)$$

where ρ is the spin density in the $2p$-orbital of the nitrogen atom, θ the angle between the applied field and the $2p$-orbital direction and B_0 is a constant which equals 48 MHz for nitrogen. Thus the diagonalized coupling tensor describing the interaction between a nitrogen nucleus and an unpaired electron in a $2p$-orbital of this nucleus should be cylindrically symmetric. The coupling parallel to the p-orbital direction would be $+2B_0$, and in the radical plane $-B_0$. The observed values shown in Table 4.4 concur reasonably well with this model, and in all cases it has been shown that the large positive anisotropic interaction is perpendicular to the radical plane. However, the negative elements of the tensor show, to varying degrees, a departure from the expected cylindrical symmetry. Measurements at 77°K on the radicals $H\dot{N}(SO_3{}^-)$ in potassium sulfamate (Rowlands, 1962) and $H_2\dot{N}{}^+$ —$SO_3{}^-$ in sulfamic acid (Rowlands and Whiffen, 1962) have indicated that at low temperatures the tensor approaches cylindrically symmetric form.

Coupling to a nitrogen atom which is adjacent to a free radical carbon has also been detected. The direct dipole–dipole interaction between the N^{14} nuclear magnetic moment and the unpaired spin density on the carbon gives rise to a small anisotropy in the coupling. The isotropic hyperfine interaction is probably negative and due to induced negative spin density on

Table 4.4 *Hyperfine interaction (in MHz) with the N^{14} nucleus*

Host crystal	Radical	Hyperfine interaction				References
		Isotropic	Anisotropic			
Dimethylglyoxime	$HON{=}C(CH_3){-}C(CH_3){=}\dot{N}^+OH$	+90	+40	−20	−20	Miyagawa and Gordy, 1959
Potassium amine disulfonate	$\dot{N}(SO_3)_2^{\,2-}$	+37	+69	−31	−37	Horsfield, Morton, Rowlands, and Whiffen, 1962
Potassium sulfamate	$H\dot{N}(SO_3)^-$	+38	+60	−28	−32	Rowlands, 1962
Betaine hydrochloride	$(CH_3)_3{-}\dot{N}^+$	+77	+92	−37	−55	Schoffa, 1964a and 1964b
Sulfamic acid	$H_2\dot{N}^+{-}SO_3^{\,-}$	+51	+52	−18	−34	Rowlands and Whiffen, 1962
Diammonium hydrogen phosphate	$H\dot{N}^+{<}$	+45	+56	−21	−35	Morton, 1963
Deuterated cytosine	$OC{-}\dot{N}{-}HC{=}CH{-}C(ND_2){=}N$	+14	+29	−14	−15	Cook, Elliott, and Wyard, 1967b
Deuterated cytosine	$OC{-}N{=}CH{-}CH{=}C(ND_2){-}\dot{N}$	+7	+15	−7	−9	Cook, Elliott, and Wyard, 1967b

the nitrogen through the large spin density on the carbon to which it is bonded, via spin polarization of the $\overset{\cdot}{)}C$—N bond.   However, these combined effects rarely give a splitting of more than 12 MHz and are usually only a contributory factor to the line width in most ESR spectra.

The N^{15} nucleus has spin $I = \frac{1}{2}$ and hence, when interacting with an unpaired electron, the resulting ESR spectrum is a doublet.   The triplet splitting of the N^{14} nucleus is different from this doublet spacing.   Thus, isotopic substitution of N^{15} can be used to observe coupling to a given nitrogen atom and this technique has been investigated by Weiner and Koski (1963).

4.4.5   HYPERFINE INTERACTION WITH THE CARBON NUCLEUS

The C^{12} nucleus has zero spin and is therefore not detectable with an ESR spectrometer.   On the other hand, the C^{13} nucleus has spin $I = \frac{1}{2}$ and thus, when interacting with a single unpaired electron, gives a two-line spectrum.   However, it has a natural abundance of only 1.1% and such a spectrum is rarely observed in irradiated organic single crystals.   An unpaired electron localized on a C^{13} nucleus will behave in a similar manner to one localized on an N^{14} nucleus and described in the previous section.   The isotropic coupling is positive (McLachlan, et al., 1960; Fraenkel, 1962; de Boer and Mackor, 1963), an unpaired electron localized in an s-orbital of a C^{13} nucleus giving a splitting of 3110 MHz.   The anisotropic hyperfine interaction should be of the form given in equation (4.24) with the constant B_0 equal to 91 MHz.   Table 4.5 lists the hyperfine interactions with the C^{13} nucleus which have been observed in organic single crystals.   The interactions are seen to conform reasonably well with the expected pattern.

ble 4.5   *Hyperfine interaction (in MHz) with the C^{13} nucleus*

lost crystal	Radical	Hyperfine interaction			References
		Isotropic	Anisotropic		
Malonic acid	$H\overset{\cdot}{C}$—$(CO_2H)_2$	+93	+120 −50	−70	McConnell and Fessenden, 1959; Cole and Heller, 1961
Glycine	H_3N^+—$\overset{\cdot}{C}H$—CO_2^-	+127	+127 −60	−67	Morton, 1964b
Glycine	$H_2\overset{\cdot}{C}$—CO_2^-	+124	+97 +9	−106	Morton, 1964b
Potassium methane disulfonate	$H\overset{\cdot}{C}(SO_3)_2^{2-}$	+126	+134 −64	−70	Horsfield, Morton, Rowlands, and Whiffen, 1962
Succinic acid	HO_2C—$(CH_2)_2$—$\overset{\cdot}{C}(OH)O^-$	+93	+134 −61	−73	Box, et al., 1965

A C^{13} coupling was first observed experimentally by McConnell and Fessenden (1959) for the radical $\dot{H}C$—$(CO_2H)_2$ in irradiated malonic acid but a coupling tensor could not be evaluated because of the low intensity of the C^{13} lines. Cole and Heller (1961) have since prepared crystals of malonic acid enriched to contain 39% C^{13} in the methylene position. They obtained well resolved spectra and were able to make a complete analysis of the coupling.

During their early work on radiation damage in glycine, Ghosh and Whiffen (1958, 1959) suggested that the radicals produced by irradiation were $\dot{N}H_2$ and H_3N^+—$\dot{C}H$—$CO_2{}^-$. This interpretation was challenged by Weiner and Koski (1963) who concluded that the radicals were $\dot{N}H_4$ and $H_2\dot{C}$—$CO_2{}^-$. Morton (1964b), using glycine enriched with 55% C^{13} on the central carbon atom, has demonstrated that both radicals show a large anisotropic coupling to the C^{13} nucleus. Neither $\dot{N}H_2$ or $\dot{N}H_4$ would show such a splitting and he concluded that the radicals were in fact H_3N^+—$\dot{C}H$—$CO_2{}^-$ and $H_2\dot{C}$—$CO_2{}^-$. These different interpretations of radiation damage in glycine illustrate the difficulty in identifying radicals even when they are aligned in a single crystal.

4.4.6 SPECTROSCOPIC SPLITTING FACTOR

The spectroscopic splitting factor or 'g-value' is a measure of the contribution of the electron's spin and orbital motion to its total angular momentum, and has a value of 2.0023 for a completely free spin. The relativity correction produces the small deviation from 2.000. Strictly, the g-value should be given a negative sign as the gyromagnetic ratio of the electron is negative. However, it is the modulus of the value which is usually quoted and this procedure will be observed in the present text. Departures from the free spin value are associated, in π-electron radicals, with spin-orbit interactions between the ground state and excited states of the radical and have been treated theoretically by McConnell and Robertson (1957). Changes in g-value are direction dependent and so require a tensor for complete analysis in single crystal studies. Measurements in the plane of the radical should give g-values greater than 2.0023, the magnitude of the shift depending on the spin-orbit coupling constant, λ, of any atom having an appreciable unpaired spin density. The g-value perpendicular to the radical plane should not depart greatly from the free spin value. Kurita (1962) has shown that in radicals of the type HO_2C—$\dot{C}H$—R, there is a linear relationship between g-value anisotropy, defined as $g_{max} - g_{min}$, and λ for the atom to which the $\dot{C}H$ carbon is bonded.

The deviations from 2.0023 in the measured g-values, do help in the identification of the radical plane, but as $g_{max} - g_{min}$ is in general less than

Table 4.6 *Principal values of g-tensor in π-electron radicals*

Host crystal	Radical	Perpendicular to plane	In plane of radical		References
Malonic acid	$H\dot{C}(CO_2H)_2$	2.0026	2.0033	2.0035	McConnell, *et al.*, 1960
Malonic acid	$H_2\dot{C}-CO_2H$	2.0020	2.0034	2.0042	Horsfield, Morton, and Whiffen, 1961b
Succinic acid	$HO_2C-CH_2-\dot{C}H-CO_2H$	2.0019	2.0026	2.0045	Pooley and Whiffen, 1961a
Glycollic acid	$HO\dot{C}H-CO_2H$	2.0017	2.0038	2.0053	Atherton and Whiffen, 1960a
Potassium glycollate	$HO\dot{C}H-COO^-$	2.0021	2.0039	2.0054	Atherton and Whiffen, 1960b
N-Acetylglycine	$H_3C-CO-NH-\dot{C}H-CO_2H$	2.0027	2.0032	2.0042	Miyagawa, *et al.*, 1960
Urea oxalate	$HO_2C-H\dot{C}OH$	2.0024	2.0047	2.0048	Rao and Gordy, 1961a
Fumaric acid	$HO_2C-RCH-\dot{C}H-CO_2H$	2.0029	2.0033	2.0043	Cook, Rowlands, and Whiffen, 1963a
Maleic acid	$HO_2C-CH_2-\dot{C}H-CO_2H$	2.0026	2.0036	2.0039	Cook, Elliott, and Wyard, 1967a
Potassium sulfamate	$H\dot{N}(SO_3)^-$	2.0037	2.0038	2.0078	Rowlands, 1962
Trifluoroacetamide	$F_2\dot{C}-\dot{C}O-NH_2$	2.0025	2.0045	2.0045	Lontz and Gordy, 1962
Sodium perfluorosuccinate	$CO_2^- -CF_2-\dot{C}F-CO_2^-$	2.0036	2.0039	2.0060	Rogers and Whiffen, 1964
Diketopiperazine	$OC-\dot{C}H-NH-CO-CH_2-NH$	2.0025	2.0040	2.0045	Miyagawa, 1961
ε-Caprolactam	$HN-\dot{C}H-(CH_2)_4-CO$	2.0025	2.0032	2.0038	Kashiwagi and Kurita, 1964
Thymidine	$OC-NR-CH_2-\dot{C}(CH_3)-CO-NH$	2.0024	2.0030	2.0042	Pruden, *et al.*, 1965

0.01, they cannot be used as a method of radical recognition.   The one exception is when an appreciable amount of the unpaired electron spin density is concentrated on a sulfur atom.   For sulfur, $\lambda = 382 \, \text{cm}^{-1}$ compared with $\lambda = 28 \, \text{cm}^{-1}$ for carbon (McClure, 1949, 1952) and work on L-cystine hydrochloride (Kurita and Gordy, 1961a), N-acetyl methionine (Cipollini and Gordy, 1962), and mercaptosuccinic acid (Hahn and Rexroad, 1963) has shown that, when a sulfur atom has a large amount of unpaired spin density, the g-value anisotropy is at least an order of magnitude larger than in radicals not containing sulfur.

Table 4.6 lists some observed principal values of the g-tensor for π-electron radicals and confirms that g-values perpendicular to the radical plane are near 2.0023 and less than those in the radical plane.

4.4.7   SECOND ORDER TRANSITIONS

Second order transitions, due to the simultaneous flipping of electron and nuclear spins, were first observed by Atherton and Whiffen (1960a) in glycollic acid, by Miyagawa and Gordy (1960) in alanine, and by McConnell, et al. (1960) in malonic acid.   When there are second order transitions, the usual selection rule $\Delta M_I = 0$ breaks down, and a second hydrogen nucleus gives rise to a pair of doublets instead of the usual single doublet, although both doublets may not be of resolvable separation or of resolvable intensity. The first two papers cited discuss the theory of second order transitions, and give formulae from which the splittings and intensities may be calculated. It is found that the spectrum depends on the strength of the magnetic field, so that when second order effects are present it is very helpful to make measurements at more than one frequency.   In particular, the two doublets are of comparable intensity when the hyperfine coupling constant is approximately twice the proton resonance frequency for the field strength being used.   For magnetic fields appreciably weaker or stronger than this, one of the doublets has negligible intensity.   Thus for alanine the second order effects were strongest at 24 GHz, and much weaker although still detectable at 9 GHz or 34 GHz.

Since the first observations, second order transitions have been observed in the ESR spectra of many organic single crystals damaged by radiation, and the relative intensities of the doublets have been found to agree with the theory.   Rexroad, et al. (1965) have recently extended the theory to include coupling cases other than a single nucleus with spin $I = \frac{1}{2}$.   They also used second order transitions to verify the α-hydrogen coupling tensor for the radical H_3N^+—$\dot{C}H$—CO_2^- previously observed in an irradiated single crystal of glycine (Ghosh and Whiffen, 1958, 1959).

Trammell, et al. (1958) have developed the corresponding theory for a hydrogen atom free radical where a nearby hydrogen nucleus, with which the free radical atom interacts only weakly through dipole–dipole coupling, flips simultaneously with the electron spin. This phenomenon of 'spin-flip' transitions leads to the appearance of a low intensity line on either side of each main spectral line, the new doublet spacing being twice the proton resonance frequency at the frequency of observation.

4.4.8   EFFECTS OF DEUTERATION

Single crystals grown from heavy water nave their labile protons, that is, those attached to nitrogen or oxygen atoms, replaced by deuterons. The deuteron has spin $I = 1$, and so gives a three-line spectrum when interacting with an unpaired electron. However, the proton has a larger magnetic moment than the deuteron and its doublet spacing is 6.51 times the triplet splitting of a deuteron in a similar position. Thus deuteration has often been used to confirm whether or not an observed interaction is with a labile proton.

The chief source of line broadening in single crystal spectra is frequently unresolved hyperfine interactions. As a deuteron gives a narrower spectrum than a proton, deuteration can sometimes be used to decrease line widths and often resolve extra structure. A good example of this technique is our interpretation of the spectra from irradiated single crystals of cytosine (Cook, Elliott, and Wyard, 1967b). One of the radicals gave a spectrum which was a broad absorption line for crystals grown from water but became up to eleven partially resolved lines for crystals obtained from heavy water. The large differences in the two sets of spectra were attributed to differences in line broadening from unresolved hyperfine interactions with the atoms of the amino group and will be discussed further in section 4.5.5.

The first suggestion that deuteration studies could be misleading was made by Pooley and Whiffen (1962), who observed the radical DO_2C—HCD—$\overset{.}{C}H$—CO_2D in irradiated succinic acid grown from heavy water. In about a third of the molecules, one of the β-protons had exchanged with a deuteron. While investigating radiation damage in deuterated α-alanine, Miyagawa and Itoh (1964) observed a reaction between the radical H_3C—$H\overset{.}{C}R$ and its host H_3C—$HC(ND_3{}^+)$—$CO_2{}^-$. The reaction proceeded very slowly at room temperature but at 150°C was complete in ten hours, the final spectrum being due to the radical D_3C—$D\overset{.}{C}R$. Morton (1964b) has shown that previous misidentifications (Ghosh and Whiffen, 1958, 1959; Weiner and Koski, 1963) of the radicals produced in irradiated glycine were due to a rapid and unexpected deuteron–proton exchange in the deuterated crystals. Thus deuterium atoms in a deuterated host crystal can exchange with hydrogen atoms of a trapped radical and this clearly indicates the need for caution when identifying radicals by deuteration studies.

4.4.9   RADIATION DAMAGE IN UNSATURATED COMPOUNDS

Many papers have shown that irradiation of saturated compounds usually results in the rupture of a bond with the consequent removal of a hydrogen atom or some other group.   Probably because of the low radical yields, only a few papers have dealt with the subject of radiation damage in unsaturated compounds.   The observed damage has sometimes been addition at the double bond, as in the case of irradiated tiglic acid (Kwiram and McConnell, 1962), furoic acid (Kwiram and McConnell, 1962; Cook, Rowlands, and Whiffen, 1963c), itaconic acid (Fujimoto, 1963), fumaric acid (Cook, Rowlands, and Whiffen, 1963c), maleic acid (Cook, Elliott, and Wyard, 1967a) and cytosine (Cook, Elliott, and Wyard, 1967b).

Irradiated tiglic acid yielded the radical HO_2C—$\overset{\cdot}{C}(CH_3)$—H_2C—CH_3, but the spin density on the free radical carbon was only 0.5.   In furoic acid, the addition was to the carbon at the five position and the spectra were interpreted in terms of a delocalized orbital for the unpaired electron.   For itaconic acid, the addition resulted in the formation of a methyl group, and this was observed to be freely rotating at room temperature but not at the temperature of liquid nitrogen.   In fumaric acid, the radical HO_2C—RCH—$H\overset{\cdot}{C}$—CO_2H dominated the spectra and there was only a small amount of the radical HO_2C—CH_2—$H\overset{\cdot}{C}$—CO_2H, while in its isomer, maleic acid, these two species were produced in nearly equal concentrations.   The α-hydrogen atoms had characteristic coupling tensors but the nature of R was unknown, except that it had no detectable interaction with the unpaired electron.   Radiation damage in cytosine produced at least three different radicals.   One of these was formed by rupture of a double bond and the subsequent addition of a hydrogen atom gave the species

$$OC—NH—\overset{\cdot}{C}H—CH_2—C(NH_2)\text{=}\overset{\cdot}{N}.$$

Heller and Cole (1962b) have shown that, in the case of glutaconic acid, the double bond was not broken, but the allyl-type radical HO_2C—$\overset{\cdot}{C}H$ =CH—$\overset{\cdot}{C}H$—CO_2H was formed.   The unpaired electron had a highly delocalized orbital and the spin density on the central carbon was smaller in magnitude and opposite in sign to that on the adjacent carbon atoms.   The same authors (Heller and Cole, 1962a) also observed irradiated potassium hydrogen maleate where a proton was removed from one of the carboxyl groups, forming the radical $\overset{\cdot}{O}CO$—$CH\text{=}CH$—CO_2^-.   The orbital of the unpaired electron extended not only over the central carbon atoms, but also over the terminal carboxyl groups.

Having discussed the experimental techniques and the interpretation of ESR single crystal spectra in terms of the types of interaction which can be observed, our investigation (Cook, Elliott, and Wyard, 1967b) of irradiated crystals of cytosine will be described as an example of the method.

4.5 ELECTRON SPIN RESONANCE OF A γ-IRRADIATED SINGLE CRYSTAL OF CYTOSINE

Cytosine has great biological significance as one of the pyrimidine bases found in both deoxyribonucleic acid and ribonucleic acid. The detailed crystal structure of cytosine monohydrate has been determined by Jeffrey and Kinoshita (1963) using X-ray methods. The crystal belongs to the monoclinic system and the dimensions of the unit cell are $a_0 = 7.801$, $b_0 = 9.844$, $c_0 = 7.683$ with $\beta = 99° 42'$, giving axial ratios:

$$a_0:b_0:c_0 = 0.792:1:0.780.$$

There are four molecules in each unit cell and the space group is $P2_1/c$. The atomic numbering system employed by Jeffrey and Kinoshita (1963) will be used in this text and is:

4.5.1   EXPERIMENTAL

Polycrystalline anhydrous cytosine, puriss grade, obtained from Fluka AG was used to grow the single crystals. The solubility of cytosine in water at 20°C is only 0.7 g per 100 ml of solvent and so small seed crystals were prepared by very slow evaporation of a saturated solution kept in a refrigerator at a temperature of about 6°C. The seeds obtained by this method measured 2 × 1 × 1 mm and showed better development of the faces than crystals grown by slow evaporation of a solution maintained at a temperature of 25°C. Cytosine was dissolved in 300 ml of distilled water to give a saturated solution at 30°C. This solution was placed in a 500 ml flask, tightly corked and cooled by putting the flask in a thermostatically controlled bath held at a temperature of about 25°C and constant to within ±0.05°C. A seed crystal was placed in the bottom of the solution and during four weeks its size increased to $6 \times 3 \times 2$ mm and its weight to 35 mg. A crystal of deuterated cytosine was prepared by a similar method, except that heavy water was the solvent. For reasons of economy, smaller quantities of solvent were used and the seeding process was repeated several times to obtain crystals of a reasonable size.

The external appearances of crystals grown from the two solvents were similar. A diagram of the crystal of cytosine monohydrate is given in Fig. 4.3. The faces were identified by comparing the angles between pairs of faces calculated from the dimensions of the unit cell and measured experimentally with an optical goniometer. All crystals which were examined

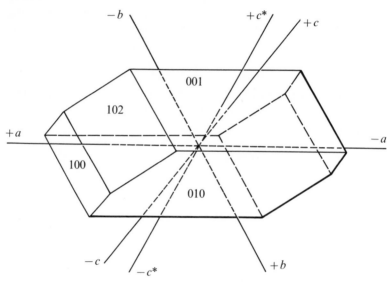

Fig. 4.3   The single crystal of cytosine monohydrate showing the choice of reference axes. The crystal of deuterated cytosine was similar to this.

showed well developed (010), ($0\bar{1}0$), (001), ($00\bar{1}$), (102), and ($\bar{1}0\bar{2}$) faces but the (100) and ($\bar{1}00$) faces were less prominent and even absent in some specimens. A set of reference axes consisting of the crystallographic a and b axes together with c^*, the third member of an orthogonal set, were chosen for the ESR measurements. These axes are also shown in Fig. 4.3. The atomic coordinates given in unit cell fractions (Jeffrey and Kinoshita, 1963) for the monoclinic system were transformed to an orthogonal system in terms of actual coordinates by the equations:

$$a = xa_0 - zc_0 \sin (\beta - 90) \qquad (4.25)$$
$$b = yb_0 \qquad (4.26)$$
$$c^* = zc_0 \cos (\beta - 90) \qquad (4.27)$$

where a, b, and c^* represent the new system, x, y, and z the old coordinates, and a_0, b_0, and c_0 the unit cell dimensions.

Before recording the ESR spectra it was necessary to know the crystal orientations at which site splitting was expected to be observed. The monoclinic system with $P2_1/c$ as space group indicated that the crystal possessed a center of symmetry and one diad axis, the b axis in Fig. 4.3. Thus, by the method described in section 4.3.4, it was shown that spectra from two magnetically distinct sites should be observed unless the main magnetic field was parallel or perpendicular to the diad axis.

The crystals were irradiated in air at room temperature to a dose of about 15 Mrad by Co^{60} γ-rays and this changed their appearances from near colourless to grey.   Colour changes have often been observed after irradiating organic crystals.   The dose rate was only 160 krad/hr and so there would have been no appreciable heating of the specimens.   The crystal of cytosine monohydrate was aligned in the ESR cavity with the aid of an optical goniometer so that one of the selected axes was perpendicular to the main magnetic field.   Room temperature spectra were recorded with an X-band (9 GHz) spectrometer at $10°$ intervals as the crystal was rotated in the magnetic field.   A similar procedure was adopted to record the spectra as the crystal was rotated about the other two axes of the orthogonal set and to record the spectra from the deuterated crystal as it was rotated about each of the three selected axes.

4.5.2   DESCRIPTION OF THE SPECTRA

The crystal of cytosine monohydrate gave two general types of spectra and these are shown in Figs. 4.4 and 4.5, where the magnetic field is parallel to the a- and c^*-axes, respectively.   The spectra were dominated by a very broad central line of varying width which split into a poorly resolved doublet when the field was within $20°$ of the c^*-axis.   However, the spectra also showed some hyperfine structure indicated by the vertical lines in Figs. 4.4 and 4.5, and the species giving rise to this structure will be labelled radical A. The radical or radicals giving rise to the broad central line will be labelled radical B.

The relative widths of the absorption lines indicated that the hyperfine structure was not due to the same radical as the central line, and several of the techniques described in section 4.3.5 were used to try to separate the spectra arising from the two species.

(a) Although there were no significant changes in the spectra after storing the crystal at room temperature for eighteen months, it was possible that annealing could preferentially destroy one of the radicals.   A crystal of cytosine monohydrate was therefore annealed for various times and at various temperatures up to 70°C.   However, above 60°C the crystal readily lost its water of crystallization, its ESR signal being completely destroyed at the same time.

(*b*) An attempt was made to produce preferentially one of the radicals by using ultraviolet radiation of the wavelength for which pyrimidines have a peak absorption, but this was unsuccessful.

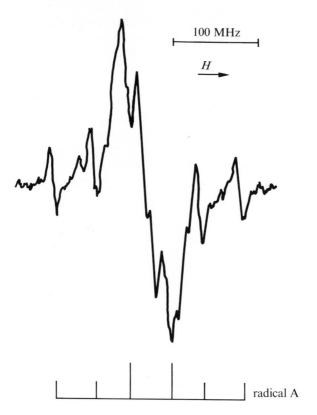

100 MHz

H

radical A

Fig. 4.4   Derivative spectrum of an irradiated single crystal of cytosine monohydrate recorded with the magnetic field parallel to the *a*-axis.

(*c*) Finally, the microwave power in the resonance cavity was increased in order to observe the power saturation of the absorption lines. Graphs of signal intensity against the square root of the microwave power are shown in Fig. 4.6 for the hyperfine structure and also the broad central line.   From these curves, it was clear that, for powers greater than one milliwatt, the central line saturated at a different rate from the hyperfine structure.

This experiment was final confirmation that at least two radical species were produced by the γ-radiation.

In general, there were six absorption lines which could be attributed to radical species A and, when reasonably well resolved, their relative intensities were near $1:1:2:2:1:1$. A detailed study of all the spectra indicated that changes in splitting between the absorption lines showed the

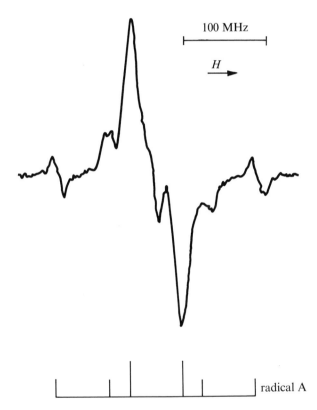

Fig. 4.5   Derivative spectrum of an irradiated single crystal of cytosine monohydrate recorded with the magnetic field parallel to the c^*-axis.

characteristic variation of the interaction between an unpaired electron and one α-hydrogen atom, superimposed on a nearly isotropic splitting of 208 MHz.   This large isotropic interaction was too great for a single β-proton and, although large anisotropic couplings with nitrogen atoms have been observed, their isotropic couplings rarely exceed 20 MHz.   Furthermore, the intensity ratio of the lines suggested that the spectra arose from coupling

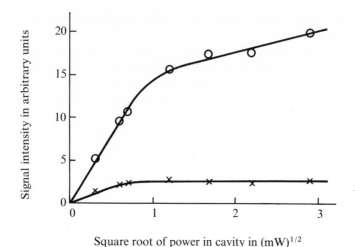

Square root of power in cavity in $(mW)^{1/2}$

Fig. 4.6   Plot of signal intensity against the square root of the power in the microwave cavity for the two radical species observed in the spectrum of cytosine monohydrate. The circles are for the broader central absorption and the crosses for the hyperfine structure of radical A.

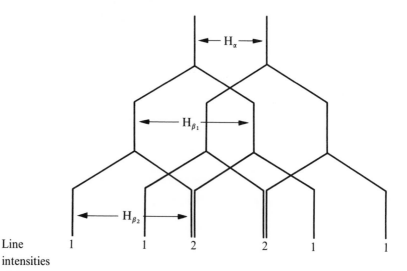

Line intensities

Fig. 4.7   Diagram showing the formation of the derivative spectrum for radical species A in an irradiated single crystal of cytosine monohydrate. The hyperfine splittings produced by interaction of the unpaired electron with one α-hydrogen atom (H_α) and two equivalent β-hydrogen atoms (H_{β_1} and H_{β_2}) result in a 6-line spectrum. The relative intensity of the lines is $1:1:2:2:1:1$.

between the unpaired electron and three protons, two of which were equivalent β-protons. The six spectral lines would then be formed as shown in Fig. 4.7.

For each plane of rotation, the α-splitting was measured as the spacing between each outer, well resolved, pair of lines. The splitting squared was plotted against the crystal's orientation in the magnetic field and a least squares method used to fit three smooth curves defined by equations (4.6), (4.7), and (4.8) to the experimental points. The square of the α-coupling tensor was therefore determined to be:

$$A = \begin{pmatrix} 3600 & 0 & -1730 \\ 0 & 1260 & 0 \\ -1730 & 0 & 5150 \end{pmatrix}. \tag{4.28}$$

This tensor is diagonalized by finding the roots of the equation:

$$\begin{vmatrix} 3600-\lambda & 0 & -1730 \\ 0 & 1260-\lambda & 0 \\ -1730 & 0 & 5150-\lambda \end{vmatrix} = 0. \tag{4.29}$$

The solution of this equation gives $\lambda = 2470$, 1260, and 6290. Thus, the diagonalized form of tensor A is:

$$\begin{pmatrix} 2470 & 0 & 0 \\ 0 & 1260 & 0 \\ 0 & 0 & 6290 \end{pmatrix}.$$

The square root of this tensor is:

$$\begin{pmatrix} 50 & 0 & 0 \\ 0 & 36 & 0 \\ 0 & 0 & 79 \end{pmatrix}.$$

The diagonal elements of this tensor are the principal values of the α-hydrogen interaction and the isotropic and anisotropic components are obtained by writing the tensor as the sum of two tensors, thus:

$$\begin{pmatrix} 50 & 0 & 0 \\ 0 & 36 & 0 \\ 0 & 0 & 79 \end{pmatrix} = \begin{pmatrix} 55 & 0 & 0 \\ 0 & 55 & 0 \\ 0 & 0 & 55 \end{pmatrix} + \begin{pmatrix} -5 & 0 & 0 \\ 0 & -19 & 0 \\ 0 & 0 & 24 \end{pmatrix}. \tag{4.30}$$

The isotropic component of the α-hydrogen interaction is therefore 55 MHz and the principal values of the anisotropic components are -5, -19, and 24 MHz. The sign of the principal values cannot be determined from the spectra but is inferred from the theory (McConnell and Chesnut, 1958;

McConnell and Strathdee, 1959) to be negative.   This sign has been incorporated in the values given for the coupling tensor in Table 4.7.

Table 4.7 *α-Hydrogen coupling tensor, in MHz, for radical species A*

Tensor in the abc* axial system	Principal values	Anisotropic compounds	
		Principal values	Direction cosines
$(-)$ $\begin{pmatrix} +58 & 0 & -13 \\ 0 & +36 & 0 \\ -13 & 0 & +70 \end{pmatrix}$	$(-)50$	$(+)5$	$(+0.84, 0.00, 0.54)$
	$(-)36$	$(+)19$	$(0.00, 1.00, 0.00)$
	$(-)79$	$(-)24$	$(-0.54, 0.00, 0.84)$
Isotropic component	$(-)55$		

The direction cosines are determined using the method described previously in section 4.3.2, as follows:

when $\qquad \lambda = 2470, \mathbf{e}_1 = l_1\mathbf{i} + m_1\mathbf{j} + n_1\mathbf{k}$

where
$$1130l_1 \quad +0m_1 - 1730n_1 = 0$$
$$0l_1 - 1210m_1 + \quad 0n_1 = 0$$
$$-1730l_1 + \quad 0m_1 + 2680n_1 = 0.$$

The solution of these three equations gives:

$$l_1 : m_1 : n_1 = 1.548 : 0 : 1.000$$

therefore $\mathbf{e}_1 = \dfrac{1}{(1.548^2 + 0^2 + 1.000^2)^{1/2}} (1.548\mathbf{i} + 0\mathbf{j} + 1.00\mathbf{k})$

$$= (0.84\mathbf{i} + 0\mathbf{j} + 0.54\mathbf{k}).$$

The direction cosines of the principal value of 50 MHz are therefore (0.84, 0.00, 0.54).   By a similar method the direction cosines for the other principal values can be determined and these are given in Table 4.7.

It remains to calculate the actual coupling tensor from the principal values and direction cosines.   This is given by:

$$\begin{pmatrix} \lambda_1 l_1{}^2 + \lambda_2 l_2{}^2 + \lambda_3 l_3{}^2 & \lambda_1 l_1 m_1 + \lambda_2 l_2 m_2 + \lambda_3 l_3 m_3 & \lambda_1 l_1 n_1 + \lambda_2 l_2 n_2 + \lambda_3 l_3 n_3 \\ \lambda_1 l_1 m_1 + \lambda_2 l_2 m_2 + \lambda_3 l_3 m_3 & \lambda_1 m_1{}^2 + \lambda_2 m_2{}^2 + \lambda_3 m_3{}^2 & \lambda_1 m_1 n_1 + \lambda_2 m_2 n_2 + \lambda_3 m_3 n_3 \\ \lambda_1 l_1 n_1 + \lambda_2 l_2 n_2 + \lambda_3 l_3 n_3 & \lambda_1 m_1 n_1 + \lambda_2 m_2 n_2 + \lambda_3 m_3 n_3 & \lambda_1 n_1{}^2 + \lambda_2 n_2{}^2 + \lambda_3 n_3{}^2 \end{pmatrix}.$$

Using the values $\lambda_1 = 50, \lambda_2 = 36, \lambda_3 = 79$

$$l_1 = 0.84, \qquad m_1 = 0.00, \qquad n_1 = 0.54$$
$$l_2 = 0.00, \qquad m_2 = 1.00, \qquad n_2 = 0.00$$
$$l_3 = -0.54, \qquad m_3 = 0.00, \qquad n_3 = 0.84$$

the actual α-hydrogen coupling tensor is calculated to be:

$$\begin{pmatrix} +58 & 0 & -13 \\ 0 & +36 & 0 \\ -13 & 0 & +70 \end{pmatrix}.$$

Although the square of the coupling tensor was determined from the experimental observations, the curves in Figs. 4.8, 4.9, and 4.10 were obtained from the actual tensor and show, for each plane of observation, the splitting itself plotted against the crystal's orientation in the magnetic field.

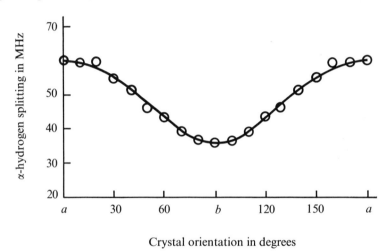

Fig. 4.8   Variation of the α-hydrogen splitting for radical species A observed in the *ab* plane. The circles represent the experimental points and the solid line is the calculated curve.

The circles represent the experimental observations and the solid lines are the calculated curves.

The space group $P2_1/c$ indicated that the spectra should have arisen from two magnetically distinct radical sites which were equivalent when the main magnetic field was parallel or perpendicular to the crystallographic *b*-axis.   The actual site splitting could only be reliably observed on the outer, well resolved, pair of lines.   At a few orientations these did become poorly resolved doublets, but generally the site splitting showed only as a broadening of the lines.   Such a small site splitting, together with the fact that the spectra recorded in the *ab* and *bc* planes were symmetrical about the axes, indicated that the A_{12} and A_{23} off-diagonal elements of the coupling tensor were negligible.   Thus, it was not necessary to determine the relative signs of these two elements.

The crystal of deuterated cytosine gave spectra very different from those which have been discussed. Radical A was still observable but the broad central absorption of species B became up to eleven partially resolved lines. These showed that, in addition to radical A, at least two other species were present. The spectra from the deuterated crystal will not be described in detail but the identification of one of the radicals observed in the spectra from species B will be discussed in section 4.5.4.

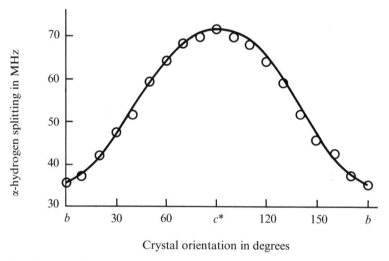

Fig. 4.9   Variation of the α-hydrogen splitting for radical species A observed in the bc^* plane. The circles represent the experimental points and the solid line is the calculated curve.

4.5.3   RADICAL SPECIES A

The principal values of the α-hydrogen coupling tensor, whose limits of error were estimated to be ± 3 MHz, are in close agreement with those generally found for carbon-centered π-electron radicals and previously listed in Table 4.1. The actual signs of the principal values could not be determined from the spectra, but there are strong theoretical grounds (McConnell and Chesnut, 1958; McConnell and Strathdee, 1959) for assuming them to be negative. The unpaired spin density on the central carbon atom was calculated from equation (4.21) to be 0.86.

If the unpaired electron interacted with one α-proton, it could be centered on either of the carbons, C_4 and C_5. It is expected (McConnell and Strathdee, 1959; Ghosh and Whiffen, 1959) that the principal axes of the coupling tensor corresponding to the least negative, intermediate, and most negative principal values will be parallel to the $\dot{C}$—H bond, normal to the radical plane and in the radical plane but perpendicular to the $\dot{C}$—H bond, respectively.   Thus the principal axis corresponding to a coupling of -36 MHz should be parallel to the $\dot{C}$—H bond.   The C_4—H_4 bond of the undamaged molecule was calculated from the atomic coordinates (Jeffrey

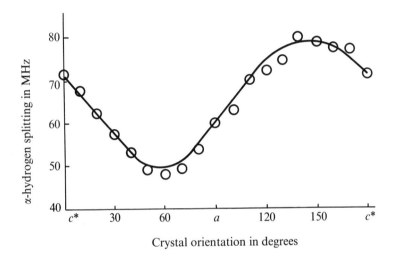

Fig. 4.10   Variation of the α-hydrogen splitting for radical species A observed in the c^*a plane. The circles represent the experimental points and the solid line is the calculated curve.

and Kinoshita, 1963) to be $25°$, and the C_5—H_5 bond to be $84°$, from this principal axis.   Hence, it seems likely that the unpaired electron is centered on carbon atom C_4, there being some rearrangement of the molecules on radical formation.

The radical was probably produced by the rupture of the double bond joining C_4 to C_5 with the addition of some fragment at C_5.   In the crystal of cytosine grown from heavy water, H_3 was replaced by deuterium and yet the spectra of radical species A still had the same overall width.   Hence there was little coupling to H_3.   This proton must therefore lie close to the nodal plane of the unpaired electron's orbital, giving only a small splitting which was less than the line width.   Therefore, both interacting β-hydrogen atoms are probably attached to C_5, a hydrogen atom being added when the double bond is fractured to give the radical:

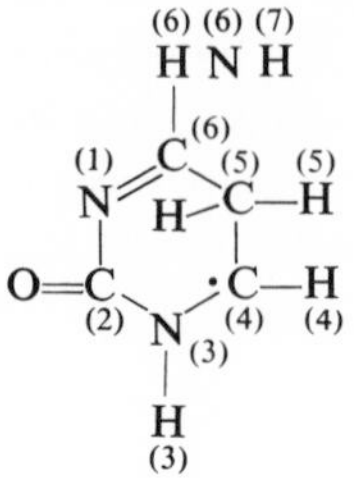

The coupling to each β-proton was almost isotropic with a value of 104 MHz, and given a positive sign on theoretical grounds (McLachlan, 1958; Lykos, 1960). It is unlikely that the two β-protons were exactly geometrically equivalent for all orientations of the crystal in the magnetic field. Slight differences in the coupling would have been masked in the spectra as the two center lines were always superimposed on the broad absorption of species B.

The direction dependence of the g-value at the center of the radical spectrum has not been investigated. However, the g-value was very nearly isotropic at 2.003 $\pm$ 0.001, as expected for a carbon-centered π-electron radical (McConnell and Robertson, 1957).

4.5.4   RADICAL SPECIES B

The radical or radicals giving rise to the broad central line could not be determined from the spectra of the irradiated cytosine monohydrate crystal owing to the lack of hyperfine structure. However, when the crystal was grown from heavy water, this single absorption line became up to eleven partially resolved lines and showed that, in addition to radical A, at least two other species were present. Only one of these could be identified and its spectra were interpreted in terms of one doublet and two triplet splittings, one of the triplets being nearly twice the size of the other. The splittings were attributed to one α-hydrogen atom and two central nitrogen atoms interacting with the unpaired electron. Such interactions would be observed if the radiation removed the deuterium attached to nitrogen atom N_3 to give:

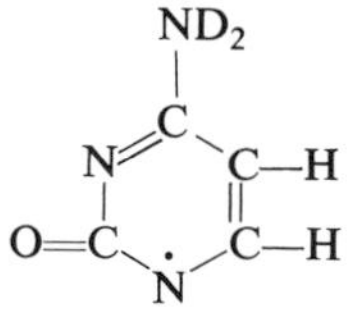

I

Seven resonance bond structures can be formed from I.

$$
\begin{array}{cccc}
\text{II} & \text{III} & \text{IV} & \text{V}
\end{array}
$$

(Structures II–V: cytosine ring resonance forms, each with ND_2 at top, ring positions showing variation of unpaired electron and charge distribution among N, O, and C atoms.)

(Structures VI, VII, VIII: further resonance forms with ND_2, N^+D_2 groups.)

Thus unpaired electron spin density can appear on the atoms N_1, N_3, N_6, O_2, and C_5. O^{16} does not have a magnetic moment and so structure II will not contribute to the ESR spectrum. However, the spectra showed interaction with only two central nitrogen atoms and the directions of the principal axes of their coupling tensors indicated that these atoms were probably N_1 and N_3. Without detailed molecular orbital calculations, it was not possible to say which nitrogen atom gave the larger splitting. The doublet arose from unpaired spin density on C_5 and consequent coupling to the α-hydrogen atom H_5. The proton attached to C_4 would be a β-hydrogen atom for an unpaired electron localized on N_3 or C_5, and the lack of observed splitting indicated that it lies close to the nodal plane of the unpaired electron's orbital. There was no detectable splitting resulting from resonance bond structures VII and VIII and hence the unpaired spin density on nitrogen atom N_6 was very small. Thus the unpaired electron of radical species B had a highly delocalized orbital and appreciable spin density appeared on alternate ring atoms.

4.5.5 CONCLUSIONS

This ESR study of radiation damage in single crystals of cytosine grown from both water and deuterium oxide has shown that at least three different radicals are produced by the radiation. Two of these species have been identified and coupling tensors evaluated for the various interactions between the unpaired electron and neighboring nuclei.

Perhaps the most surprising result of this investigation has been the great differences between the spectra observed from the normal and deuterated crystals of cytosine.   A broad central absorption line in the case of the former became up to eleven partially resolved lines when the crystal was grown from deuterium oxide.   Although resonance bond structures VII and VIII did not give detectable ESR splittings, their very presence may explain the differences between the two sets of spectra.   An unpaired electron localized on N_6 will have large anisotropic interactions with the two α-hydrogen atoms H_6 and H_7.   Even with a very small unpaired spin density on N_6, these interactions could be large enough to broaden each individual line so that all hyperfine structure is blurred out of the spectrum.   The proton has a larger magnetic moment than the deuteron and its doublet spacing is 6.51 times the triplet splitting of a deuteron in a similar position.   Thus, when hydrogen atoms H_6 and H_7 are replaced by deuterium, the overall splitting decreases and could become less than the width of the individual lines.   The hyperfine structure would then be observed.   Furthermore, for unpaired spin density on N_1 or C_5, H_6 and H_7 are γ-hydrogen atoms.   Investigations

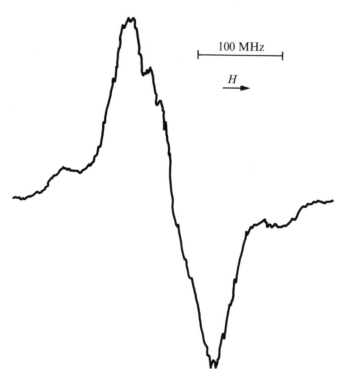

Fig. 4.11   Derivative spectrum of an irradiated polycrystalline sample of cytosine.

of γ-proton couplings in glutaric (Horsfield, Morton, and Whiffen, 1961a) and adipic (Morton and Horsfield, 1961b) acids have shown their splittings to be less than 9 MHz. However, with two such protons, a combined splitting of 15 MHz could be produced and, together with a very small unpaired spin density on N_6, would probably broaden the absorption lines sufficiently to prevent resolution of the hyperfine structure. Deuteration would reduce the γ-proton splittings to around 5 MHz and hence the hyperfine structure could be resolved.

The spectrum from an irradiated polycrystalline sample of anhydrous cytosine is shown in Fig. 4.11. The large anisotropies in the α-proton coupling produced a scrambling effect in the spectrum and all the hyperfine structure of radical species A was blurred out. This is a good example of the advantages in using single crystals to study the effects of radiation on organic compounds.

ACKNOWLEDGEMENTS

This work forms part of the research program of the Physics Department, Guy's Hospital Medical School, London and was supported by the British Empire Cancer Campaign. We are grateful to Professor C. B. Allsopp for his interest and support and to Dr. J. P. Elliott for many helpful discussions.

REFERENCES

Abragam, A., and Pryce, M. H. L., 1951, *Proc. R. Soc.* A, **205**, 135.

Akasaka, K., Ohnishi, S., Suita, T., and Nitta, I., 1964, *J. chem. Phys.*, **40**, 3110.

Atherton, N. M., and Whiffen, D. H., 1960a, *Molec. Phys.*, **3**, 1; 1960b, ibid., **3**, 103.

Atkin, R. H., 1956, *Mathematics and Wave Mechanics* (London: Heinemann Ltd.), Ch. 3.

Bleaney, B., and Stevens, K. W. H., 1953, *Rep. Prog. Phys.*, **16**, 108.

de Boer, E., and Mackor, E. L., 1963, *J. chem. Phys.*, **38**, 1450.

Bowers, K. D., and Owen, J., 1955, *Rep. Prog. Phys.*, **18**, 304.

Box, H. C., and Freund, H. G., 1964, *J. chem. Phys.*, **40**, 817.

Box, H. C., Freund, H. G., and Lilga, K. T., 1963, *J. chem. Phys.*, **38**, 2100; 1965, ibid., **42**, 1471.

Cipollini, E., and Gordy, W., 1962, *J. chem. Phys.*, **37**, 13.

Cole, T., and Heller, H. C., 1961, *J. chem. Phys.*, **34**, 1085.

Cole, T., Heller, H. C., and McConnell, H. M., 1959, *Proc. natn. Acad. Sci., U.S.A.*, **45**, 525.

Cook, J. B., Elliott, J. P., and Wyard, S. J., 1967a, *Molec. Phys.*, **12**, 185; 1967b, ibid., **13**, 49.

Cook, R. J., Rowlands, J. R., and Whiffen, D. H., 1962, *Proc. chem. Soc.*, p. 252; 1963a, *J. chem. Soc.*, p. 3520; 1963b, *Molec. Phys.*, **7**, 31; 1963c, ibid., **7**, 57.

Delbousquet, M. X., 1964, in *Electronic Magnetic Resonance and Solid Dielectrics*, Ed. R. Servant and A. Charru (Amsterdam: North Holland Publ. Co.), p. 176.

Derbyshire, W., 1962, *Molec. Phys.*, **5**, 225.

Fermi, E., 1930, *Z. Phys.*, **60**, 320.

Fischer, H., 1965, *Magnetic Properties of Free Radicals*, Landolt-Börnstein Tables. Group II, Vol. I. (Berlin: Springer-Verlag).

Fraenkel, G. K., 1962, *Pure Appl. Chem.*, **4**, 143.

Frosch, R. A., and Foley, H. M. 1952, *Phys. Rev.*, **88**, 1337.

Fujimoto, M., 1963, *J. chem. Phys.*, **39**, 840.

Ghosh, D. K., and Whiffen, D. H., 1958, in *Chemical Society Symposium, Bristol* (London: Chemical Society, p. 168), 1959, *Molec. Phys.*, **2**, 285.

Gordy, W., Ard. W. B., and Shields, H., 1955, *Proc. natn. Acad. Sci., U.S.A.*, **41**, 983.

Hahn, Y. H., and Rexroad, H. N., 1963, *J. chem. Phys.*, **38**, 1599.

Heller, H. C., 1962, *J. chem. Phys.*, **36**, 175.

Heller, H. C., and Cole, T., 1962a, *J. Am. chem. Soc.*, **84**, 4448; 1962b, *J. chem. Phys.*, **37**, 243.

Heller, H. C., and McConnell, H. M., 1960, *J. chem. Phys.*, **32**, 1535.

Henn, D. E., and Whiffen, D. H., 1964, *Molec. Phys.*, **8**, 407.

Holden, A. N., Kittel, C., Merritt, F. R., and Yager, W. A., 1950, *Phys. Rev.*, **77**, 147.

Horsfield, A., and Morton, J. R., 1962, *Trans. Faraday Soc.*, **58**, 470.

Horsfield, A., Morton, J. R., Rowlands, J. R., and Whiffen, D. H., 1962, *Molec. Phys.*, **5**, 241.

Horsfield, A., Morton, J. R., and Whiffen, D. H., 1961a, *Molec. Phys.*, **4**, 169; 1961b, ibid., **4**, 327; 1961c, ibid., **4**, 425; 1961d, *Nature, Lond.*, **189**, 481; 1961e, *Trans. Faraday Soc.*, **57**, 1657; 1962, *Molec. Phys.*, **5**, 115.

Jaseja, T. S., and Anderson, R. S., 1961, *J. chem. Phys.*, **35**, 2192; 1962a, ibid., **36**, 1098; 1962b, ibid., **36**, 2727.

Jeffrey, G. A., and Kinoshita, Y., 1963, *Acta Cryst.*, **16**, 20.

Kashiwagi, M., and Kurita, Y., 1963, *J. chem. Phys.*, **39**, 3165; 1964, ibid., **40**, 1780.

Katayama, M., 1962a, *J. chem. Phys.*, **37**, 2143; 1962b, *J. molec. Spectrosc.*, **9**, 429.

Katayama, M., and Gordy, W., 1961, *J. chem. Phys.*, **35**, 117.

Kurita, Y., 1962, *J. chem. Phys.*, **36**, 560.
Kurita, Y., and Gordy, W., 1961a, *J. chem. Phys.*, **34**, 282; 1961b, ibid., **34**, 1285.
Kwiram, A. L., and McConnell, H. M., 1962, *Proc. natn. Acad., Sci., U.S.A.*, **48**, 499.
Lin, W. C., and McDowell, C. A., 1961a, *Molec. Phys.*, **4**, 333; 1961b, ibid., **4**, 343.
Lin, W. C., and McDowell, C. A., 1963, *Can. J. Chem.*, **41**, 9.
Livingston, R., Zeldes, H., and Taylor, E. H., 1955, *Discuss. Faraday Soc.*, **19**, 166.
Lontz, R. J., and Gordy, W., 1962, *J. chem. Phys.*, **37**, 1357.
Lykos, P. G., 1960, *J. chem. Phys.*, **32**, 625.
McClure, D. S., 1949, *J. chem. Phys.*, **17**, 905; 1952, ibid., **20**, 682.
McConnell, H. M., and Chesnut, D. B., 1958, *J. chem. Phys.*, **28**, 107.
McConnell, H. M., and Fessenden, R. W., 1959, *J. chem. Phys.*, **31**, 1688.
McConnell, H. M., and Giuliano, C. R., 1961, *J. chem. Phys.*, **35**, 1910.
McConnell, H. M., Heller, H. C., Cole, T., and Fessenden, R. W., 1960, *J. Am. chem. Soc.*, **82**, 766.
McConnell, H. M., and Robertson, R. E., 1957, *J. phys. Chem.*, Ithaca, **61**, 1018.
McConnell, H. M., and Strathdee, J., 1959, *Molec. Phys.*, **2**, 129.
McLachlan, A. D., 1958, *Molec. Phys.*, **1**, 233.
McLachlan, A. D., Dearman, H. H., and Lefebvre, R., 1960, *J. chem. Phys.*, **33**, 65.
Miyagawa, I., 1961, *Tech. Rep. Inst. Solid State Phys. Univ. of Tokyo*, Ser. A., No. 27.
Miyagawa, I., and Gordy, W., 1959, *J. chem., Phys.*, **30**, 1590; 1960, ibid., **32**, 255.
Miyagawa, I., and Itoh, K., 1962, *J. chem. Phys.*, **36**, 2157; 1964, ibid., **40**, 3328.
Miyagawa, I., Kurita, Y., and Gordy, W., 1960, *J. chem. Phys.*, **33**, 1599.
Morton, J. R., 1963, *J. Phys. Chem. Solids*, **24**, 209; 1964a, *Chem. Rev.*, **64**, 453; 1964b, *J. Am. chem. Soc.*, **86**, 2325; 1964c, *J. chem. Phys.*, **41**, 2956.
Morton, J. R., and Horsfield, A., 1961a, *J. chem. Phys.*, **35**, 1142; 1961b, *Molec. Phys.*, **4**, 219.
Orton, J. W., 1959, *Rep. Prog. Phys.*, **22**, 204.
Phillips, F. C., 1946, in *An Introduction to Crystallography* (London: Longmans, Green and Co.).
Pooley, D., and Whiffen, D. H., 1961a, *Molec. Phys.*, **4**, 81; 1961b, *Trans. Faraday Soc.*, **57**, 1445; 1962, *J. chem. Soc.*, p. 366.
Pruden, B., Snipes, W., and Gordy, W., 1965, *Proc. natn. Acad. Sci., U.S.A.*, **53**, 917.

van Roggen, A., van Roggen, L., and Gordy, W., 1956, *Bull. Am. phys. Soc.*, **1**, 266.

Rao, D. V. G. L. N., and Gordy, W., 1961a, *J. chem. Phys.*, **35**, 362; 1961b, ibid., **35**, 764; 1962, ibid., **36**, 1143.

Rao, D. V. G. L. N., and Katayama, M., 1962, *J. chem. Phys.*, **37**, 382.

Rexroad, H. N., Hahn, Y. H., and Temple, W. J., 1965, *J. chem. Phys.*, **42**, 324.

Rogers, M. T., and Whiffen, D. H., 1964, *J. chem. Phys.*, **40**, 2662.

Rowlands, J. R., 1961, *J. chem. Soc.*, p. 4264; 1962, *Molec. Phys.*, **5**, 565.

Rowlands, J. R., and Whiffen, D. H., 1961, *Molec. Phys.*, **4**, 349; 1962, *Nature*, Lond., **193**, 61.

Schoffa, G., 1964a, in *Electronic Magnetic Resonance and Solid Dielectrics*, Ed. R. Servant and A. Charru (Amsterdam: North-Holland Publ. Co.), p. 185; 1964b, *J. chem. Phys.*, **40**, 908.

Schonland, D. S., 1959, *Proc. phys. Soc.*, **73**, 788.

Stone, E. W., and Maki, A. H., 1962, *J. chem. Phys.*, **37**, 1326.

Tamura, N., Collins, M. A., and Whiffen, D. H., 1966a, *Trans. Faraday Soc.*, **62**, 1037; 1966b, ibid., **62**, 2434.

Trammell, G. T., Zeldes, H., and Livingston, R., 1958, *Phys. Rev.*, **110**, 630.

Tsvetkov, Yu, D., Rowlands, J. R., and Whiffen, D. H., 1964, *J. chem. Soc.* p. 810.

Uebersfield, J., and Erb, E., 1956, *C. r. hebd. Séanc. Acad. Sci., Paris*, **242**, 478.

Ueda, H., 1964, *J. chem. Phys.*, **40**, 901.

Venkataraman, B., and Fraenkel, G. K., 1955, *J. chem. Phys.*, **23**, 588.

Weidner, R. T., and Whitmer, C. A., 1953, *Phys. Rev.*, **91**, 1279.

Weil, J. A., and Anderson, J. H., 1958, *J. chem. Phys.*, **28**, 864.

Weiner, R. F., and Koski, W. S., 1963, *J. Am. chem. Soc.*, **85**, 873.

Weissman, S. I., 1956, *J. chem. Phys.*, **25**, 890.

Whiffen, D. H., 1961, in *Free Radicals in Biological Systems*, Ed. M. S. Blois, H. W. Brown, R. M. Lemmon, R. O. Lindblom, and M. Weissbluth (New York: Academic Press), p. 227; 1962, *Pure appl. Chem.*, **4**, 185.

Zavoisky, E., 1945, *J. Phys. U.S.S.R.*, **9**, 245.

Zeldes, H., Trammell, G. T., Livingston, R., and Holmberg, R. W., 1960, *J. chem. Phys.*, **32**, 618.

CHAPTER FIVE

ELECTRON SPIN RESONANCE OF RADICALS IN IRRADIATED HYDROGEN-- OXYGEN SYSTEMS IN THE SOLID STATE

Thomas E. Gunter

Donner Laboratory, University of California, Berkeley, U.S.A.

5.1 INTRODUCTION

The radiation chemistry of aqueous solutions and of hydrogen peroxide solutions is discussed in such a vast number of papers published throughout the last half century that no one could hope to deal with them all. Indeed, even the much more specialized field of ESR investigations of irradiated aqueous and hydrogen peroxide systems has become so extensive that one must specialize still further, in a paper of this length, in order to be able to discuss any of the details of the subject. Hence, in this paper attention has been focussed on concrete identification and description of the effective spin-Hamiltonian parameters of several of the more common free radical species, predicted by radiation chemists from radiation yield data, and found by ESR spectroscopists in irradiated, frozen samples. A brief discussion and comparison of radical yields in these species is also included.

Those species discussed at length, which have been identified in irradiated frozen solutions, and whose effective spin-Hamiltonian has been determined are the hydrogen atom, the OH radical, the solvated electron, and the HO_2 radical.

5.2 A BRIEF DISCUSSION OF THE RADIATION CHEMISTRY OF AQUEOUS SOLUTIONS AND THE PART PLAYED BY ESR

The existence of free radicals in irradiated aqueous solutions was hypothesized by radiation chemists several decades ago to explain radiation yields of the end products of radiation induced reactions. Hence, radiation chemistry provides first, a large amount of indirect evidence for the existence of particular types of free radicals in irradiated aqueous solutions, and second, radiation yield data for these radicals.

It has long been observed that when an aqueous solution is irradiated with light particles, such as electrons, the water changes very little, while the solute may be greatly changed by the radiation (Fricke and Brownscombe, 1933). With heavy particles, in contrast, the water itself extensively decomposes into hydrogen gas, oxygen gas, and hydrogen peroxide (Dale, *et al.*, 1949). Results of this type lead to the idea that intermediate species formed by the radiation are responsible for part of the radiation damage (Weiss, 1944). Obviously, since the whole solution is irradiated in the case of light-particle radiation, a large portion of the radiation must be absorbed in the water. The indirect action hypothesis (Fricke and Brownscombe, 1933; Allen, 1961) then explains the apparent lack of effect in the water by saying that water, upon receiving energy from the radiation, becomes 'activated' or, in the modern point of view, decomposes into chemically active free radicals. These radicals in turn interact with the solute causing most of the chemical changes observed. Those remaining then disappear due to recombination with each other.

It is usually assumed that radiation somehow breaks up the H_2O

159

molecule into H and OH radicals. In the case of irradiation by light particles, the density of these radical pairs along the track is small and the radicals have a very good chance of recombining with each other to form H_2O. With heavy-particle radiation, on the other hand, the density of radical pairs along the tracks is much greater and, correspondingly, the chance of combination of H and OH with like radicals to form H_2 and H_2O_2 is much greater.

Radiation chemical data is often given quantitatively in terms of radiation yield, G, which is defined as the number of molecules, atoms, or ions formed by radiation per 100 eV of radiation energy absorbed by the solution. With light-particle radiation in H_2O, one works with G_{H_2}, $G_{H_2O_2}$, G_H, and G_{OH}, whereas with heavy particles G_{O_2H} must also be dealt with (Allen, 1961).

Experimental data from radiation yield experiments usually take the form of yields for stable molecular species and ionic complexes (when certain ionic salts are added to the solution). Reaction mechanisms are postulated which involve radicals as intermediates, and radical yields are calculated. A simple example of this is a study of the reactions which are thought to go on in a Fricke dosimeter. $FeSO_4$ is put into an acid solution in which atmospheric oxygen is dissolved. The solution is then irradiated by Co^{60} γ-rays, for example. Somehow during the irradiation, H_2O is assumed to have been broken up into H and OH.†

Since H_2 and H_2O_2 are formed by combination of H and OH respectively with like radicals, for material balance we have the relation:

$$G_H + 2G_{H_2} = G_{OH} + 2G_{H_2O_2}. \tag{5.1}$$

Fe^{3+} can be observed in the solution because of its strong absorption at 3050 Å in the ultraviolet and its concentration can be measured by comparison to a standard.

We then postulate that the following reactions take place in the irradiated solution:

$$Fe^{2+} + OH \rightarrow FeOH^{2+} \tag{5.2}$$

$$Fe^{2+} + H_2O_2 \rightarrow FeOH^{2+} + OH \tag{5.3}$$

and

$$Fe^{2+} + H + O_2H^+ \rightarrow Fe^{3+} + H_2O_2. \tag{5.4}$$

(*Note:* $H^+ + O_2 = O_2H^+$ due to atmospheric oxygen in acid solution.)

Then

$$G_{Fe^{3+}} = G_{OH} + 2G_{H_2O_2} + 3G_H \tag{5.5}$$

or

$$G_{Fe^{3+}} = 2G_{H_2} + 4G_H \tag{5.6}$$

and

$$G_H = \tfrac{1}{4}(G_{Fe^{3+}} - 2G_{H_2}). \tag{5.7}$$

† The discussion used is based on yield equations set up by Dainton (1959) and yield values given by Allen and Rothschild (1957) and by Allen (1961) in a more detailed treatment of radiation chemistry in the oxidation of Fe^{2+}.

Let us use the experimentally measured values of $G_{Fe^{3+}} = 15.5$ (Allen, 1957, 1961) and $G_{H_2} = 0.45$ (Allen, 1957; Hochanadel and Lind, 1956) in our example. Then $G_H = \frac{1}{4}(15.5 - 0.9) = 3.65$. It is desirable to supplement the above type of result with direct physical proof of the existence of the hypothesized free radicals.

Electron spin resonance (ESR) provides an excellent experimental tool to use in radical identification. Free radicals by their very definition are molecular or atomic species with an odd number of electrons. Since they must then contain an unpaired orbital electron, free radicals are invariably paramagnetic. Electron spin resonance is sensitive only to paramagnetic species and is little affected by the nonmagnetic molecules in the sample.

ESR allows one to obtain several types of data about free radicals. It is possible to specifically identify some radical species by their ESR spectra. This can be done if the number and relative intensities of the lines can be predicted through a knowledge of the hyperfine interactions. (The simplest example of this is the case of a system with spin $= \frac{1}{2}$ which contains a single proton. Since each of the electron Zeeman states are split into two hyperfine levels by interaction with the proton, and since transitions involving a proton spin-flip are forbidden, only two absorption lines are allowed between the four states and an ESR doublet is the resulting spectrum.)

Regardless of whether or not the radical can be identified through its spectrum, the spin concentration may be determined by calculating the area under its absorption curve and comparing it to that of a standard whose spin concentration is known. The radiation yield for the radical may then be calculated.

5.3   WHY FROZEN AQUEOUS SAMPLES ARE USED IN ESR STUDIES

Most of the work on irradiated hydrogen–oxygen systems has been carried out at liquid nitrogen temperature (77°K) and a smaller amount has been carried out at liquid helium temperature (4.2°K). In order to see why the ESR work on free radicals in aqueous solutions is usually done at low temperatures, let us consider the problem of using the ESR technique to study radicals produced in liquid water at, say 300°K.

The first severe problem with liquid water as the object of a study of radiation produced free radicals, is radical lifetime. Although the exact lifetimes of the radicals of interest (say OH, H, O_2H, and e_{sol}^- as a start) at 300°K are unknown in aqueous solution, a good order of magnitude guess is around one microsecond. Hence in the water system, either a steady state radical concentration, maintained by continuous irradiation, must be set up, or the radicals must be studied immediately after a strong pulse of radiation by electronic gating techniques.

The second problem with the water system is its property of having large dielectric losses at microwave frequencies. Because of 'loading' of the microwave cavity usually used in ESR detection, the size of the sample which can be used is greatly restricted. Hence detection difficulties are greatly increased. (For a detailed consideration of this problem see the paper by Stoodley (1963).)

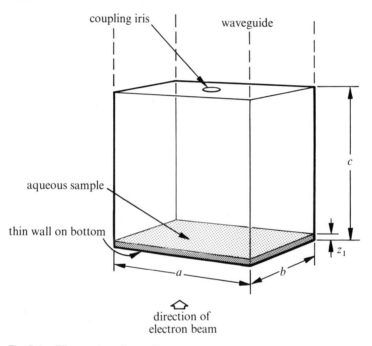

Fig. 5.1 TE_{101} rectangular cavity.

Let us look at the problem as it would be set up in a typical experimental system using say a TE_{101} rectangular cavity. In this cavity the sample is to be placed in the bottom (as shown in Fig. 5.1) in a region of low microwave electric field intensity and high microwave magnetic field intensity.

To see how much the sample size is restricted by dielectric losses we may use the results of Feher (1957). Feher has shown that maximum signal voltage out of an ESR cavity in which the sample gives dielectric losses can be obtained when the microwave power lost to the dielectric is one-half the microwave power dissipated in the cavity walls. This then determines the amount of sample which should be used for maximum detection sensitivity for an aqueous sample. Electric and magnetic field equations for the TE_{101} cavity are given by Moreno (1958) and may be written as

$$E_y = \frac{\omega a}{\pi v_c} B_0 \sin \frac{\pi x}{a} \sin \frac{\pi z}{c} \cos \omega t, \qquad H_z = - B_0 \cos \frac{\pi x}{a} \sin \frac{\pi z}{c} \sin \omega t$$

$$E_x = E_z = 0, \qquad H_x = B_0 \frac{ka}{\pi} \sin \frac{\pi x}{a} \cos \frac{\pi z}{c} \sin \omega t$$

$$H_y = 0. \tag{5.8}$$

Since in steady state the energy held by the cavity is constant with time, calculations may be simplified by choosing the time in the calculation such that the simplest field expressions result.

Since the microwave field energy is given by

$$\frac{1}{8\pi} \int (E^2 + H^2) \, dV$$

where dV is an element of volume of the cavity, the energy stored in the cavity would be

$$\left(\frac{\omega a}{\pi v_c}\right)^2 \frac{B_0^2}{8\pi} \int dV \left\{ \sin^2 \frac{\pi x}{a} \sin^2 \frac{\pi z}{c} \right\} = \frac{B_0^2}{8\pi} \frac{abc}{4} \left(\frac{\omega a}{\pi v_c}\right)^2. \tag{5.9}$$

The power dissipated in the dielectric is given by

$$\frac{\omega}{8\pi} \int_{\text{sample}} dV \epsilon'' |E|^2 = \frac{\omega \epsilon''}{8\pi} \left(\frac{\omega a}{\pi v_c}\right)^2 B_0^2 \int_{\text{sample}} dV \left\{ \sin^2 \frac{\pi x}{a} \sin^2 \frac{\pi z}{c} \right\}$$

$$= B_0^2 \frac{\omega \epsilon''}{8\pi} \left(\frac{\omega a}{\pi v_c}\right)^2 \frac{\pi}{6} abc \left(\frac{z_1}{c}\right)^3. \tag{5.10}$$

Hence from Feher's condition for loading of the cavity, the optimum sample thickness z_1, is obtained when

$$\frac{\omega \epsilon''}{8\pi} \left(\frac{\omega a}{\pi v_c}\right)^2 \frac{\pi abc}{6} \left(\frac{z_1}{c}\right)^3 = \frac{1}{2} \frac{1}{8\pi} \frac{abc\omega}{4 Q_0 (2\pi)} \left(\frac{\omega a}{\pi v_c}\right)^2 \tag{5.11}$$

(the power lost in the dielectric equals one-half the power lost in the cavity walls). In the above, v_c is the velocity of light, k is the magnitude of the wave vector, ω is the microwave angular frequency, a, b, and c are the cavity dimensions, and ϵ'' is the imaginary part of the dielectric constant. As an example, let the microwave frequency be 9.5 GHz and the temperature be 300°K.

Then, using $a = 2.285$ cm, $b = 1.143$ cm, $c = 2.53$ cm, and ϵ'' as determined from information given by Collie, *et al.* (1948a, 1948b) to be 32, and if Q_0, the quality factor of the unloaded cavity, is taken as 7500,

$$\left(\frac{z_1}{c}\right)^3 = \frac{3}{8\pi^2 \epsilon'' Q_0} \tag{5.12}$$

or the sample thickness is

$$z_1 = 1.55 \times 10^{-2} \text{ cm.}$$

In order to see how large the radiation dose rate should be in order to produce a detectable number of radicals in such a small sample, let us make the following assumptions:

1. The radiation is by a beam of 6 MeV electrons.
2. The radicals of interest have a lifetime of 10^{-6} sec.
3. The radiation yield for the radicals of interest is 3.
4. 10^{14} radicals can be detected by an ESR spectrometer for this type of aqueous sample.

Each of the 6 MeV electrons would be expected to yield an energy to the sample of

$$\Delta E = E_0(1 - e^{-\mu z_1}) \tag{5.13}$$

where μ is the stopping power of water for 6 MeV electrons, and E_0 is the initial beam energy, 6 MeV. μ may be computed from information given by Evans (1955) to be 2.05 cm^{-1}. Hence

$$\Delta E = 6\{1 - \exp(2.05 \times 1.55 \times 10^{-2})\} = 0.192 \text{ MeV.}$$

A radiation yield of 3 means that approximately 33 eV are required to produce a radical. The electron beam then could be expected to produce $192 \times 10^3/33 = 5.78 \times 10^3$ radicals per electron. Therefore, if the lifetime of a radical is taken to be one microsecond, the electron beam necessary to produce a steady state concentration of 10^{14} radicals is

$$\frac{10^{14}}{5.78 \times 10^3} \frac{\text{electrons}}{\mu\text{sec}} = 1.73 \times 10^{16} \frac{\text{electrons}}{\text{sec}}$$

or 2.77×10^{-3} amps.

This means that one might be able to detect a very weak signal from free radicals produced in liquid water if a strong radiation beam current (of 6 MeV electrons) of about 3 mA were used. Because of such problems as electronic interference in the ESR spectrometer produced by the radiation source, water vapor loading of the cavity, etc., this estimate is probably optimistic.   ESR on radicals in irradiated liquid water would hence be a possible, but difficult, study.

It is much easier to study frozen samples at or below liquid air temperature.   At these temperatures radical lifetimes for at least some of the radicals of interest are extremely long (months or longer).   In addition, the imaginary part of the dielectric constant of H_2O decreases considerably with temperature so that much larger samples can be used.

Another approach has been to study free radicals produced in the gas phase where, simply due to separation of the radicals, their lifetimes are greatly increased.   For study, these radicals are usually collected on a cold finger.

Experiments providing examples of each of these techniques with frozen and gaseous samples will be described later.

5.4   ESR STUDIES ON IRRADIATED ACIDS AND BASES

5.4.1   THE HYDROGEN ATOM

The first free radical identification to be made in irradiated, frozen aqueous solution by ESR techniques was that of atomic hydrogen by Livingston, *et al.* (1954, 1956).

The samples used were frozen acid solutions of $HClO_4$, H_2SO_4, and H_3PO_4 irradiated with Co^{60} γ-rays at 77°K, using a 23 GHz paramagnetic resonance spectrometer.   The spectra thus obtained showed a broad spectrum near spectroscopic $g = 2$, composed roughly of one broad and one narrower line and a much wider split doublet with a total splitting averaging 505.4 Oe centered near the free electron g-value.   When the above acid solutions were deuterated, that is, the protons replaced by deuterons, the wide-spaced doublet was replaced by a triplet.   The H_2SO_4 case is shown in Fig. 5.2.   (The spectra shown here were taken by Henriksen (1964) at X-band frequency, using X-ray irradiated H_2SO_4 solution at 77°K.)   The doublet shown here was identified as that of the hydrogen atom, first, because of the change of the spectrum from doublet to triplet with substitution of $I = 1$ deuterons for $I = \frac{1}{2}$ protons, and second, because the observed splittings were in close agreement with splittings predicted using atomic beam and nuclear resonance values for the proton and deuteron moments.

The Hamiltonian of the hyperfine interaction may be written as:

$$\mathcal{H}_{hfs} = \frac{3(\mu_s \cdot \mathbf{r})(\mu_I \cdot \mathbf{r})}{r^5} - \frac{(\mu_s \cdot \mu_I)}{r^3} + \frac{8\pi}{3} \delta(\mathbf{r})(\mu_s \cdot \mu_I) \qquad (5.14)$$

where μ_s = electron magnetic moment operator

μ_I = nuclear magnetic moment operator

$\mathbf{r}$ = radius from nucleus to electron.

Symmetry arguments may be used to show that the dipole–dipole part of the above interaction gives zero contribution to the splitting when averaged over all space with the hydrogen atom $1s$ distribution function, ψ_{1s}^2, as the weighting function. Because of the Dirac delta function, however, the same is not true for the Fermi–Segré term in the above interaction.

0.45 M H_2SO_4

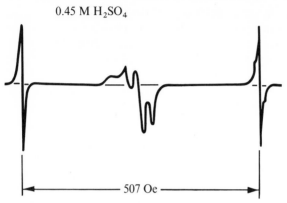

507 Oe

Fig. 5.2 5×10^5 rad X-irradiated H_2SO_4 solutions. Irradiation and detection were at 77°K.

The hydrogen atom $1s$ wave function may be written as:

$$\psi_{1s}(r) = \left(\frac{1}{4\pi}\right)^{1/2} \left(\frac{1}{a_0}\right)^{3/2} 2\, e^{-r/a_0} \tag{5.15}$$

where a_0, the Bohr radius for the $1s$ shell, $= 0.529 \times 10^{-8}$ cm.

If the electron Zeeman interaction is included, in order to write the effective spin-Hamiltonian for the hydrogen atom system, one may write:

$$\mathcal{H}_{\text{hfs}} = g\beta(\mathbf{S \cdot H}) - \frac{8\pi}{3}\left(\frac{1}{4\pi}\right)\left(\frac{1}{a_0}\right)^3 4g\beta\gamma_H\hbar(\mathbf{S \cdot I}) \tag{5.16}$$

where g = free electron g-factor or 2.0023
β = Bohr magneton, 9.27×10^{-21} ergs/Oe
γ_H = proton gyromagnetic ratio, $4.258 \times 2\pi$ MHz/kOe or 2.79 nuclear magnetons.

The resonance equation for the doublet follows directly from the above giving the energy difference between the $m_s = \frac{1}{2}$ and $-\frac{1}{2}$ states:

$$h\nu + g\beta H - \frac{8}{3}\frac{1}{a_0{}^3} g\beta\gamma_H\hbar m_I \tag{5.17}$$

where m_I is the component of nuclear spin along the z-axis along which the electron spin is quantized, and m_s is correspondingly the component of the electron spin along the z axis. The field positions of the doublet lines are obtained by putting in the values $\pm\frac{1}{2}$ for m_I. Hence:

$$H_{\pm} = \frac{h\nu \pm \frac{4}{3}(1/a_0^3)g\beta\hbar\gamma_H}{g\beta} \tag{5.18}$$

or

$$\Delta H = \frac{8}{3}\frac{\gamma_H\hbar}{a_0^3} = H_+ - H_-$$

Therefore, upon substitution of values for the quantities in the above equation, one finds:

$$\Delta H = \frac{8}{3}\frac{4.258 \times 10^3 \,(\text{Oe sec})^{-1} \, 6.625 \times 10^{-27} \, \text{erg sec}}{(0.529)^3 \, 10^{-24} \, \text{cm}^3}$$

$$= 507 \text{ Oe since } \text{Oe}^2 = \text{erg/cm}^3$$

This problem could be turned around so that one might say that a hyperfine splitting of 505.4 Oe implies a proton magnetic moment of 2.784 nuclear magnetons.

Livingston, *et al.*, measured a splitting between the central line and both the high and low field lines in the deuterium atom triplet averaging 77.5 Oe. This means an average separation of high and low field lines of 155 Oe.

The expected splitting for the deuterium atom may be found by substituting

$$\gamma_D = 0.857 \text{ nuclear magnetons} = 0.655 \times 2\pi \text{ MHz/kOe}$$

$$I = 1, m_I = 1, 0, -1$$

into equation (5.17) above.

The line position for the deuterium atom lines then follows similarly to equation (5.18) for the proton line position giving

$$H = \frac{h\nu + m_I\frac{8}{3}(g\beta\gamma_D\hbar/a_0^3)}{g\beta}. \tag{5.19}$$

Or if ΔH_{10} refers to the separation of the high field line from the central line and ΔH_{0-1} to that of the central line from the low field line, one has

$$\Delta H_{10} = \Delta H_{0-1} = \frac{8}{3}\frac{g\beta\gamma_D\hbar}{a_0^3}. \tag{5.20}$$

Hence the ratio of hydrogen atom to deuterium atom hyperfine splittings is given by the ratio of magnetic moments, μ_H/μ_D, or gyromagnetic ratios, γ_H/γ_D.   The result is the expected hyperfine triplet with a predicted oversplitting of 156 Oe or 78 Oe between each pair of nearest lines.

A comparison of the values of proton and deuteron magnetic moments calculated from the results of Livingston, *et al.*, with molecular beam measurements of the same magnetic moments by Nafe and Nelson (1948) and with the currently accepted values is given in Table 5.1.

Table 5.1

Magnetic moment in units of nuclear magnetons	Livingston, *et al.* (1954, 1956)	Nafe and Nelson (1948)	Currently accepted values (Lindgren, 1963)
Proton	2.784	2.7896	2.79277
Deuteron	0.852	0.8564	0.85741

At about the same time that Livingston, *et al.* published the results discussed above, Smaller, *et al.* (1954) and later Matheson and Smaller (1955) published a study on neutral ice.   This sample, irradiated by Co^{60} γ-rays, was studied with a 350 MHz ESR spectrometer at both 77°K and 4.2°K. Smaller, *et al.* did not observe the hydrogen atom doublet reported by Livingston, *et al.* but reported a quite different spectral doublet near $g = 2$ which they sought to identify as the hydrogen atom.   This spectrum has since been thought to be due to the OH radical.   The fact that the 507 Oe doublet cannot be seen in neutral ice irradiated at 77°K has been confirmed by several experiments.

Both Piette, *et al.* (1959) using an X-band ESR spectrometer and electron irradiation at 4.2°K, and Rexroad and Gordy (1962) using a K-band system and Co^{60} γ-rays at 4.2°K, confirmed in neutral ice samples the hydrogen atom spectrum observed by Livingston in acidic samples at 77°K.   The rest of the spectrum observed in each case, centered near the free electron g-value, within an overall spread of about 150 Oe, varied with the technique used.

Piette, *et al.* also observed the 507 Oe hyperfine doublet in electron irradiated solid hydrogen at 4.2°K.   No other lines were observed in this sample.

At present very little doubt can remain that the 507 Oe doublet is correctly identified as due to atomic hydrogen.

5.4.2   THE SOLVATED ELECTRON

Henriksen (1964) not only verified that the atomic hydrogen spectrum could be found in strong acids at 77°K, but also showed that in spite of the hydrogen atom not being trapped in neutral polycrystalline ice at 77°K, it could be found in electron irradiated alkaline solutions at this temperature (see Fig. 5.3).   These results and their explanation represent another success of ESR studies on free radicals in irradiated aqueous solutions.

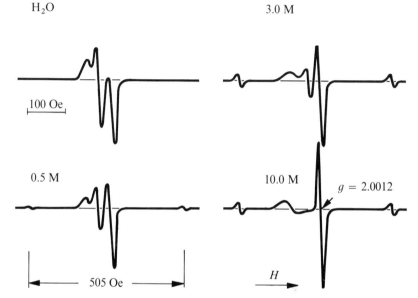

Fig. 5.3   The qualitative ESR spectra of water and aqueous solutions of NaOH at different concentrations. The solutions were irradiated at 77°K. Radiation dose, 5×10^5 rad ; sweep rate 126 Oe/min.

In 1953 Samuel and Magee posed the question of the part played by a stabilized electron in the formation of hydrogen atoms in radiation induced reactions.   If the formation of hydrogen atoms and hydroxyl radicals in irradiated water takes place through the following reactions:

$$H_2O = H_2O^+ + e^- \qquad (5.21)$$

$$H_2O^+ = OH + H^+ \qquad (5.22)$$

$$H_2O + e^- = OH^- + H \qquad (5.23)$$

one should be able to discuss conditions under which the electron is stabilized in the solution.   Samuel and Magee say that an electron should become free of its parent ion if its kinetic energy becomes greater than the Coulomb energy of binding to this parent ion.   Writing this condition as:

$$\frac{e^2}{\varepsilon r} < kT \qquad (5.24)$$

if $e = 4.80 \times 10^{-10}$ e.s.u.

   $k = 1.38 \times 10^{-16}$ ergs/degree

   $T = 300°$K

   $\epsilon = 3$ for times shorter than the relaxation time of water (Samuel and Magee, 1953)

$$r_s = \frac{e^2}{\epsilon kT} = \frac{(4.80 \times 10^{-10})^2}{3 \times 1.38 \times 10^{-16} \times 300} \tag{5.25}$$

$$= 1.85 \times 10^{-6} \text{ cm} = 185 \text{ Å at } 300°\text{K or } 17°\text{C}$$

one acquires an expression for a radius r_s, such that if the electron becomes separated from its parent ion by a distance greater than r_s it becomes essentially 'free'; that is, the electron becomes thermalized, if its separation from its parent ion becomes so large that (5.24) holds.

At temperatures nearer the freezing point the value of r_s should be smaller, perhaps as low as 115 Å. Considering a random walk collision process for a secondary electron of energy 10 eV, Samuel and Magee determined that the maximum separation of the average secondary electron from its parent ion is around 18 Å, which would be far too short to allow the electron to become free. Their conclusion then was that the electron intermediary process of atomic hydrogen formation in H_2O should not be observable and that H_2O should break up into radicals according to the equation:

$$H_2O = H_2O^+ + e^- \rightarrow H_2O^* \rightarrow H + OH. \tag{5.26}$$

This theory would then predict equal numbers of H and OH radicals formed by the initial water decomposition, and the same initial spatial distribution.

Lea (1946), and later Platzman (1953) added further thoughts to the theory of water decomposition. Lea noted that cloud chamber photographs showed that regardless of the figures from a random walk calculation, electrons separated a far greater distance than 18 Å from their parent ion. When the delta-ray tracks in vapor were decreased by the ratio of vapor density to liquid density in an effort to adjust for the shorter mean path between collisions, 150 Å became a typical maximum separation to expect in liquid water. He concluded then that some electrons would be freed and would go on to produce hydrogen atoms through reaction (5.23).

Platzman pointed out that equation (5.23) is energetically unfavorable unless one allows the electron to hydrolyze water in the process. He added that the time even a slow electron could be expected to remain in the vicinity of a water molecule was 10^{-13} sec, whereas the electric dipole relaxation time for water is of the order 3×10^{-11} sec, and hence he did not expect reaction (5.23) to go forward except in acid solution where it takes the form:

$$H^+ + e^- = H. \tag{5.27}$$

Platzman's reasoning leads to the conclusion that one should be able to see a single resonance line from an 'almost free' electron at low temperature in alkaline solutions, if equations (5.21) and (5.22) are prominent reactions in irradiated H_2O.

Henriksen's reasons for identifying the line seen in Figs. 5.3 and 5.4 as due to 'solvated electrons' are:

(a) The ESR spectrum is a single line near the free electron g-value, as expected.

(b) This spectrum is present only in alkaline solutions and is independent of the cation used.

(c) Upon deuteration the line narrows a bit due to the smaller magnetic moment of the deuteron, but it remains a single line near the free electron g-value.

(d) A similar ESR line is seen in a solution of Na dissolved in liquid ammonia where a solvated electron has long been thought to exist.

(e) The color of the irradiated alkaline solution is blue just as with Na in liquid ammonia.

It is interesting to note that the maximum yields of solvated electron plus hydrogen atom in alkaline solution are equivalent to the maximum yield of hydrogen atom in acid solution in the case of glassy samples.   This may be evidence that the atomic hydrogen seen in acid solutions is produced largely through reaction (5.27).

In view of the hydrogen atom spectra seen in strong alkaline solution, Henriksen concludes that both the Samuel–Magee and the Lea–Platzman processes take place.   Henriksen's maximum yield data for solvated electron and hydrogen atom spectra in alkaline solutions (seen in Table 5.3) suggest that the Lea–Platzman process is the predominant one, however.

The broad low field hump seen in Fig. 5.4 is thought by Henriksen to be probably due to O^- radical ion.   This interpretation is consistent with the work of Ersov, et al. (1963) and with that of Moorthy and Weiss (1964). Moorthy and Weiss, who made further studies of irradiated alkaline solutions, support Henriksen's identification of the solvated electron line in the resulting ESR spectra.

5.5 OH IN IRRADIATED ICE AND CRYSTAL HYDRATES

The ESR spectrum of the OH radical has been identified in irradiated neutral ice and in irradiated crystals containing waters of hydration at $77°K$

(Gunter and Jeffries, 1964; Gunter, 1965, 1966, 1967; Brivati, *et al.*, 1965; Dibdin, 1966).

Whatever causes the resonance lines near $g = 2$, henceforth called the central resonance spectrum, in irradiated neutral ice at 77°K, it must obviously be a radical or radical ion containing hydrogen, oxygen, or both. H, OH, O_2H, H_2O^+, H_2O^-, O^-, and any of these in combination with an

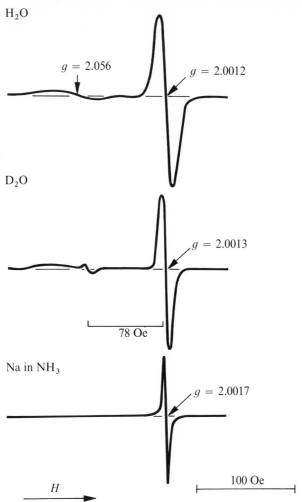

H_2O

$g = 2.056$ $g = 2.0012$

D_2O

$g = 2.0013$

78 Oe

Na in NH_3

$g = 2.0017$

100 Oe

H

Fig. 5.4   The qualitative ESR spectra for irradiated solutions of NaOH (10M) in H_2O and D_2O. The bottom curve is the reson-ance line observed for the solvated electrons formed when Na is dissolved in liquid ammonia. All spectra were recorded at 77°K at a sweep rate of 47 Oe/min.

H_2O molecule are possible candidates for this resonance.   Of these, only the spectrum of atomic hydrogen had previously been positively identified and found not to contribute at all to the central resonance lines.   In order to evaluate the identification of the spectrum under consideration, it is necessary to look at the expected spectra for the above radicals and radical ions.

Molecular radicals trapped in solid matrices usually show spin only paramagnetism.   This means that if one looks at the Zeeman interaction in the form

$$H_z = \beta(\mathbf{L} + 2\mathbf{S})\cdot\mathbf{H} \qquad (5.28)$$

the $\mathbf{L}$ term contributes little to the observed paramagnetism.   Often the cause of this in the case of molecular radicals trapped in a solid matrix is that hydrogen bonding binds the radical rather tightly to the matrix in which it is held.   This hydrogen bonding has the same effect as the strong crystal fields which produce spin only paramagnetism in the iron group compounds; i.e., strong bonding of the paramagnetic center to the lattice, through a noncentral interaction, implies nonconservation of orbital angular momentum.   Therefore, $\mathbf{L}$ is not an effective operator in equation (5.28).   This effect is known as 'quenching of $\mathbf{L}$'.   Spin-orbit interaction 'lifts' this quenching of $\mathbf{L}$ in higher order considerations.   If the interaction causing nonconservation of orbital angular momentum is hydrogen bonding, for example, and is of the order of several thousand wave numbers in magnitude, and if the coefficient of the $\mathbf{L} \cdot \mathbf{S}$ coupling interaction is of the order of one hundred wave numbers, the spectroscopic splitting tensor g may be expected to have principal values, which may differ from the free electron g-value, 2.0023.   This difference should be of the order of the ratio of the spin-orbit coupling energy to hydrogen bonding energy.   Under the assumptions made of the magnitudes of the interactions involved this could give a contribution as large as 0.1 to the g-value.   A calculation of this effect for OH in ice will be discussed in more detail later.

An $S = \frac{1}{2}$ ground state is usually found in free radicals.   The reason is that free radicals, by definition, contain an odd number of electrons, all of which are paired except the one in the highest populated orbital.   This single unpaired electron spin gives a $S = \frac{1}{2}$ ground state.

The OH radical should show an effective spin of $\frac{1}{2}$ when trapped in a solid matrix.   The hyperfine interaction for the single proton in OH should split each of the Zeeman lines and give a doublet, since $\Delta m_I = 0$ is required by a selection rule.   Here m_I is the quantum number of the z component of nuclear spin angular momentum.   The splitting of this doublet cannot be calculated without knowledge of the wave function of the unpaired electron.   As will be discussed later, however, it can be approximately predicted from previous work on the OH radical.

Similarly, the O_2H radical would be expected to show a hyperfine doublet. The splitting of O_2H is expected to be less than that in OH due to greater average separation of electron and proton spins. This is because the unpaired electron is localized primarily on the oxygen atom farthest from the hydrogen.

Figure 5.5 shows that the expected ESR spectrum of a system of effective spin $S = \frac{1}{2}$ and two equivalent protons is a triplet of $1:2:1$ intensity ratios. This is the case for both the water ions, $H_2O^\pm$. O^- radical ion ion having no proton should show a singlet spectrum.

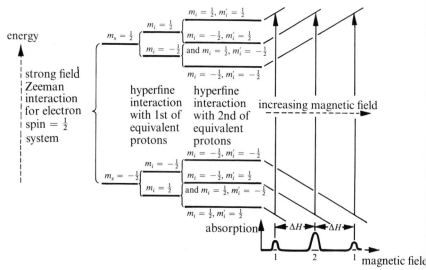

Fig. 5.5   Energy level splitting and resulting line spectrum of an $S = \frac{1}{2}$ electron spin system interacting with two equivalent protons and a strong magnetic field.

Since the dipole–dipole part of the hyperfine interaction falls off as $1/r^3$ the radicals which contain bound waters should show only a very small splitting from the protons in the bound water because they have, in general, a larger separation between the electron spin and the protons. This splitting would probably be smaller than the line width of the unhydrated radical and hence not be seen.

The ESR spectrum in irradiated, neutral ice at $77°K$ has been thought by many researchers to be due to OH radical, either by itself or with another radical. One of the first systematic studies of the resonance near $g = 2$ in irradiated, neutral ice was made by Siegel and co-workers (Siegel, et al., 1960, 1961; Judeikis, et al., 1962; Siegel, 1963), who worked with Co^{60} irradiated neutral ice using an X-band ESR spectrometer. Siegel interpreted the spectrum observed in ice (similar to that seen in Figs. 5.6 and 5.7) as a doublet at $g = 2.008$ with a hyperfine splitting of 41.5 Oe and a low field hump. Upon deuteration (Fig. 5.6b) Siegel found what was interpreted as a triplet at the same g-value as the previous doublet with a 6.5 Oe splitting, and again with a low field hump. The ratio of line splittings in these two cases is $41.5/6.5 = 6.38$, which is very near the magnetic moment ratio for the proton and deuteron μ_p/μ_d of 6.5. Figure 5.6 gives a splitting ratio

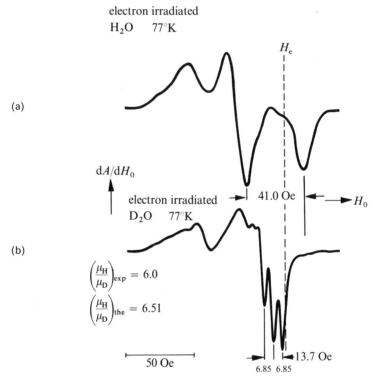

Fig. 5.6 (a) Derivative of absorption vs. field for electron irradiated polycrystalline ice at 77° K. (b) Derivative of absorption vs. field for electron irradiated polycrystalline heavy ice at 77°K.

of $41.0/6.85 = 6.0$ from measurements made at this laboratory. It will be recalled from the hyperfine calculation above that splittings change by the magnetic moment ratio upon isotopic substitution. Primarily on this basis Siegel sought to identify the sources of these spectra as OH and OD respectively.

If the doublet seen by Siegel is OH, it should show an isotropic hyperfine splitting near 26.7 Oe, the isotropic hyperfine splitting found for OH in the gaseous phase (Radford, 1962).   This point will be discussed in detail later.

A study of the ESR spectra of irradiated single crystal ice would seem at first to be a valuable source of information about the effective spin-Hamiltonian of radicals formed in irradiated ice.

McMillan, *et al.* (1960) have reported a study of irradiated single crystal ice.   They assign a doublet with $g_{\parallel} = 2.0127$, $g_{\perp} = 2.0077$, a, the isotropic or contact hyperfine interaction, $= 41.3$ Oe, $B_{\parallel} = 12$ Oe, and

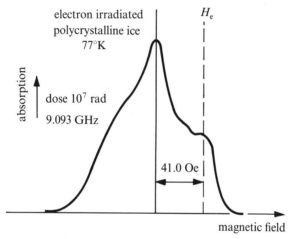

Fig. 5.7   Absorption vs. field for electron irradiated polycrystalline ice at 77°K.

$B_{\perp} = -6$ Oe, to the OH radical.   The B's are the parallel and perpendicular parts of the dipole–dipole interaction between electron and proton.   With a single crystal, this effective spin-Hamiltonian would predict a high field line almost stationary in magnetic field value upon crystal rotation.   The low field line is predicted to be 53 Oe from the high field line in the parallel case and 35 Oe from it in the perpendicular case.   In polycrystalline ice the same effect spin-Hamiltonian would show a strong high field line and a weak, broad low field line.   Therefore this effective spin-Hamiltonian does not agree with the polycrystalline spectrum.

In addition, the contact interaction given by McMillan, *et al.*, 41.3 Oe, is in poor agreement with that determined for OH in the vapor phase, 26.7 Oe, as will be discussed later.

Finally, from their spectral data, McMillan, *et al.* assign the radical axis to the directions from the center toward each of the corners of the hexagon of the ice lattice, that is, the OH radicals are all taken to lie in the plane perpendicular to the optic axis of the ice crystal.   This might be expected if ice had simple hexagonal symmetry.   However, the hexagonal space group symmetry of ice is $D_{6h}^4 - C6/mmm$ (Barnes, 1929; Peterson and Levy, 1957) as is shown in Fig. 5.8.   The radical axis given by McMillan, *et al.* makes an angle of $90°$ with one of the original hydrogen bond directions and $19°$ with the six other original hydrogen bond directions.   Intuitively, it

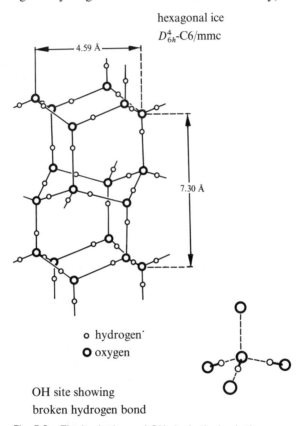

hexagonal ice
D_{6h}^4-C6/mmc

o hydrogen˙
O oxygen

OH site showing
broken hydrogen bond

Fig. 5.8   The ice lattice and OH site in the ice lattice.

would appear more likely for OH in ice to lie along one of the original hydrogen bond directions because in this orientation the radical would be held in place and hence stabilized by hydrogen bonding.   There are seven hydrogen bond directions in the ice lattice.   One of them, that along the optic axis, occurs twice as often as any of the other six.

In order to see what ESR spectrum might be expected for OH in single crystal ice, it is necessary to study the theory of this radical in some detail.

The structural form of hexagonal ice is the tridymite structure shown in Fig. 5.8. Lattice dimensions at $0°C$, as given by Lonsdale (1958), are $a = 4.523$ Å and $c = 7.367$ Å. The O—H—O length or oxygen–oxygen separation along the optic axis is 2.760 Å, and the O—H length for the separation of an oxygen atom from one of its two hydrogen atoms is 0.98 Å, again at $0°C$.

Each oxygen atom may be thought of as at the center of a tetrahedron. The corners of the tetrahedron are other oxygen atoms. The protons forming hydrogen bonds between each oxygen and its four nearest neighbor oxygens are so arranged that there are two protons 0.98 Å away from each oxygen and two other protons 1.78 Å away from each oxygen.

From the work of Pauling (1939), Lennard-Jones and Pople (1951), and Schneider (1955) it is possible to build a picture of the hydrogen bond as a bond which is essentially electrostatic in nature. The work of Coulson and Danielson (1954) leads to the conclusion that such an electrostatic picture of the hydrogen bond is likely to lead to errors of only a few per cent in g-value calculations for the case of OH hydrogen bonded into the ice lattice as is depicted in Fig. 5.8.

A picture of an H_2O dissociation in which OH is produced may then be made. Consider the H_2O to undergo dissociation through either the Samuel–Magee or the Lea–Platzman process. At the time of formation of OH either a proton or a hydrogen atom leaves the immediate area of the dissociation. The majority of the OH radicals are then stabilized by hydrogen bonding at the site of the H_2O from which the OH was formed.

Since the bonding has been shown to be primarily ionic in nature, it is natural to seek to use the crystal field theory pioneered by Stevens (1952) and discussed in the book by Judd (1963) to determine the spectroscopic splitting tensor for OH in ice.

The electronic ground state of OH has been determined to be a $^2\Pi_{3/2}$ state. The first electronic excited state has also been determined to be a $^2\Sigma$ state some 3×10^4 wave numbers above the ground state. It is important to note that in the work of Dousmanis, $et\ al.$ (1955) and of Radford (1961, 1962) the OH ground state wave function may be considered as simply a wave function for a system with an orbital angular momentum quantum number of one, symmetric about some center of symmetry along the molecular axis.

This allows a picture of the 'hydrogen bonding' interaction for OH in ice to be represented by a strong term of C_{3v} symmetry having the strength of three hydrogen bonds and a weaker term of σ_v symmetry due to the strains induced by the broken bond.

These two symmetries define the x, y, and z directions for a given OH radical in the following way. The C_3 axis of the C_{3v} symmetry interaction determines the z direction, which is along the OH molecular axis. The σ_v symmetry causes the π orbital of the unpaired electron to be orientated in a preferred direction. This direction is then defined as the x direction.

While the magnitude of the σ_v symmetry term would be very difficult to determine from theory with any great accuracy, it is reasonable to expect the magnitude of this term to have an energy equivalent of approximately the strength of one hydrogen bond.

Using crystal field theory, the crystal field interaction Hamiltonian may be set up as

$$V_{CF} = V_1[3L_z^2 - L(L + 1)] + V_2[L_+^2 + L_-^2]. \qquad (5.29)$$

In the above, V_1 is an interaction energy equivalent to three hydrogen bonds or about 3×6.5 kcal/mole† ≈ 6873 cm^{-1}. V_2 may be estimated to have a magnitude of 1145 cm^{-1}. In the form written above, both V_1 and V_2 are negative quantities.

It should be noted that for each of the seven inequivalent OH sites in ice, there are now three sites. Each of the three sites has the same direction g_z but the directions g_x and g_y depend on the direction of the lattice defect term of σ_v symmetry with respect to the radical axis. Since $(g_y - g_x)\beta H \leq$ (the ESR line width) for the case of OH lines in ice, an approximation procedure may be undertaken which allows one to ignore the complicated details of the theory in the x, y plane and account for the behavior of the ESR lines at this orientation with an 'average' $g_\perp$. Since the details of the theory are 'averaged out' in this approach, one would expect the observed spectra to show details, especially in line shape, near the perpendicular orientation, which are not accounted for by this simplified theory.

Consider a single set of three sites as mentioned above (i.e., the sites owing their inequivalence to the direction of the interaction). For two special orientations of the magnetic field such a group of three sites finds itself in an orientation of higher symmetry. The first occurs when the external field is along the x axis of one radical site (i.e., along a lobe of the OH π orbital) and hence makes an angle of $60°$ with the x axis of each of the other two sites in this set of three. The second occurs when the field is along the y axis of one of the radical sites. In these orientations two of the sites which are inequivalent at an arbitrary orientation become equivalent. If an equal distribution of radicals among the three inequivalent sites at an arbitrary orientation is assumed, the two lines observed when the magnetic field is in either of the special orientations discussed above should have an intensity ratio of $2:1$.

† This value is arrived at by taking the average of what appears to be the most reliable references to hydrogen bond strength in ice from the review of this subject in *The Hydrogen Bond* by Pimentel and McClellan (1960).

Where the separation of two lines is small with respect to their line width, the assumption of Gaussian line shape allows one to estimate the position of the zero of the absorption derivative for this case where one of the lines has twice the number of radicals as the other. To lowest order in line separation with respect to line width this is given by

$$g = \frac{3g'g''}{2g'' + g'} \tag{5.30}$$

where g' is the g-value of the more intense line, g'' is the g-value of the less intense line, and g is the g-value of the 'composite' line made up of a superposition of the other two. To higher orders the corrections become more complicated and involve the line shape function itself.

Since the two orientations discussed above for OH represent extrema for the composite line in the x, y plane, and since these extreme line positions recorded at 9 GHz should be separated by less than the experimental precision of line position measurement, the average of these two extrema provides a reasonable estimate of the experimentally observed $g_\perp$.

The spin-orbit interaction V_{S-O} which partially lifts the quenching of L due to hydrogen bonding, may be written as

$$V_{S-O} = \Lambda \mathbf{L} \cdot \mathbf{S} = \Lambda[L_z S_z + \tfrac{1}{2}(L_+ S_- + L_- S_+)]. \tag{5.31}$$

The value of Λ used is that found from the work of Dousmanis, et al. (1955), for OH in the gas phase, $\Lambda = -139.7 \, \text{cm}^{-1}$.

Perturbation theory (Gunter, 1966, 1967) yields the value of g_x, g_y, and g_z as

$$\begin{aligned}
g_x &= g_e - 4\eta - 2g_e\phi^2 = 2.0136 \\
g_y &= g_e - 2g_e\phi^2 + 4\phi\eta = 2.0016 \\
g_z &= g_e - 4\phi - g_e\eta^2 - 4\phi\eta = 2.0631
\end{aligned} \tag{5.32}$$

where ϕ and η are defined by

$$\phi = \frac{1}{2}\left(\frac{\Lambda}{4|V_2|}\right)$$

$$\eta = \frac{1}{2}\left(\frac{\Lambda}{3|V_1| + 2|V_2|}\right).$$

The predicted values of $g_\parallel$ and $g_\perp$ for OH in ice, correct to 2nd order corrections, are calculated to be

$$g_\parallel = 2.0631$$

and

$$g_\perp = 2.0063$$

where it must be remembered that the value of $g_\parallel$ was used in setting up the interaction Hamiltonian and hence is forced to agree with the experimental results.

H. E. Radford (1961, 1962) has studied the OH radical produced by microwave discharges in water vapor using ESR techniques. While Radford's work is directed toward a physical understanding of the OH radical and is not a study of radicals produced by radiation, it can be used in identifying OH radical spectra in samples where OH is produced by radiation.

OH free radical in the vapor phase was analyzed theoretically by Radford following the theory of Van Vleck (1929) and of Dousmanis, et al. (1955). The theory was extended to cover the strong field Zeeman and hyperfine interactions.

This theory may be briefly outlined as follows. Optical and microwave absorption data had shown OH to be in a $^2\Pi_{3/2}$ ground state. Wave functions for OH correct to the electronic, vibrational, rotational, and fine structure interactions were determined by considering a case between Hund's cases (A) and (B). g-Values were determined by considering the Zeeman interaction as a perturbation on a system with the above described wave functions. The hyperfine interaction was treated as a perturbation on the states correct to the Zeeman interaction as described above, and was used in a form given by Frosch and Foley (1952):

$$\mathscr{H}_{hfs} = a(\mathbf{I} \cdot \mathbf{L}) - (b + c)I_z S_z + \tfrac{1}{2}b(I_+ S_- + I_- S_+) \tag{5.33}$$

where a, b, and c are coefficients which must be determined by experiment. Radford gives the values

$$b(\text{OH}) = -119.0 \pm 0.4 \text{ MHz}$$

and

$$c(\text{OH}) = 133.2 \pm 1.0 \text{ MHz}$$

for the quantities of interest to this study as determined by his experiment.

It might be noted that the excellent agreement between experiment and theory in Radford's work, in which agreement is found to the experimental precision of about 3 parts in 10^5, inspire confidence in the correctness of the analysis and results.

If one takes the hyperfine interaction in the form shown in equation (5.14) and makes the substitutions

$$\boldsymbol{\mu}_s = g\beta\mathbf{S}, \qquad \boldsymbol{\mu}_I = \gamma\hbar\mathbf{I}, \qquad a = (8\pi/3)\,\delta(r)$$

one obtains the form

$$\mathscr{H}_{hfs} = g\beta\gamma\hbar \left[\frac{3(\mathbf{S} \cdot \mathbf{r})(\mathbf{I} \cdot \mathbf{r})}{r^5} - \frac{\mathbf{S} \cdot \mathbf{I}}{r^3} + a(\mathbf{S} \cdot \mathbf{I}) \right]. \tag{5.34}$$

Notice that this interaction may be written in tensor form as

$$\mathcal{H}_{\text{hfs}} = g\beta\gamma\hbar\mathbf{S} \begin{vmatrix} \dfrac{3x^2 - r^2}{r^5} + a & \dfrac{xy}{r^5} & \dfrac{xz}{r^5} \\[2ex] \dfrac{xy}{r^5} & \dfrac{3y^2 - r^2}{r^5} + a & \dfrac{yz}{r^5} \\[2ex] \dfrac{xz}{r^5} & \dfrac{yz}{r^5} & \dfrac{3z^2 - r^2}{r^5} + a \end{vmatrix} \mathbf{I}$$

where $\mathbf{S}$ is now looked upon as a row vector and $\mathbf{I}$ as a column vector. In the principal axis system this interaction then takes the form

$$\mathcal{H}_{\text{hfs}} = g\beta\gamma\hbar\mathbf{S} \begin{vmatrix} a - \dfrac{1}{r^3} & 0 & 0 \\[2ex] 0 & a - \dfrac{1}{r^3} & 0 \\[2ex] 0 & 0 & a + \dfrac{2}{r^3} \end{vmatrix} \mathbf{I}. \tag{5.35}$$

It is clear at this point that the sum of the eigenvalues of this matrix gives $3a$ or $8\pi\,\delta(r)$. This value which is related to the probability of finding the electron at the site of the proton depends primarily upon the electronic interactions in the OH system and hence should be characteristic of the type of radical. Hydrogen bonding of the radical to the matrix in a solid would perturb this value but not greatly, since hydrogen bonding energy (of the order of 10^3 wave numbers) is small with respect to electronic or Coulombic energy (of the order of 10^4 or 10^5 wave numbers). Vibration and rotation would perturb this value slightly in the gaseous state.

It might be noted in the case of the above tensor that diagonalization is not really necessary in order to obtain the above result. Since the tensor is real, its trace must be independent of the axis system chosen, and hence the diagonal sum equaling $8\pi\,\delta(r)$ follows directly from the first form of the tensor shown.

One would expect then that the value of the Fermi–Segré or isotropic part of the hyperfine interaction would be similar for OH in the gaseous state and for OH hydrogen bonded in a solid matrix such as ice, or calcium or lithium sulfates, because the strength of this interaction is determined by the probability of finding the electron at the site of the proton. Hence perturbations which greatly affect this splitting must compare in strength with the Coulomb interaction.

The isotropic hyperfine splitting calculated from Radford's data is given by $b + c/3 = 74.6$ MHz using the values of b and c quoted above.

(Note that one must use the b and c values quoted by Radford in his second paper on OH (1962). The values given for these quantities in the first paper are calculated by making an assumption which turns out to be incorrect and which can be eliminated by the use of additional data found in the experiments discussed in the second paper.)   The field splitting equivalent to 74.6 MHz is

$$\frac{74.6 \times 10^6 h}{g\beta} = \frac{74.6 \times 6.625}{2 \times 0.9273} \, 10^{-1} = 26.7 \text{ Oe}.$$

If the hyperfine interaction is written in the form

$$\mathscr{H}_{\text{hfs}} = A_z(I_z S_z) + A_x(I_x S_x) + A_y(I_y S_y) \tag{5.36}$$

where the A's are the principal values of the hyperfine interaction tensor (note that the above form assumes that the x, y, and z directions are along the principal axes of this tensor), the values of the A's obtained from Radford's data are

$$A_z = (b + c) = 14.2 \pm 1.4 \text{ MHz} = 5.07 \text{ Oe}$$
$$A_x = A_y = b = -119.0 \pm 0.4 \text{ MHz} = -42.5 \text{ Oe}.$$

The hyperfine interaction, written in this form, includes both the Fermi contact interaction and electron–proton dipole–dipole interactions. The influence of the crystal field interaction on the electron orbitals might be expected to give a larger variation in the dipole–dipole part of the hyperfine interaction between the cases of OH in the gaseous phase and in OH trapped in the ice matrix than would be expected for the isotropic contact interaction.

Gunter and Jeffries (1964) and Gunter (1965, 1966, 1967) have carried out another study of irradiated single crystal ice. ESR spectra were recorded at a sample temperature of 77°K in this study after electron irradiation at 77°K. The observed spectra consistently showed the necessary rotation symmetries (for example, a 60 degree symmetry was observed for spectra taken with the H field in the plane perpendicular to the optic axis) and were consistent even to the smaller details between samples.   Eight different crystal samples were studied, in which rotation of the crystal was about the optic axis, in order to verify that lack of good spectral resolution was not due to imperfect or twinned crystals.

Due to the inherent complexity of ice spectra observed in the single crystal ice case (see Fig. 5.9), it was thought useful to study irradiated H_2O in the form of waters of hydration in simple hydrated crystals.   In those hydrated crystals which have a smaller number of sites for waters of hydration, it was hoped that a smaller number of radical sites would also be found.

Studies have now been carried out on several systems containing waters of hydration.   Crystals which contain a large number of inequivalent water sites, such as $MgSO_4 \cdot 7H_2O$ and $CdSO_4 \cdot 6H_2O$ show the same type of spectral complexity as is seen in ice itself.   When simpler hydrates such as $CaSO_4 \cdot 2H_2O$ and $Li_2SO_4 \cdot H_2O$ were studied after irradiation by electrons at $77°K$, the number of inequivalent radical sites was much smaller and the

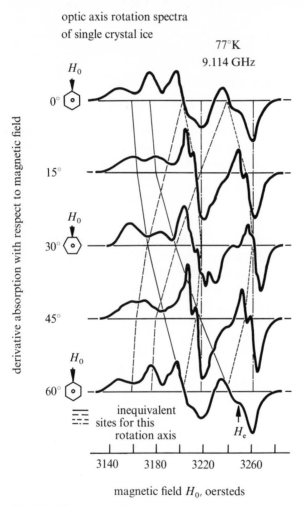

Fig. 5.9   Single crystal ice spectra.

individual spectral lines were easy to resolve (Gunter and Jeffries, 1964; Gunter, 1965, 1966, 1967).

Irradiated calcium and lithium sulfates were first studied by Wigen and Cowen (1960).   The spectra reported in electron irradiated samples of these salts showed two important types of centers.   The first gave an isotropic line near the free electron g-value and was attributed to a trapped electron; the second gave anisotropic lines varying in hyperfine splitting from a few Oe to a maximum of 21 Oe.   These lines were attributed to a hole on the sulfate oxygen which is hydrogen bonded to a water molecule.

The study currently underway at this laboratory forces a change in the interpretation of the irradiated sulfate spectra.   The experimental hyperfine splittings found in this study differ by more than a factor of two from those reported by Wigen and Cowen.

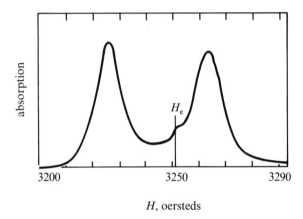

H, oersteds

Fig. 5.10   The equal line intensity doublet and trapped electron line found in $CaSO_4 \cdot 2H_2O$ irradiated by electrons at 77°K. $H_{\text{parallel}}(010)$; 9.1110 GHz.

The isotropic splitting found from the $CaSO_4 \cdot 2H_2O$ anisotropic line spectrum shown in Fig. 5.10 as an equal line intensity doublet is 24.1 Oe, as can be seen from the spin-Hamiltonian data in Fig. 5.11.   The corresponding isotropic splitting found from the $Li_2SO_4 \cdot H_2O$ anisotropic line spectrum shown in Figs. 5.12 and 5.13 is 22.0 Oe.

The satisfactory agreement for the value of the isotropic hyperfine splitting for OH in the gaseous phase and OH hydrogen bonded to oxygen in the irradiated sulfates (as shown in Table 5.2) gives very strong support for the identification of these centers in the irradiated sulfates as OH radical.

Additional support for this identification is obtained from a study of deuterated lithium sulfate, $Li_2SO_4 \cdot D_2O$ where the triplet from each OD radical is as shown in Fig. 5.14.   It should also be noted that the members of the doublets in the irradiated sulfates are of equal line intensity as is required for a hyperfine doublet.

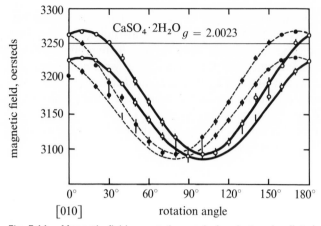

Fig. 5.11   Magnetic field vs. rotation angle for electron irradiated $CaSO_4 \cdot 2H_2O$ at 77°K. The spin-Hamiltonian parameters are $g_{\parallel} = 2.1108$, $g_{\perp} = 2.0028$, $A_z = 3.3$ Oe, $A_x = -43$ Oe, $A_y = -32.5$ Oe.

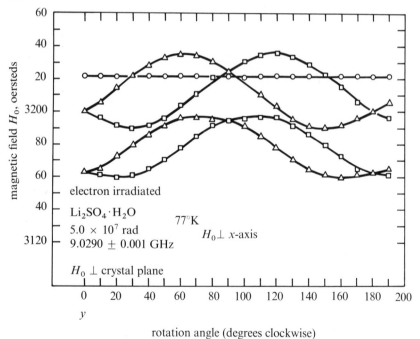

Fig. 5.12   Magnetic field vs. rotation angle for electron irradiated $Li_2SO_4 \cdot H_2O$ at 77°K for rotation about x-axis. The spin-Hamiltonian parameters are $g_1 = 2.0072$, $g_2 = 2.0057$, $g_3 = 2.0667$; $A_x = -24$ Oe, $A_y = -46$ Oe, $A_z = 4.0$ Oe (good to approx. 1 Oe). (Note: Z-axis ≡ crystal b-axis, y- axis ≡ crystal c-axis; then axes x, y, z form a right-handed ortho-system.)

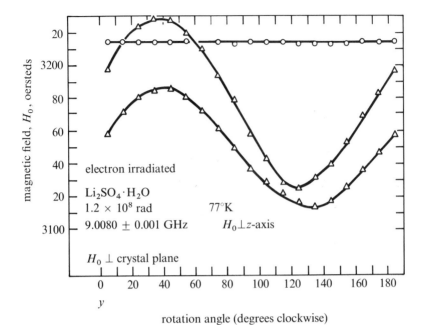

Fig. 5.13   Magnetic field vs. rotation angle for electron irradiated $Li_2SO_4 \cdot H_2O$ at 77°K for rotation about z-axis ($\equiv$ crystal b-axis). The spin-Hamiltonian parameters are the same as those in Fig. 5.12.

In the irradiated sulfates, in addition to the OH lines and the weak isotropic line, first seen by Wigen and Cowen, very weak hydrogen atom lines were also observed even at 77°K. The observed splittings are 513 Oe for the irradiated calcium sulfate case and 506.5 Oe for the irradiated lithium sulfate case. It should be noted that at X-band frequencies these lines do not appear to be centered quite at the free electron g-value. This is because 3000 Oe is not sufficient to allow one to assume he is working in the 'strong field' region and the complete Breit–Rabi expression must be used to accurately predict line positions.

Table 5.2

Sample	Isotropic hyperfine splitting (Oe)
1. OH in vapor (Radford, 1962)	-26.7
2. $CaSO_4 \cdot 2H_2O$ (Gunter and Jeffries, 1964)	-24.1
3. $Li_2SO_4 \cdot H_2O$ (Gunter, 1965, 1966, 1967)	-22.0
4. $Li_2SO_4 \cdot D_2O$ (Gunter, 1965, 1966, 1967)	-3.39 or $-22.0/6.5$
5. Ice (Gunter, 1965, 1966, 1967)	-26.3
6. Ice (Brivati, 1965)	-28.7

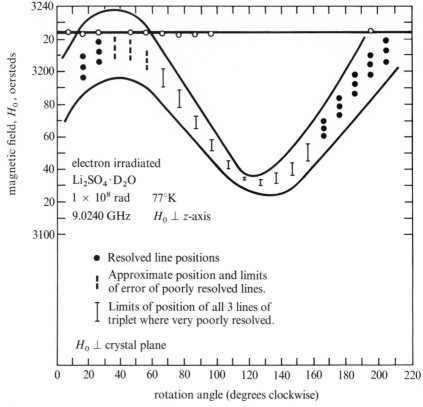

Fig. 5.14   Magnetic field vs. rotation angle for electron irradiated $Li_2SO_4 \cdot D_2O$ at 77°K for rotation about z-axis ($\equiv$ crystal b-axis). The solid lines represent the corresponding positions of the OH doublet in irradiated $Li_2SO_4 \cdot H_2O$. Spin-Hamiltonian parameters are $g_1 = 2.0072$, $g_2 = 2.0057$, $g_3 = 2.0667$, $A_x = -3.7$ Oe, $A_y = -7.1$ Oe, $A_z = 0.61$ Oe.

The system of the irradiated sulfates is hence a very interesting one which allows one to observe three very important products of H_2O disintegration, a trapped electron, OH radical, and the hydrogen atom, through spectra which are completely resolved with respect to line overlap, in the same experimental sample.   It would seem to be a very worthwhile experiment to measure the radiation yields of these species, at say 4.2°K, in these crystals.   These experiments are now in progress.

Since information on the positions in the irradiated sulfate crystals at which the OH radicals are trapped comes from the ESR data itself, and since the effective crystal fields at these locations remain unknown except as partly determined by the ESR spectra, a theoretical estimate of the spectroscopic splitting tensor is not feasible in the irradiated sulfate case.

Because one would expect OH to be held by four hydrogen bonds in the irradiated ice case, the quenching of the orbital angular momentum would be expected to be more complete in the ice case than for OH in the irradiated crystals.   The spin-Hamiltonian parameters

$$g_\parallel = 2.0615 \pm 0.01 \qquad A_z = 7 \pm 5 \text{ Oe}$$
$$g_\perp = 2.0095 \pm 0.005 \qquad A_x = A_y = -43 \pm 5 \text{ Oe}$$

were determined from the ice spectral data.   The algebraic sign, which was not determined by the experiment was taken to agree with the corresponding sign found by Radford.   These spin-Hamiltonian parameters which are in good agreement with those predicted for OH in ice are shown on the single crystal ice spectral data given in Fig. 5.9 as a series of lines representing the hyperfine doublets due to various inequivalent sites in this crystal.   The agreement of the experimental spin-Hamiltonian parameters with the predicted values is considered good in view of the 10–20 Oe maximum derivative line width of the spectral lines.

It should be noted that $g_\parallel$ has been modified since the publication of the spin-Hamiltonian parameters of Gunter (1965) in order to obtain a better fit to the data.   Brivati, *et al.* (1965) and Dibdin (1966) have recently published results from studies of irradiated single crystal ice giving spin-Hamiltonian parameters in agreement with those given above.

The spin-Hamiltonian parameters given by Brivati, *et al.*, are

$$g_\parallel = 2.05 \pm 0.01 \qquad A_z = 0 \pm 7 \text{ Oe}$$
$$g_\perp = 2.008 \pm 0.001 \qquad A_x = A_y = 43 \pm 2 \text{ Oe.}$$

Since these parameters agree with those given above to within about the precision of measurement, they will not be discussed separately below.

This effective spin-Hamiltonian, which differs from that given by McMillan, *et al.*, is thought to be correct, because (1) it assumes OH to be bound along the original hydrogen bond directions, (2) it is in good agreement with the predicted effective spin-Hamiltonian, (3) it fits the single crystal spectra data as well as could be expected for spectra of such complexity.

Irradiated H_2O has been studied in forms other than the polycrystalline ice, single crystal ice, and water of hydration forms mentioned above. Marx, *et al.* (1963) have studied electron irradiated, amorphous ice condensed from water vapor at 77°K and the condensate of irradiated water vapor also condensed at 77°K.   In the case of amorphous ice the observed spectrum is described as a slightly asymmetrical quartet with the central lines well resolved and separated by 27 Oe and the lateral (outside) lines split by 58 Oe from each other and not completely resolved from the central two.

This spectrum is quite different from that seen in polycrystalline ice. The spectrum is attributed to OH radical subject to crystal fields (in this case hydrogen bonding) quite different from that in polycrystalline ice.

In condensed, irradiated H_2O vapor still another type of spectrum was observed. In the H_2O case a broad line slightly split so as to indicate a possible hyperfine doublet was observed. The high field part of this spectrum slowly disappears with increasing temperature leaving a singlet which disappears above $150°K$. The corresponding D_2O vapor experiment shows a well-resolved doublet. Again on increasing the temperature the high field component of the spectrum disappears. In both cases the condensate was blue in color, with the blue color disappearing above $150°K$ with the low field line.

OH was observed by optical spectroscopy in the gas phase, but is not thought to be present in the condensate.

The explanation given by Marx, et al. for their spectral observations is as follows. The less stable part of the spectrum (high field) is attributed to a solvated electron formed by interaction of secondary electrons with 'quasi-liquid', mobile water molecules at the surface of the condensate. The electron 'solvated' at the condensate surface is then trapped into the vitreous matrix.

The low field line is ascribed to O_2H which is thought to be formed by a reaction of OH with H_2O_2 according to the equation

$$OH + H_2O_2 \rightarrow HO_2 + H_2O. \tag{5.37}$$

H_2O_2 is thought to be formed by recombination of OH radicals. These reactions are viewed as taking place like the solvation of the above discussed electrons in the 'quasi-liquid', mobile layer at the surface of the condensate. This identification and reaction scheme for the low field line is postulated because of the similarity of the spectral results to spectra ascribed to HO_2 in experiments on H_2O_2 to be discussed later, and because the disappearance temperature for the radical species is similar to that of HO_2 in the irradiated H_2O_2 experiments.

It was noted by Marx, et al. that the total number of radicals remained constant through the range of temperature at which the high field line disappears. This is taken as evidence that the reaction

$$e^- + H_2O_2 \rightarrow OH^- + OH \tag{5.38}$$

takes place at this transition temperature and that the OH radical thus produced goes on to form O_2H as described before.

It would seem that work on amorphous ice and an irradiated water vapor condensate at lower temperature, say $4.2°K$, might allow one to verify some of the hypotheses of Marx, et al. This would be true if the lower temperature allowed one to inhibit at least to a measurable extent the reactions for destruction of OH radical, and if an identifiable spectrum for OH could be found as a result.

5.6   THE IRRADIATED H_2O_2–H_2O SYSTEM

Smith and Wyard (1960, 1961a, 1961b, 1961c) have studied another irradiated hydrogen–oxygen system, H_2O_2 in H_2O, extensively.

In order to obtain as much information as possible from the polycrystalline spectrum, Searl, *et al.* (1959, 1960, 1961) determined analytically and with the aid of a computer the expected shape of an ESR line for a polycrystalline substance which shows a singlet with a large g-value anisotropy when in single crystal form.   Their results are shown graphically in Fig. 5.15.

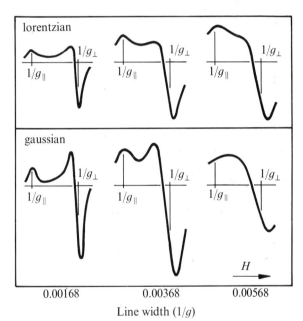

Fig. 5.15   First derivative of absorption in polycrystalline substances. The curves are shown for sweeping with field. For all the curves $g_{\parallel}$ = 2.039 and $g_{\perp}$ = 2.006. The line widths are in units of $1/g$.

The assumptions made in the calculations were the following:

(*a*) The line shape is either Gaussian or Lorentzian.
(*b*) The line width is rotation invariant.
(*c*) $g^2 = g_{\parallel}^2 \cos^2 \theta + g_{\perp}^2 \sin^2 \theta$.

By applying calculations of ESR polycrystalline line shape based on the above assumptions to ESR spectra of H_2O_2 irradiated by u.v. and by ionizing radiation of varying LET (see section 3.1, p. 63) using both glassy and polycrystalline samples, the principal values of the g and hyperfine tensors were obtained.   An example of a spectrum for which some of these calculations were made and the corresponding spectral data is given in Figs. 5.16 and 5.17.

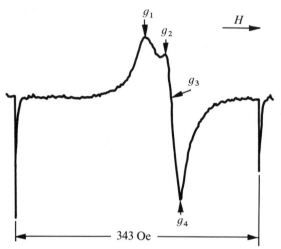

Fig. 5.16   Primary radical produced by u.v. in 87% hydrogen peroxide at 90°K.

The characteristics of the ESR spectra obtained from irradiated H_2O_2 depend on several experimental variables such as type of radiation used, structure and technique of production of the sample, and temperature history of the sample after irradiation.   The interpretation of the experimental spectra is also dependent to some extent on the above variables.

In the case of ultraviolet irradiation of H_2O_2 glasses, with a wavelength of around 3100 Å, a broad resonance spectrum is seen at liquid oxygen temperature (see Fig. 5.16).   After annealing at around 140°K for several minutes the observed spectrum is greatly narrowed, and effective spin-Hamiltonian parameters can be determined.   In addition, in very concentrated H_2O_2 in H_2O polycrystalline samples, ultraviolet light produces a quite different spectrum which decays in about one hour at 77°K (Wyard and Smith, 1963).

With low LET ionizing radiation on the other hand, the initial width of the spectrum seen at liquid nitrogen or liquid oxygen temperature is not so broad as that seen after a comparable low dose of ultraviolet irradiation.

After annealing at around 140°K spectral changes occur in the glassy samples similar to those observed in the u.v. irradiated glassy samples.   The spectrum observed after these annealing-induced changes is like that observed after annealing the u.v. irradiated samples (see Fig. 5.17).

If glassy samples irradiated by either u.v. or ionizing irradiation are carefully annealed further at around 150°K, still another spectrum appears which disappears completely at around 210°K (Wyard and Smith, 1963).

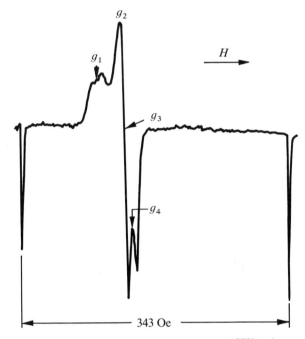

Fig. 5.17   Secondary radical produced by u.v. in 87% hydrogen peroxide at 90°K warmed up to 138°K and then measured at 90°K.   Spin-Hamiltonian   parameters   are g_1 = 2.0023, g_2 = 2.0065, g_3 = 2.0350, $A_\perp$ = 12.5 Oe, $A_\parallel$ = 14.2 Oe.

Experiments have been carried out at 4.2°K on electron and u.v. irradiated samples.   The experimental results were essentially the same as those found at 77°K.   With tritium B irradiated polycrystalline samples, weak hydrogen atom lines were seen at 4.2°K.

Polycrystalline samples have also been studied.   In these, the exact spectral shape depends on the technique used for forming the sample which determines the amount of preferred orientation (Smith and Wyard, 1961c).

An interpretation of the above results differs somewhat from the case of u.v. irradiation to that of ionizing radiation.   In the u.v. case, it is thought that the H_2O_2 molecule is broken up initially into two OH radicals which each react with one of the surrounding H_2O_2 molecules through the reaction

$$OH + H_2O_2 \rightarrow HO_2 + H_2O. \tag{5.39}$$

The spectrum of the short-lived species seen in H_2O_2 just after u.v. irradiation at 77°K could be due to OH.

For ionizing radiation, on the other hand, it is thought that H_2O_2 may not break up immediately into two OH radicals. The initial species are probably e^-, H_2O^+, and $H_2O_2{}^+$. Secondary reactions occurring soon after the primary ones could then produce both OH and O_2H, with the OH reacting quickly with H_2O_2 to produce more HO_2 as in reaction (5.39) above. Any hydrogen atom produced by a reaction of e^- with an H_2O would be expected, due to the very high rate constant (Schwarz, 1962) of the reaction

$$H + H_2O_2 \rightarrow H_2O + OH \tag{5.40}$$

to produce OH which would then react by (5.39) above to give HO_2.

The spectrum common to all the irradiated H_2O_2 glasses after annealing at 140°K is attributed to HO_2. The reasons for this are as follows: (a) This spectrum is produced by u.v. which is known to break up H_2O_2 into two OH radicals. Hence the spectrum is either OH or something derived from it. (b) In liquid solutions OH has been shown to react with H_2O_2 to give HO_2 by reaction (5.39) above. (c) Measurements on polycrystalline H_2O_2–H_2O samples which have the crystal axis frozen in a preferred direction have shown that the axis of symmetry of the radical observed is parallel to the O—O orientation in the H_2O_2 molecule (Smith and Wyard, 1961c).

Optical spectroscopy on the irradiated H_2O_2 system, which should have shown OH absorption bands if OH was indeed present at the concentration of the radicals observed in irradiated H_2O_2, failed to show such bands (Smith and Wyard, 1961d). This may be taken as additional support for the identification of the radical species seen by ESR spectroscopy in irradiated H_2O_2 not as OH, but as the species derived from OH, HO_2.

The spectrum seen in the H_2O_2 glasses after annealing at 150°K is thought to be HO_3 produced by the reaction

$$OH + O_2 \rightarrow HO_3. \tag{5.41}$$

The irradiated H_2O_2 system has some rather interesting features not usually found in free radical systems. In particular, in the case of u.v. irradiated samples where H_2O_2 is thought to break up directly into pairs of OH radicals, a pair of HO_2 radicals can be produced with a separation of less than 4 Å. The radiation yield for H_2O_2 is quite high with respect to the total number of radicals produced, giving a G (number of radicals per

100 eV of absorbed radiation energy) of 10 at $77°K$, for example, as against a G of 0.6 for the OH spectrum of ice under comparable conditions. The observed local concentrations are greater than one would expect from random distribution of the radicals.

This shows up experimentally in two ways. First, as would be expected from spin–spin interaction, a high local concentration shows up as a broad line spectrum. Hence measurement of the line width allows one to estimate local free radical concentration (Wyard, 1965).

Second, a large spin–spin interaction can produce another effect related to the 'pair states' observed in dilute ferromagnetic materials. In order to see this connection, let us consider a perturbation interaction due to spin–spin interaction of the form

$$H_{\text{pert}} = -\sum_{i,\,j\text{ near}} \frac{J_{ij}}{2} (S_i \cdot S_j) \tag{5.42}$$

without concerning ourselves about whether this comes from exchange terms as in the ferromagnetic case or from dipole–dipole interaction. (The arguments given below will follow to first order perturbation theory if the complete form of the dipole–dipole interaction is used as well as from an interaction of the above type.) S_i and S_j are spin quantum numbers for the ith and jth spins.

If n' is used as the number of spins near the ith spin, and if one makes the simplifying assumption that each of these has an interaction coefficient $J_{ij} = J$, one can rewrite equation (5.42) above as

$$H_{\text{pert}} = -\frac{n'}{2} J(S \cdot S') \tag{5.43}$$

for each spin, where S is the spin quantum number for the spin of interest and S' is that of one of its neighboring spins. Now, $(S \cdot S')$ can be written as

$$\left(\frac{S_+ S'_-}{2} + \frac{S_- S'_+}{2} + S_z S'_z \right) \tag{5.44}$$

where S'_+ and S'_- are the usual raising and lowering operators

$$S_+ = S_x + iS_y$$
and
$$S_- = S_x - iS_y$$

and S_z is the z component of the spin angular momentum operator.

The spin wave functions, α for $S_z = \frac{1}{2}$, and β for $S_z = -\frac{1}{2}$ can be used to describe the state of the two neighboring spins. If in a pair of spin wave functions, the first symbol of the pair describes the state of spin S

discussed above, and the second describes the state of spin S', four orthogonal wave functions can be chosen which describe the possible states of the coupled spin systems in terms of the α's and β's. These are $\alpha\alpha$, $(\alpha\beta + \beta\alpha)/\sqrt{2}$, $\beta\beta$, and $(\alpha\beta - \beta\alpha)/\sqrt{2}$. The first three describe a two-radical system whose three states look like a system with spin equal to one; the last term describes a system with spin equal to zero. This means that the spin wave functions which describe a two-radical state are made up of single radical spin wave functions in such a way that it shows characteristics of either $S = 1$ or $S = 0$ wave functions. Second order transitions between the $M_s = 1$ and $M_s = -1$ levels are allowed. Hence it may be possible to detect $|\Delta M_s| = 2$ transitions between the levels of the coupled system.

In the above, M_s represents the quantum number for the z component of spin angular momentum.

Such a $\Delta M_s = 2$ transition is observed in the irradiated H_2O_2 system (Wyard, 1962) and since the ratio of its transition probability to that of the usual $\Delta M = 1$ transition depends on the strength of the spin–spin interaction, one can use this ratio as a measurement of local concentration of the radicals.

Both the line width and the $\Delta M = 2$ transition techniques have been used by Wyard (1964) with irradiated H_2O_2 giving consistent results. Local concentrations as high as 0.1 M have been found after irradiation by carbon ions having an average LET of 310 keV/μ.

Table 5.3

Radical species	Type of matrix	Temp. at ESR det. ($^\circ$K)	Yield $\left(\dfrac{\text{radicals}}{100 \text{ eV}}\right)$	Type of radiation	Observer
H	Ice	4.2	0.9	Co^{60} γ-rays	Siegel, et al. (19
H	Frozen 7 molar H_2SO_4	77	2.7	220 kV X-rays	Henriksen (196
H	Frozen 9 molar NaOH	77	0.1	220 kV X-rays	Henriksen (196
OH	Ice	4.2	0.8	Co^{60} γ-rays	Siegel, et al. (19
OH	Ice	77	0.6	Co^{60} γ-rays	Siegel, et al. (19
OH	Ice	77	0.6	6 MeV electrons	Gunter (1965, 1 1967)
e^-	Frozen 16 molar NaOH	77	2.6	220 kV X-rays	Henriksen (196
O_2H	H_2O_2—H_2O	77	10.0	6 MeV electrons	Wyard and Smi (1963)

5.7   RADIATION YIELDS MEASURED BY ESR TECHNIQUES

Table 5.3 shows a condensation of results from yield measurements made by ESR techniques on some of the radical species discussed above.

5.8   CONCLUSION

Studies on irradiated frozen solutions such as those discussed above have yielded convincing identifications of the ESR spectra produced by the hydrogen atom, the OH radical, the solvated electron, and HO_2 radical and possible identifications of other species such as O^- radical ion and HO_3.   Effective spin-Hamiltonian parameters have been determined for the hydrogen atom, OH radical hydrogen bonded into several matrices, the solvated electron in alkaline solutions, and HO_2 in hydrogen peroxide glasses.   With further work on positive identification of those species whose identification is now based somewhat on guess work, and with further measurements of radical yields such as those of the OH radical, hydrogen atom, and trapped electron in irradiated crystal hydrates at $4.2°K$, a greater contribution can be made by the ESR spectral studies to the understanding of the transfer of initial radiation energy through free radical species to the final damage sites in biological materials.

ACKNOWLEDGEMENTS

The author wishes to acknowledge the help of Prof. C. D. Jeffries, Prof. C. A. Tobias, Dr. T. Henriksen, and Prof. S. J. Wyard with the study of the OH radical discussed in this paper.   He also wishes to thank Dr. T. Henriksen, Prof. S. J. Wyard, and Dr. K. H. Langley for reading and criticizing the manuscript.

REFERENCES

Allen, A. O., 1961, *The Radiation Chemistry of Water and Aqueous Solutions* (Princeton: D. Van Nostrand Co., Inc.), pp. 24–30.
Allen, A. O., and Rothschild, W. G., 1957, *Radiat. Res.*, **7**, 591.
Barnes, W. H., 1929, *Proc. R. Soc.* A, **125**, 670.
Brivati, J. A., Symons, M. C. R., Tinling, D. J. A., Wardale, H. W., and Williams, D. D., 1965, *Chem. Communs*, **1**, 402.
Collie, C. H., Hasted, J. B., and Ritson, D. M., 1948a, *Proc. phys. Soc.*, **60**, 71; 1948b, ibid., **60**, 145.
Coulson, C. A., and Danielson, U., 1954, *Ark. Fys.*, **8**, 239.
Dainton, F. S., 1959, *Radiat. Res. Suppl.*, **1**, 1.

Dale, W. M., Gray, L. H., and Meredith, W. J., 1949, *Phil. Trans. R. Soc.* A., **242**, 33.

Dibdin, G. H., 1966, *Nature*, Lond., **209**, 394.

Dousmanis, G. C., Sanders, T. M., and Townes, C. H., 1955, *Phys. Rev.*, **100**, 1735.

Ersov, B. G., Pikaef, A. K., and Glazumov, P. J., 1963, *Dokl. Akad. Nauk. SSSR*, **149**, 363.

Evans, R. D., 1955, *The Atomic Nucleus* (New York: McGraw-Hill Book Co.), Ch. 18.

Feher, G., 1957, *Bell Syst. tech. J.*, **36**, 449.

Fricke, H., and Brownscombe, E. R., 1933, *Phys. Rev.*, **44**, 240.

Frosch, R. A., and Foley, H. M., 1952, *Phys. Rev.*, **88**, 1347.

Gunter, T. E., 1965, *UCRL 16613*, 82; 1966, University of California, Berkeley: Thesis; 1967, *J. chem. Phys.*, **46**, 3818.

Gunter, T. E., and Jeffries, C. D., 1964, *UCRL 11387, Suppl.* 8.

Henriksen, T., 1964, *Radiat. Res.*, **23**, 63.

Hochanadel, C. J., and Lind, S. C., 1956, *A. Rev. phys. Chem.*, **7**, 83.

Judd, B. R., 1963, *Operator Techniques in Atomic Spectroscopy* (New York: McGraw-Hill Book Co.).

Judeikis, H. S., Flournoy, J. M., and Siegel, S., 1962, *J. chem. Phys.*, **37**, 2272.

Lea, D. E., 1946, *Actions of Radiations on Living Cells* (Cambridge: University Press).

Lennard-Jones, J., and Pople, J. A., 1951, *Proc. R. Soc.* A, **205**, 155.

Lindgren, I., 1963, *Proceedings of the Conference on Perturbed Angular Correlations* (Uppsala).

Livingston, R., Zeldes, H., and Taylor, E. H., 1954, *Phys. Rev.*, **94**, 725; 1956, *Discuss. Faraday Soc.*, **19**, 166.

Lonsdale, K., 1958, *Proc. R. Soc.* A, **247**, 424.

Marx, R., Leach, S., and Horani, M., 1963, *Sixth International Symposium on Free Radicals* (Cambridge), Section AF.

Matheson, M. S., and Smaller, B., 1955, *J. chem. Phys.*, **23**, 521.

McMillan, J. A., Matheson, M. S., and Smaller, B., 1960, *J. chem. Phys.*, **33**, 609.

Moorthy, P. N., and Weiss, J. J., 1964, *Phil. Mag.*, **10**, 659.

Moreno, T., 1958, *Microwave Transmission and Design Data* (New York: Dover Pub. Inc.), p. 200.

Nafe, J. E., and Nelson, E. B., 1948, *Phys. Rev.*, **73**, 718.

Pauling, L., 1939, *The Nature of the Chemical Bond* (Ithaca: Cornell University Press).

Peterson, S. W., and Levy, H. A., 1957, *Acta Cryst.*, **10**, 70.

Piette, L. H., Rempel, R. C., Weaver, H. E., and Flournoy, J. M., 1959, *J. chem. Phys.*, **30**, 1623.

Pimentel, P. G., and McClellan, A. L., 1960, *The Hydrogen Bond* (San Francisco: W. H. Freeman and Co.), pp. 213, 214.

Platzman, R. L., 1953, *Natn. Acad. Sci. Res. Coun. Publs*, **305**, 34.

Radford, H. E., 1961, *Phys. Rev.*, **122**, 114; 1962, ibid., **126**, 1035.

Rexroad, H. N., and Gordy, W., 1962, *Phys. Rev.*, **125**, 242.

Samuel, A. H., and Magee, J. L., 1953, *J. chem. Phys.*, **21**, 1080.

Schneider, W. G., 1955, *J. chem. Phys.*, **23**, 26.

Schwarz, H. A., 1962, *J. phys. Chem., Ithaca*, **66**, 255.

Searl, J. W., Smith, R. C., and Wyard, S. J., 1959, *Proc. phys. Soc.*, **74**, 491; 1960, *Bull. Ampère 9ᵉ année fasc. spécial*, p. 236; 1961, *Proc. phys. Soc.*, **78**, 1174.

Siegel, S., 1963, *J. chem. Phys.*, **39**, 390.

Siegel, S., Baum, L. K., Skolnik, S., and Flournoy, J. M., 1960, *J. chem. Phys.*, **32**, 1249.

Siegel, S., Flournoy, J. M., and Baum, L. H., 1961, *J. chem. Phys.*, **34**, 1782.

Smaller, B., Matheson, M. S., and Yasaitis, E. L., 1954, *Phys. Rev.*, **94**, 202.

Smith, R. C., and Wyard, S. J., 1960, *Bull. Ampère 9ᵉ année fasc. spécial*, p. 224; 1961a, *Nature*, Lond., **189**, 211; 1961b, ibid., **191**, 897; 1961c, *J. chem. Phys.*, **35**, 2254; 1961d, *Fifth International Symposium on Free Radicals* (Uppsala), Paper 66.

Stevens, K. W. H., 1952, *Proc. phys. Soc.* A, **65**, 209.

Stoodley, L. G., 1963, *J. Electron. Control*, **14**, 531.

Van Vleck, J. H., 1929, *Phys. Rev.*, **33**, 467.

Weiss, J., 1944, *Nature*, Lond., **153**, 749.

Wigen, P. E., and Cowen, J. A., 1960, *J. Phys. Chem. Solids*, **17**, 26.

Wyard, S. J., 1962, *Bull. Ampère 11ᵉ année fasc. spécial*, p. 388; 1964, *UCRL 11387 Suppl.*, 1; 1965, *Proc. phys. Soc.*, **86**, 587.

Wyard, S. J., and Smith, R. C., 1963, *Sixth International Symposium on Free Radicals* (Cambridge), Paper AD1.

CHAPTER SIX

THE MECHANISMS FOR RADIATION DAMAGE AND REPAIR IN SOLID BIOLOGICAL SYSTEMS AS REVEALED BY ESR SPECTROSCOPY

Thormod Henriksen

Norsk Hydro's Institute for Cancer Research, Montebello, Norway

6.1   INTRODUCTION

When chemical and biological systems are exposed to ionizing radiation, a sequence of events is started.   The early processes in the physico-chemical stage have so far mostly escaped our attention due to lack of experimental methods.   We have therefore relatively little information about the processes leading to the radiation inactivation of enzymes, the mechanisms underlying the action of the radioprotective compounds, and the processes for energy migration within and between macromolecules.   In the subsequent discussion it will be pointed out how ESR spectroscopy can be used to study certain radical reactions which may be of importance for our understanding of the mechanisms by which radiation energy is absorbed and transformed in biological systems in the solid state.

Numerous experiments have been carried out which clearly demonstrate that the observed radiation effect in a solid system can be influenced by the presence of another substance.†   Thus, the observed effect can be either enhanced or reduced, i.e., we have either a sensitization or a protection.   The fact that the observed radiation effect can be modified by irradiating the studied substance as part of a molecular mixture is probably due to an energy migration from one part of the irradiated system to the other.

One ESR experiment which clearly demonstrated that radiation energy can migrate in a solid biological system was presented several years ago by Gordy and his group at Duke University (Gordy, et al., 1955; Gordy and Shields, 1958).   In an extensive study of amino acids and proteins they found that only irradiated substances exhibited ESR patterns.   The protein spectra consisted mainly of two types of resonances in spite of the fact that the constituent amino acids exhibited a large variety of different resonance patterns.   The conclusion of this experiment was that radiation energy, which initially is absorbed evenly throughout the protein molecule, can be subsequently transferred in some way or other to two different sites in the molecule.

Transfer of radiation energy from one part of a macromolecule to another seems also to be of great importance for the inactivation of enzymes.   Thus, the different mechanisms proposed for radiation inactivation include some type of energy transfer to the active site of the enzyme molecule (see for example Augenstein, 1963; Augenstein, et al., 1964; Braams, 1963).

The purpose of the present paper is to demonstrate how ESR spectroscopy makes it possible to follow some of the early processes in the physico-chemical stage in irradiated solid, biological systems.   The different mechanisms proposed for the radiation inactivation of solid enzymes as well

† See Norman and Ginoza, 1958; Alexander and Toms, 1958; Braams, et al., 1958; Wilson, 1959; Braams, 1960; Gordy and Miyagawa, 1960; Henriksen and Pihl, 1961; Brustad, 1961; Libby, et al., 1961; Ormerod and Alexander, 1962, 1963; Henriksen, et al., 1963b; Butler and Robins, 1962; Pihl and Sanner, 1963, 1964.

as for the action of radioprotective substances in the solid state will be discussed.

6.2 THE ELECTRON STRUCTURE OF THE PROTEIN MOLECULE

6.2.1 GENERAL REMARKS

Almost all the ESR experiments, dealing with transport of radiation energy, have been carried out with reference to proteins and/or mixtures of proteins and radioprotective substances.   In order to discuss these experiments and the mechanisms for energy migration, it is worthwhile to review briefly what is known about protein structure and especially the electron structure of proteins.   (For a more extensive discussion of protein structure see, for example, *Brookhaven Symposia in Biology*, 1960; Low and Edsall, 1956; Pauling, *et al.*, 1951; Pullman and Pullman, 1963).

In order to build up a protein molecule we start out with about twenty different amino acids.   These building stones are held together by the carboxyl group in one amino acid being bonded to the amino group in another;

$$\left[NH_2 - \underset{\underset{H}{|}}{\overset{\overset{R_i}{|}}{C}} - COOH \right]_n \xrightarrow{-H_2O} NH_2 - \underset{\underset{H}{|}}{\overset{\overset{R_1}{|}}{C}} - CO - NH - \underset{\underset{H}{|}}{\overset{\overset{R_2}{|}}{C}} - CO -$$

The individual amino acids can be distinguished from each other by the side group, R_i.   This group can vary from a simple hydrogen atom as in glycine to relatively complicated groups as, for example, in tryptophan.   The proteins consist of long chains of amino acids.   The sequence and number of amino acids in these peptide chains is usually called the primary structure of the proteins.   After the pioneering work of Sanger and his group (Sanger, 1956; Sanger and Thompson, 1953a, 1953b; Sanger and Tuppy, 1951a, 1951b) the sequence of amino acids have now been determined completely for a few proteins, and large fractions of the polypeptide-chains for other proteins are also known (Hirs, *et al.*, 1960; Sŏyrm, 1962).   As our knowledge about the primary structure increases it should become possible to study the principles behind the construction of the proteins.   One may ask, for instance, whether there are certain amino acid sequences that occur frequently in the proteins whereas others are forbidden (Sŏyrm, 1962).

6.2.2 THE PEPTIDE BOND

When the sequence and number of amino acids are known we have a flat, two-dimensional protein molecule.   In order to obtain a three-dimensional molecule we must look into the folding of the peptide chains and their superfolding in three-dimensional space.   The electron distribution and the structure of the peptide bond represent a key to the understanding of the protein structure.   Most of our knowledge about the structure of the peptide bond has been derived from X-ray diffraction experiments (see Corey and Pauling, 1953; Pauling and Corey, 1951a, 1951b; Pauling, *et al.*, 1951; Pullman and Pullman, 1963).

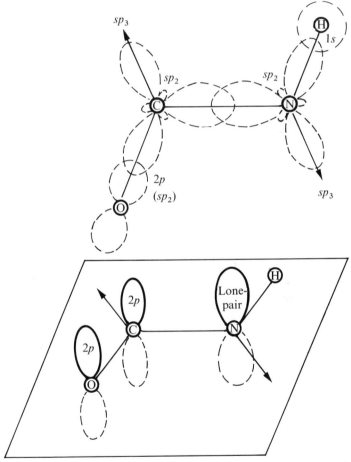

Fig. 6.1   The electron structure of the peptide bond. The upper drawing is entirely in the plane of the paper. The dashed curves represent the carbon and nitrogen sp_2 hybrid orbitals, the hydrogen $1s$ orbital, and the oxygen $2p_x$ orbital. The sp_3 orbitals which belong to the adjacent carbon atoms are not shown. In the lower drawing the peptide group atoms are placed in a plane (the fully drawn parallelogram). The Π-orbitals represented by the carbon and nitrogen $2p_y$ orbitals as well as the nitrogen lone pair are perpendicular to this plane.

In Fig. 6.1 an attempt is made to describe the electron distribution of the peptide bond. Both the carbon and the nitrogen atom in the peptide group are bonded to asymmetrical carbon atoms in two different amino acid residues by σ-bonds. Three of the four valence electrons of carbon form sp_2 hybrid orbitals which give rise to three planar σ-bonds. The last electron is in a $2p$ orbital perpendicular to the plane of the σ-bonds (Fig. 6.1, lower part). Oxygen has six valence electrons. One is involved in a σ-bond with carbon, whereas another one, in a $2p_y$ orbital perpendicular to the σ-bond, takes part in a π-bond with carbon. The last four electrons form two lone pairs. The possibility should be considered that we also have sp_2 hybridization for oxygen. This will, however, not influence the bonding to the carbon atom, but will change the lone pair orbitals from $2s$ and $2p$ to sp_2 hybrid orbitals.

Different possibilities exist for the nitrogen atom in the peptide bond. For example, three of the electrons may be in $2p$ orbitals and thus form bonds in all three dimensions, whereas the last two form a $2s$ lone pair. However, the actual distribution seems to be that three electrons are in sp_2 hybrid orbitals which give three planar σ-bonds. The last two form a lone pair in an orbital with the same orientation as the two other π-electrons in the peptide group (Fig. 6.1, lower part). From this electron distribution the following important conclusions can be drawn:

(a) The peptide group is planar.
(b) The peptide group forms a small system with four delocalized π-electrons.
(c) The C—N bond has a considerable double bond character which also can be deduced from the bond length of 1.32 Å.
(d) The peptide group can be in either a *cis* or a *trans* form. The *trans* form is the most stable and is usually found in the proteins.

The electron distribution of the peptide group and the conclusions derived from it will be used in the subsequent discussion. It should be noticed that historically these conclusions were first derived from experimental work (Corey and Pauling, 1953; Pauling and Corey, 1951a, 1951b).

6.2.3   THE THREE-DIMENSIONAL PROTEIN MOLECULE

When the peptide chain is fully stretched we have a repetition length of 7.27 Å (Fig. 6.2). In spite of the fact that the peptide group forms a plane there is a possibility for rotation at the asymmetrical carbon atom. This will lead to a folding of the peptide chain. This folding results in what is usually called the secondary structure of the protein molecule. Pauling and Corey (Pauling and Corey, 1951a, 1951b; Corey and Pauling, 1953) in their pioneering work used X-ray diffraction methods and studied the folding of synthetic polypeptides where all the side groups (R_i in Fig. 6.2) are identical.

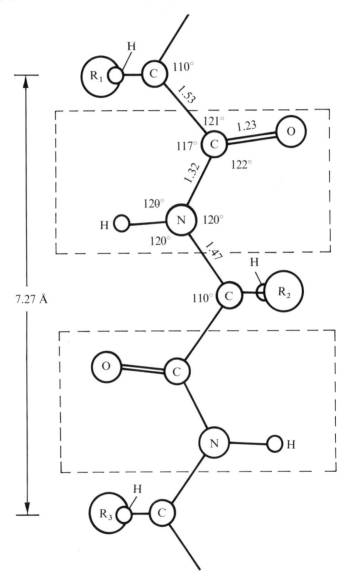

Fig. 6.2   The dimensions of the fully stretched peptide chain. The two different dashed-rectangles indicate two parallel peptide planes. In an actual peptide chain these planes are usually not parallel. (After Pauling and Corey, 1951a, b).

According to the X-ray diffraction patterns, the polypeptides were divided into an α- and a β-structure. The β-structure, which is the simplest one, consists of parallel peptide chains held together by hydrogen bonds (Fig. 6.3, bottom structure). This structure sometimes forms a sheet which can be folded. The α-structure is a helix. When we keep in mind that the peptide group is planar and furthermore that the hydrogen bond length is approximately 2.8 Å, there are only a few possibilities for constructing a helix. Pauling and Corey propose two types—one with 3.7 residues per turn and another with 5.1 residues per turn. Only the first one, which is usually called the α-helix, has been found in native proteins. There is one important difference between the α- and β-structure which may be significant in the subsequent discussion of energy transfer. In the α-structure the hydrogen bonds are parallel to the helix and hold together amino acids within the same peptide chain (Fig. 6.3), whereas in the β-structure we have interchain hydrogen bonds.

The superfolding of the peptide chains in the three-dimensional space form the tertiary structure of the proteins. The stabilization of the tertiary structure is due to —S—S— bonds, hydrogen bonds, hydrophobic bonds, electrostatic forces between positively and negatively charged groups, and van der Waals forces.

The most powerful tool in the study of the tertiary structure is the X-ray diffraction method. As early as twenty-five years ago the first X-ray diffraction patterns of proteins were presented, but due to the complexity of these patterns relatively little structural information could be derived. However, new possibilities were opened in 1953 when Perutz (Green, et al., 1954) started to build heavy atoms, such as mercury, into specific sites in the protein molecule. These modified proteins gave diffraction patterns different from those of normal proteins, and it was possible to use the method of isomorphous replacement and thus determine the relative phases of the reflections.

It is well known that the tedious but brilliant work of Kendrew and Perutz[†] has resulted in excellent pictures of the myoglobin and hemoglobin molecules. Thus, in the case of myoglobin, data now exist with a resolution down to 2 Å, and it is possible to deduce that about 75% of the 152 amino acids form eight different α-helices. In the case of hemoglobin, Muirhead and Perutz (1963) have shown that the structure changes during conversion from the reduced to the oxidized form. In the reduced form, the two β-peptide chains have moved slightly away from each other and thus increased the distance between the two heme groups by approximately 7 Å.

[†] Kendrew, et al., 1958; Kendrew, et al., 1960; Perutz, et al., 1960; Muirhead and Perutz, 1963.

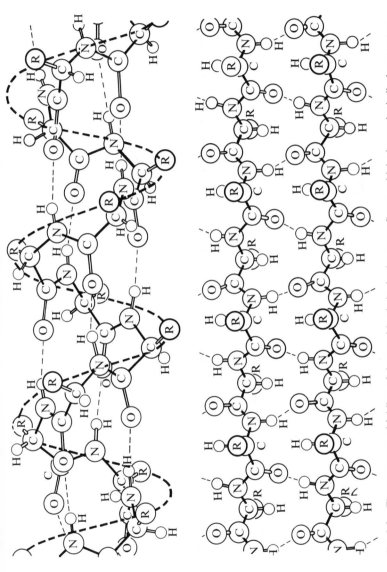

Fig. 6.3   The two types of folding of the peptide chain. In the upper figure, which shows the helical α-structure, the hydrogen bonds form intrachain bonds whereas in the β-structure (bottom figure) they hold together different peptide chains.

6.2.4   CONCLUSION

Valuable information now exists about the primary, secondary, and tertiary structure of proteins, and it should be possible in the near future to correlate structural information with radiation damage.

So far we know relatively little about the electron structure of the protein molecules.   It was mentioned above that the peptide groups form small systems with four delocalized π-electrons.   Furthermore, we have four amino acids with aromatic side chains, namely, phenylalanine, histidine, tyrosine, and tryptophan.   These groups, together with the peptide bonds, form small islands of π-electron structures in an otherwise saturated system.   A first attempt to describe the electron distribution in the saturated system was recently made by Del Re, et al. (1963).   They used a method to describe the σ-bonds which is equivalent to the Hückel method for π-electrons.   The method is semi-empirical and leads to the distribution of charge in the molecules.

The nuclear spin resonance (NMR) technique can also give some information about the electron distribution.   Thus, the position of the resonance line (proton shift) depends upon the electron distribution around the particular proton.   It appears that the charge distribution calculated by Del Re, et al. (1963) for the amino acids is in good agreement with the experimental results obtained by the NMR technique.

Of special interest with regard to the following discussion of radiation damage to the protein molecules is the possibility of a more general delocalization of electrons.   An important question is if there exists some type of connection between the islands of delocalized π-electrons which could give rise to an electronic conduction in the protein molecules.

6.3   MECHANISMS FOR ENERGY MIGRATION IN PROTEINS

6.3.1   GENERAL REMARKS

Several different hypotheses have been proposed for the migration of energy in organic molecules.   Thus, the hypothesis of conduction bands in proteins is relatively old and was first mentioned by Jordan (1938).   It was, however, Szent-György who explicitly proposed some type of energy transport in biological systems by a conduction mechanism similar to that found for crystals and semiconductors (Szent-György, 1941a, 1941b).   It is not the purpose of the present paper to review all the work on energy migration. Here we will concentrate especially on the migration of radiation energy in solid proteins exposed to ionizing radiation and discuss the different mechanisms with reference to ESR spectroscopy.[†]

[†] Blumenfeld and Kalmanson, 1958a, 1958b, 1961; Gordy and Miyagawa, 1960; Henriksen, 1963; Henriksen, et al., 1963b; Patten and Gordy, 1961.

6.3.2   ELECTRON CONDUCTION ALONG THE HYDROGEN BONDS

The first possibility for electron transport takes into consideration a possible delocalization effect of the hydrogen bond. A hydrogen bond which can be characterized by a lone pair on the one side and an electron pair with a proton on the other side seems to form a flip-flop conjugating mechanism. In the language of the valence bond theory the dipole N—H will give the hydrogen atom a positive charge which will disturb the electron distribution on the oxygen atom. Thus, the total wave function will contain structures such as:

$$\rangle N \overset{-}{-} \overset{+}{H} \text{---} \overset{-}{O} \text{---} \quad \text{and} \quad \rangle \overset{-}{N} \text{---} H \text{---} \overset{+}{O} \text{---}$$

where there is some conduction along the bond.

In Fig. 6.4 an attempt is made to visualize these conduction channels. In the helix structure the channels are parallel to the helix whereas in the β-structure they go from one peptide chain to the other.

The first theoretical discussion of the possibility of electron conduction across the hydrogen bond came from Evans and Gergely (1949). They used the method of linear combination of atomic orbitals. They used known parameters for the peptide bond, but had to introduce an unknown exchange integral for the hydrogen bond. Their calculations lead to the conclusion that energy bands exist in proteins and that the energy gap between the highest filled and the lowest empty bands was approximately 3 eV.

A number of experiments have been presented[†] which demonstrate that electric conduction in proteins follows the semiconductor formula:

$$\rho(T) = \rho_0 \exp(E/kT)$$

where $\rho(T)$ is the resistivity as a function of the temperature and E is the apparent activation energy. The observed activation energies for solid proteins seem to fall in the range 1–3 eV[‡] which is surprisingly like the theoretical value calculated by Evans and Gergely for electron conduction along the hydrogen bonds.

Two Russian scientists, Blumenfeld and Kalmanson (1958a, 1958b, 1961), studied the production of free radicals in proteins by the ESR technique. They reported that the yield of radicals in native proteins was several orders of magnitude less than that found for the constituent amino acids. Furthermore, they reported that when the proteins were heat-denatured in solution and subsequently irradiated in the dry state, the radical yield increased to become comparable to that for the individual amino acids. The

[†] Baxter, 1943; Brillouin, 1962; Cardew and Eley, 1959; Eley, 1962; Garrett, 1959; King and Medley, 1949.

[‡] Baxter 1943; Cardew and Eley, 1959; Garrett, 1959; King and Medley, 1949.

explanation they offered for these experiments is very interesting. Thus, they adopted the idea that the hydrogen bond system seems to offer some possibilities for electron conduction from one peptide group to the other (see Fig. 6.4). They assumed that the ESR spectra represented positive holes

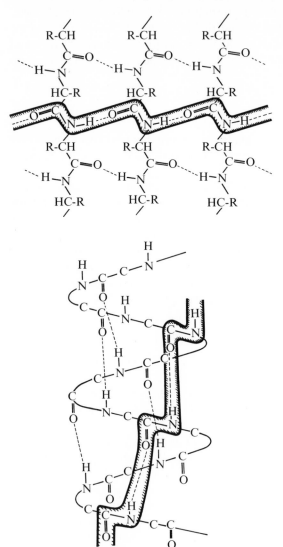

Fig. 6.4 This is an attempt to visualize the proposed conduction channels in proteins represented by electron migration along the hydrogen bonds.

produced by the ionization processes.   Consequently, in native proteins the electrons, which were knocked out by the ionization processes, were assumed to enter the system of conduction bands, migrate within the proteins to the positive holes, and then recombine, with the result that no ESR signal was observed.   By heat treatment of the proteins in solution it was assumed that this net of hydrogen bonds was broken down, with the result that the electrons could no longer migrate within the protein molecules.   However, a large number of ESR experiments carried out in other laboratories† have shown that when solid proteins are irradiated in vacuum at room temperature, the yield of radicals, measured in G-values (number of radicals per 100 eV of absorbed radiation energy), is in the range 1.0–7.0 which is of the same order of magnitude as that for the constituent amino acids.   Furthermore, experiments carried out in our Laboratory (Henriksen, et al., 1963a) show that there are no drastic changes in the radical yield when the proteins are heat-denatured in solution.   This means that Blumenfeld and Kalmanson's results are completely different from those reported by other groups, and no explanations for these differences can be offered.   It should be pointed out that the protein radicals seem to be much more sensitive to oxygen than those found in amino acids.   The possibility, therefore, exists that oxygen accidentally was present in the Russian experiments and that the oxygen effect changes drastically from native to denatured proteins.

The conclusion of the above experiments and discussion is that there is no evidence from ESR for an electron migration along the hydrogen bonds. This conclusion may be of some interest with regard to the semiconductor properties of the proteins.   The conduction experiments which resulted in activation energies of the same order of magnitude as that calculated by Evans and Gergely were taken as support for an electronic conduction along the hydrogen bonds.   However, several other studies, both experimental and theoretical, seem to be incompatible with this mechanism.   Thus it was found‡ that the activation energies depend largely upon the water content in the proteins as well as upon the addition of small amounts of dyestuffs. These observations have led to speculations about electronic or ionic conduction.

More recently, Suard, et al. (1961) in a theoretical work used the self-consistent field method to calculate the electronic states in the proteins. They found that the energy gap between the highest filled and the lowest empty bands is about 5 eV instead of 3 eV as calculated by Evans and Gergely. This large energy gap seems, therefore, to exclude the model of intrinsic, electronic conductivity across the hydrogen bonds.   We should, however,

---

† Henriksen, 1963; Henriksen, et al., 1963a; Hunt, et al., 1962; Hunt and Williams, 1964; Müller, 1963; Ormerod and Alexander, 1962.

‡ Davis, et al., 1960; Eley, 1962; Peersen and Ore, 1964; Riehl, 1957; Rosenberg, 1962.

bear in mind that these calculations have been made on idealized systems not taking into consideration impurities, absorbed water, etc.

6.3.3 INTRAMOLECULAR MIGRATION OF RADIATION ENERGY

The ESR experiments on solid proteins have shown that there is some type of energy transfer from one part of a protein molecule to another. The mechanisms proposed for this transport include both intra- and intermolecular migration of radiation energy. In order to discuss these two possibilities in more detail let us briefly summarize the more important experimental observations.

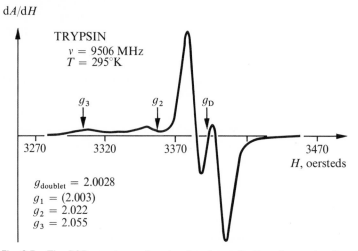

Fig. 6.5   The ESR spectrum of an irradiated protein. Trypsin was irradiated in vacuum, at room temperature, with 6.5 MeV electrons, and the first derivative of the absorption spectrum is given. A 9.5 GHz spectrometer was used. The microwave frequency was measured by a wavemeter, and the magnetic field by a proton resonance fieldmeter. The principal g-values for the sulfur radical represent maxima and zero point in the derivative curve.

It was pointed out already in Gordy's first paper (Gordy, *et al.*, 1955) that when proteins were irradiated at room temperature, in vacuum, only two main types of resonance were observed. In Fig. 6.5 a typical example of the protein spectra is presented. Trypsin was irradiated at room temperature with 6.5 MeV electrons and the first derivative of the absorption spectrum is given. The pattern is composite, consisting of a doublet which is very sensitive to microwave saturation, and a broad resonance.

The ESR center giving rise to the broad resonance has a large anisotropy. Since this resonance is similar to that found for polycrystalline sulfur compounds such as cysteine, cystine, cysteamine, and several others, Gordy and Shields (1958) ascribed the resonance to a sulfur radical where the unpaired electron is localized mainly on the sulfur atom in the cysteine residue. Organic sulfur radicals of this type have been studied in irradiated, single crystals of cystine dihydrochloride (Kurita and Gordy, 1961).   It was found that the three principal g-values are all different and have the values $g_1 = 2.003, g_2 = 2.025, g_3 = 2.053$.   Kneubühl (1960) has theoretically calculated the line shape for a polycrystalline sample containing a radical with three different g-values.   It appears that the principal values correspond to maxima and zero point in the derivative curve.   This means that it is possible to get a rough estimation of the g-values from polycrystalline spectra such as the one presented in Fig. 6.5 (Henriksen, 1962).   For trypsin two of the principal g-values have been determined whereas the third one is masked by the doublet.   Since the data in Fig. 6.5 are in excellent agreement with the results obtained for organic sulfur radicals, we conclude that the broad resonance in the protein spectra is due to sulfur radicals.

The spectroscopic g-factor for the doublet is, in the case of trypsin, 2.0028 (see Fig. 6.5).   For other proteins slightly different values have been obtained, but the variation is small.   The splitting between the two lines is approximately 17 Oe.   In Gordy's first papers (Gordy, et al., 1955; Gordy and Shields, 1958) it was suggested that the doublet was due to a radical in which the unpaired electron was localized on the oxygen atom taking part in the hydrogen bond, and that the unpaired electron could interact with the proton.   This interpretation has also been adopted by other groups (Blumenfeld and Kalmanson, 1958a, 1958b, 1961; Pulatova, et al., 1961).   However, studies on irradiated dipeptides and polypeptides† have led us to the conclusion that the doublet may be ascribed to a radical in which the unpaired electron is localized mainly in a π-orbital, on an α-carbon atom in the protein backbone;

The main evidence for this interpretation is as follows:

(a) In the polycrystalline state the spectra of irradiated dipeptides, like glycylglycine and acetylglycine, are similar to the protein doublet.   Both the g-factor and the hyperfine splitting are the same.   When single crystals of these dipeptides are irradiated the ESR results can be adequately explained

† Box, et al., 1963; Drew and Gordy, 1963; Gordy and Shields, 1960; Katayama and Gordy, 1961; Lin and McDowell, 1961; Miyagawa, et al., 1960.

by assuming the following radical:

The principal g-values are different, but the variation is small and the average value is found to be 2.0032 (Katayama and Gordy, 1961; Miyagawa, *et al.*, 1960).   The doublet splitting varies with the orientation of the crystal. This variation can be explained by assuming a hyperfine interaction consisting of a Fermi term of 18 Oe and an anisotropic dipole–dipole term similar to that calculated for a $\rangle$CH fragment by McConnell and Strathdee (1959).   Gordy and co-workers assumed a spin density on the carbon atom of approximately 70% of its full value.   With reference to proteins this probably means that the electron is delocalized and that its orbital also includes the adjacent peptide groups.

(*b*) In proteins such as silk, for instance, some type of orientation— as is possible with single crystals—may be achieved.   In an ESR work on oriented silk Gordy and Shields (1960) found that the results could be explained by assuming the backbone-type radical.   They used a Fermi term of 17 Oe and an anisotropic term similar to that calculated by McConnell and Strathdee.   It was then possible to calculate the shape of the silk doublet for silk strands parallel and perpendicular to the magnetic field.   The good correlation between the calculated and observed spectra strongly support the backbone type radical.

It is clearly seen that the backbone-type radical can be formed at each amino acid residue by breaking off the side chain.   Since in glycine only a hydrogen atom has to be removed, it has been suggested that this is the most reasonable place for the unpaired electron.   Support for this assumption was obtained in an experiment where a series of proteins were irradiated. With the assumption that the cysteine and glycine residues are of special importance, as far as the formation of the protein radicals are concerned, it seems reasonable to expect that the extent of the formation of the sulfur-resonance and the doublet somehow depend upon the content of cysteine and glycine residues.   Thus, there was found to be a good correlation between the extent of the sulfur-resonance and the ratio of half cystine residues to glycine residues (Henriksen, *et al.*, 1963a).

In a study on polyamino acids Drew and Gordy (1963) found that for about half of these substances the room temperature spectra could be ascribed to free radicals formed by the loss of an H atom from the α-carbon in the polypeptide chain.   For the other polyamino acids a side-chain radical was proposed.   It is interesting to note that for the amino acids glycine, sarcosine, leucine, and glutamic acid, the main resonance consisted of a doublet with approximately 18 Oe splitting.   With regard to proteins these results seem to imply that we also have to take some of the other amino acid residues into consideration when we discuss the backbone-type radical (Patten and Gordy, 1964).

The conclusion of the above discussion is that when proteins are irradiated and examined at room temperature only a very limited number of radical sites seems possible.   Since the initial energy absorption takes place evenly throughout the molecule this would imply that the absorbed radiation energy somehow must migrate to these specific sites.   Information about this migration can be obtained in experiments carried out at low temperatures.   Thus, it was relatively early discovered that when the proteins were irradiated at 77°K the ESR spectra were completely different from those at room temperature (Henriksen, *et al.*, 1963a; Patten and Gordy, 1961).   This is demonstrated for trypsin in Fig. 6.6.   The protein spectra

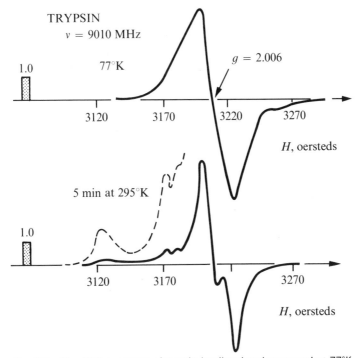

Fig. 6.6   The ESR spectrum of trypsin irradiated and measured at 77°K. After the first measurement (upper figure) the sample was annealed for 5 min. at room temperature and then again measured at 77°K. The dashed curve represents measurement at high gain. The relative spectrometer sensitivity is otherwise given by the columns to the left.

observed after irradiation at 77°K are usually poor in hyperfine structure and consist mainly of a broad single peak with a g-value of approximately 2.006–2.008.   When the samples subsequently are annealed at higher temperatures and again measured at 77°K, spectral changes are observed, demonstrating that secondary radical reactions take place.   Our knowledge about these reactions is very limited.   However, a few things can be deduced from the spectra.   The total number of radicals usually decreases in these reactions (Henriksen, 1962; Henriksen, *et al.*, 1963a).   Second, few, if any, sulfur radicals of the type discussed above, seem to be present at low temperatures.   These sulfur radicals are formed rather slowly unless the temperature exceeds about 280°K.

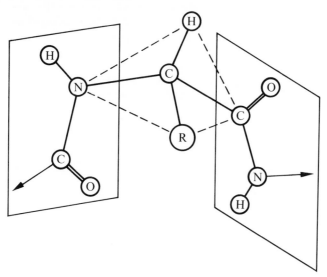

Fig. 6.7   Migration of electrons or electron holes along the protein backbone includes a charge migration from one peptide plane to the other across the asymmetrical carbon atom.

From these relatively few experimental facts, we can try to discuss the mechanisms for the formation of the secondary protein radicals and consequently for the migration of radiation energy.   Gordy and his co-workers (Gordy and Miyagawa, 1960; Patten and Gordy, 1961) have proposed an intramolecular migration of electrons.   Thus, they assume that the formation of the secondary radicals takes place in two separate phases.   The first phase involves the random formation of electron holes by the ionization processes.   The low temperature spectra (Fig. 6.6) are assumed to reveal this primary phase.   In the second phase, the electron or the electron hole is assumed to migrate within the protein molecule to the specific trapping sites.

At these sites new radicals are formed by breaking off an atom like the hydrogen atom.   The migration itself is assumed to occur along the backbone of the protein from one peptide group to another via the asymmetrical carbon atom by a hyperconjugation.   An attempt to visualize this is presented in Fig. 6.7.   This migration, if it occurs, will depend upon the orientation of the two peptide planes to each other.   It is clear from Fig. 6.1 that maximum migration will take place when the two planes are parallel.   With increasing temperature the molecular motions and twisting of the planes will increase and this was assumed to give a more efficient migration.

This migration of electrons in the protein molecule, which differs from the above-mentioned migration across the hydrogen bonds, has also been assumed by Augenstein, *et al.* (1964) to account partly for the radiation inactivation of solid enzymes (see below).   These authors believe that the temperature dependence of the migration has an activation energy of approximately 2.2 kcal/mole.

6.3.4   INTERMOLECULAR MIGRATION OF RADIATION ENERGY

Based on our ESR results an alternative hypothesis has been proposed for the formation of the protein radicals which includes an inter-molecular transport of radiation energy (Henriksen, 1962; Henriksen and Pihl, 1961; Henriksen, *et al.*, 1963a, 1963b) (see also Fig. 6.13).   In this hypothesis it is assumed that the ESR centers initially formed are a mixture of several different species, i.e., both positive and negative ions formed by the ionization processes, as well as radical fragments formed by rupture of chemical bonds.   In the next phase these radicals are assumed to be involved in secondary reactions both with each other and with neighboring intact molecules, or with other groups within the same molecule with the result that the secondary radicals are formed.

If the present hypothesis is applied to proteins we should first observe a mixture of radicals (Fig. 6.6).   Second, these radicals will react and form the two types of resonances observed at room temperature (Fig. 6.5).   So far it is not possible to distinguish this hypothesis from Gordy's intramolecular migration theory.   However, according to the present model it should be possible to influence the secondary reactions (step II in Fig. 6.13) and partly intercept them by, for example, adding foreign substances to the protein.   In such mixtures we would expect that some of the radicals initially formed in the protein molecule will interact with the added substance with the result that the unpaired electron becomes transferred to this molecule, and, of course, vice versa.   Consequently, in molecular mixtures we would expect some type of pecking order; i.e., by adding certain substances to the protein a protection would take place, whereas in other cases a sensitization would result.

Molecular mixtures of proteins and small molecular compounds have been studied by different groups.† The mixtures are usually prepared by mixing and subsequently freeze-drying solutions of the respective substances. Irradiation is carried out at a temperature which is low enough to prevent most of the secondary reactions. Subsequently, the mixture is heat-treated and the secondary reactions are followed by ESR spectroscopy. A typical example of such an experiment is shown in Fig. 6.8. The enzyme glyceraldehyde-3-phosphate dehydrogenase (GAPDH) is mixed with the thiol

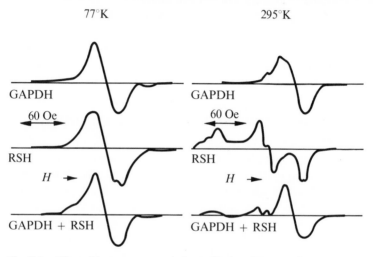

Fig. 6.8   Effect of heat treatment on the qualitative spectrum of a mixture of GAPDH (90% by weight) and RSH (10%). The samples were irradiated with X-rays in the solid state at 77°K and the spectra recorded at this temperature before and after heat treatments up to 295°K. For comparison, the corresponding spectra of the individual components, similarly treated, are included. (Data taken from Henriksen, et al., 1963b.)

cysteamine (RSH) which is known to give protection against ionizing radiation *in vivo*. The substances were irradiated singly and in mixtures consisting of 90% enzyme and 10% thiol by weight. The irradiation temperature was 77°K and all ESR measurements were carried out at this particular temperature which ensures that the observed qualitative spectral changes are due to secondary radical reactions. After the first measurement the samples were annealed for a few minutes at room temperature. As shown in Fig. 6.8 the spectra of the two components at 77°K are very similar. Whereas annealing to 295°K gave almost no change in the spectrum of

† Gordy and Miyagawa, 1960; Henriksen, *et al.*, 1963b; Libby, *et al.*, 1961; Ormerod and Alexander, 1962, 1963; Pihl and Sanner, 1964.

GAPDH the spectrum of RSH changed completely to become a typical sulfur pattern, i.e., sulfur radicals are formed. Heat treatment of the mixture resulted as well in the formation of sulfur radicals. This finding raises the question whether the occurrence of the sulfur radicals in the mixture can be accounted for by the sulfur radicals induced in the RSH alone. In order to answer this question is is necessary to calculate the absolute number of sulfur radicals formed.

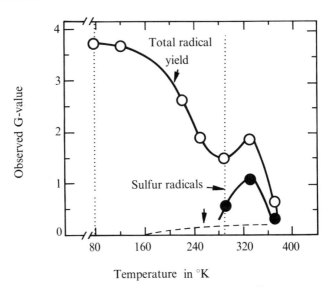

Fig. 6.9   Radical yield in a mixture of GAPDH (90% by weight) and RSH (10%) as a function of the annealing temperature. Conditions as in Fig. 6.8. The number of sulfur radicals was obtained from an analysis of the spectra. The dashed line represents the expected total yield of sulfur radicals in the mixture, on the assumption that this is equal to the weighted average of the sulfur yields for the two components irradiated separately. The dotted vertical lines indicate the irradiation temperature and the room temperature. (Data taken from Henriksen, et al., 1963b.)

In Fig. 6.9 the total yield of radicals in the mixture as a function of the annealing temperature is presented. The yield of sulfur radicals, obtained from an analysis of the spectra, is also given. This analysis appears to be a simple procedure since the major portion of the sulfur resonance is localized at lower magnetic field values than the resonance of most hydrocarbon radicals (Henriksen, 1962). The sulfur resonance of irradiated cysteine was used to carry out this analysis. The dashed line in Fig. 6.9 represents the expected number of sulfur radicals calculated on the basis of the sulfur radicals formed in RSH alone.   It follows that the number of sulfur radicals actually formed in the mixture becomes approximately four to five times as high as that expected.   Consequently, the two components of the mixture must somehow interact to increase the formation of sulfur radicals.   Results similar to those presented here have been obtained for a number of other molecular mixtures (Henriksen, et al., 1963b).   In all cases, the number of sulfur radicals is larger than can be accounted for on the basis of the sulfur radicals formed in the two components when irradiated alone.

Since the sulfur resonance found in irradiated proteins is indistinguishable from that of RSH, it is not possible from the above experiments to decide whether the additional unpaired spins on sulfur atoms reside in the thiol, in the protein (GAPDH contains eight SH groups per molecular weight 10^5) or in both substances.   The most plausible explanation would seem to be that interactions between the two components of the mixture have resulted in a transfer of unpaired spins from the protein molecule to the sulfur of the added thiol.   In order to clear up this point we must look in more detail into the structure of the sulfur radical and its ESR pattern.

In work on a single crystal of cystine dihydrochloride, Kurita and Gordy (1961) suggested that the unpaired spin of the sulfur radical

$$\begin{array}{c} H \\ | \\ R-C-S\cdot \\ | \\ H \end{array}$$

is in a π-orbital with the sulfur $3p$ orbital as the principal component.   It is further assumed that configurations where the unpaired electron is in nonbonding sp_2 hybrid orbitals, or in a σ-bonding orbital, contribute to a certain extent.   This mixing of configurations leads to the anisotropy in the g-factor (Pryce, 1950), and the π-character of the sulfur $3p$ orbital gives rise to an isotropic interaction of the unpaired electron with the protons in the CH_2 group adjacent to the sulfur.   If the unpaired electron interacts with both protons four hyperfine lines would appear in the most general case.   A triplet is the result of an equivalent interaction.   However, if the rotation of the CH_2 group is restricted, one of the two protons may be in a more favorable position with regard to an interaction with the unpaired electron, and a doublet may result.   The latter situation seems to occur for the sulfur radical.   Thus, for a single crystal a doublet with a splitting of 9 Oe is observed, although for a polycrystalline sample this hyperfine structure is smeared out at room temperature.   However, when the observation temperature is below about 160°K a splitting is also observed for polycrystalline samples.   In the middle of the resonance a doublet appears as demonstrated in Fig. 6.10 for cysteine observed at 77°K. Consequently, sulfur radicals of the type R—CH$_2$—S· which include protein sulfur radicals, seem to exhibit a temperature dependent hyperfine splitting. If, therefore, a compound is chosen where the hydrogen atoms on the carbon adjacent to the sulfur is substituted by another group this hyperfine structure should change. Thus, in agreement with expectation, no doublet is found for penicillamine where the H atoms have been substituted by methyl groups as shown in Fig. 6.10. This finding implies that it is possible to use thiols of low molecular

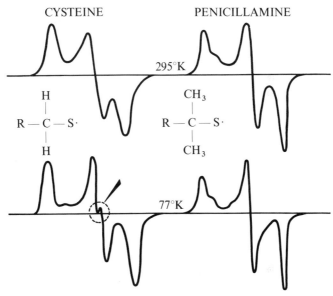

Fig. 6.10   The qualitative ESR spectra of cysteine and penicillamine. The samples have been irradiated at room temperature and the spectra recorded at 295°K (the upper spectra) and 77°K. The doublet splitting observed for cysteine at 77°K is observable below about 160°K and the resolution increases with decreasing temperature. The sulfur radicals formed in proteins exhibit a resonance with a temperature dependent hyperfine splitting similar to that in cysteine.

weight in the molecular mixtures so that the sulfur radicals in the thiol can be distinguished from those in the protein.

In Fig. 6.11 the results are presented for a mixture of bovine serum albumin (90%) and penicillamine (10%). The results show that in this mixture the majority of the unpaired spins eventually become localized on the sulfur of the penicillamine. When the total number of ESR centers in the mixture was calculated from the observations made prior to heat treatment it was found that it was equal to the sum of those induced for the two

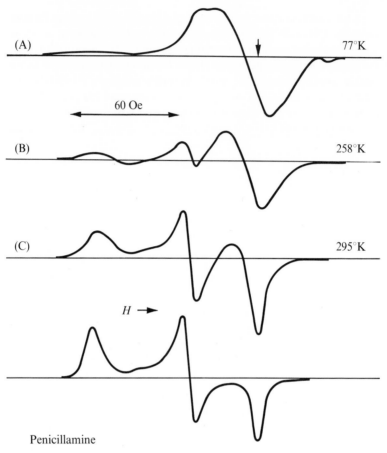

(A)   77°K

← 60 Oe →

(B)   258°K

(C)   295°K

$H \rightarrow$

Penicillamine

Fig. 6.11   Effect of heat treatment on the qualitative ESR spectra of a mixture of bovine serum albumin (90% by weight) and penicillamine (10%). Conditions as in Fig. 6.8. The bottom spectrum of penicillamine is directly comparable to that shown in C. (Data taken from Henriksen, *et al.*, 1963b.)

components irradiated separately (Henriksen, *et al.*, 1963b).   The results for a series of mixtures of bovine serum albumin and RSH are given in Fig. 6.12.   It appears that the yield for the mixture is equal to or slightly larger than the weighted average of those for the two components.   These results demonstrate that at 77°K, ESR centers are formed in both components, and furthermore that the added thiol has a negligible influence at this temperature.   The subsequent heat treatment results in a transfer of spins from the protein to the added thiol.

Since the molecular mixtures are made up by mixing the freeze-drying solutions of the two components, it is necessary to ascertain whether or not the thiols are bonded to the proteins.   This was tested by preparing mixtures of proteins with S^{35} labeled cysteamine.   The freeze-dried mixture was redissolved in water, and the protein-bound radioactivity was measured (Henriksen, *et al.*, 1963b).   The results showed that the transfer of unpaired spins involved almost exclusively RSH that was not covalently bonded to the protein.

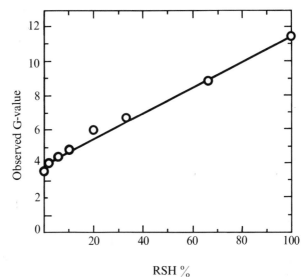

RSH %

Fig. 6.12   The radical yield at 77°K of bovine serum albumin–RSH mixtures as a function of their composition. Mixtures with increasing content of RSH were irradiated at 77°K and measured at this temperature before any heat treatment. (Data taken from Henriksen, *et al.*, 1963b.)

6.3.5   CONCLUSION

The ESR experiments on solid proteins have clearly demonstrated that the radicals which are present at room temperature are not the primary radicals formed by ionizing radiation.   We have discussed both an intra- and an intermolecular mechanism for the formation of the secondary radicals.   The above experiments on molecular mixtures demonstrate that the intermolecular mechanism for transport of radiation energy may take place in a solid system.   However, this does not exclude Gordy's intramolecular migration of electrons or some other type of intramolecular transformation.   The conclusion is that the amount of experimental information is too small to decide whether the secondary radicals are formed by the intermolecular mechanism, by some type of intramolecular transformation, or by both types of processes.

In order to get more information about the initial ESR centers and the processes occurring prior to the formation of the secondary radicals (steps I and II in Fig. 6.13, p. 230), it would be of great interest to carry out experiments on single crystals irradiated at low temperatures and subsequently heat treated. A first attempt in that direction was recently reported by Akasaka, *et al.* (1964), and by Box and Freund (1964). Both groups irradiated single crystals of cystine dihydrochloride at 77°K. Akasaka, *et al.* concluded that the well-known sulfur radicals were formed by a two-step intramolecular transformation of the initial radical which was assumed to be a cystine molecule with an ionized S—S bond.

6.4 MECHANISMS FOR ENZYME INACTIVATION AND RADIO-PROTECTION IN THE SOLID STATE

6.4.1 GENERAL REMARKS

In spite of the large number of radiation experiments on solid enzymes we have very little information about the mechanisms underlying the loss of enzymatic activity. We know that the radio-sensitivity can be changed by adding other substances to the solid proteins.[†] However, in order to produce any effect the added substances have to be present in the system during irradiation. This seems, therefore, to imply that the key to the understanding of the radioprotective substances is the early physico-chemical processes. Our purpose is, therefore, to study the processes responsible for the concentration of enough radiation energy to destroy the active site of the enzyme molecule, and to discover in which phase and to what extent the protective substances interfere with these processes. In the following discussion we will try to present some of the mechanisms proposed for the radiation inactivation of solid enzymes, and especially to discuss the correlation between the production of free radicals and the biological damage.

6.4.2 INACTIVATION MECHANISMS

A. *THE TARGET THEORY*

For several years the well-known target theory has been used to describe the radiation inactivation of solid enzymes. (For a general discussion of the target theory see for example refs.[‡]) The virtue of this theory was that it opened up possibilities for determining the dimensions, such as the volume and the cross-section, of the irradiated object. It was assumed that a hit or an absorption event must take place within the actual target. In the case of

[†] Alexander and Toms, 1958; Braams, 1960; Braams, *et al.*, 1958; Brustad, 1961; Butler and Robins, 1962; Norman and Ginoza, 1958; Pihl and Sanner, 1963; Wilson, 1959.
[‡] Lea, 1947; Timoféeff-Ressovsky and Zimmer, 1947; Zimmer, 1961.

enzymes it was generally agreed that the enzyme molecule was inactivated whenever a primary ionization takes place within the molecule itself. In several experiments with fast ionizing particles good agreements were obtained between the target dimensions calculated by this hypothesis and those obtained by other methods.[†]

In the target theory the primary absorption event is directly correlated with the observable biological damage, and no attempts are made to describe either the intermediate species formed or the early secondary reactions. It is assumed that the action of radiation responsible for the biological damage occurs at the site of the hit, i.e., in the target itself. The above-mentioned experiments which clearly demonstrated that radiation energy can migrate in a biological system, and especially the experiments which show that the radiosensitivity can be changed in molecular mixtures, seem therefore difficult to reconcile with the target theory in its original form. Furthermore, it has also been found that enzyme inactivation depends upon the irradiation temperature (Brustad, 1964; Pollard, et al., 1952; Setlow, 1952). Since it is assumed that the primary absorption event is independent of the target temperature this may be explained as a temperature effect on the early secondary reactions. Consequently, with the methods now available for studying intermediates in the physico-chemical stage, such as ESR spectroscopy, thermoluminescence, and flash radiolysis, it seems possible to take another step and either extend the old target theory or introduce some other models.

B. AUGENSTEIN, BRUSTAD, AND MASON'S MECHANISM

The first systematic study on the effect of the irradiation temperature on the inactivation of solid enzymes was recently reported by Brustad (1964). Trypsin was irradiated with a number of heavily charged particles in the temperature range 10–420°K. After exposure the samples were brought to room temperature, dissolved in an aqueous solution, and the enzymatic activity measured. Since the inactivation curve for trypsin with respect to the radiation dose is exponential, the parameter used for the radiosensitivity may either be the reciprocal of the D_{37} dose[‡] or the apparent inactivation cross-section. Brustad found that the apparent inactivation cross-section was independent of the irradiation temperature up to 100°K. Above this level the cross-section increased with increasing temperature. The total variation between the low temperature region and room temperature was of the order 2 to 3. (An example is shown in Fig. 6.17.) The results were

[†] Dolphin and Hutchinson, 1960; Ore, 1957; Pollard, et al., 1955; Pollard and Whitmore, 1957.

[‡] The dose corresponding to inactivation of 63% of the enzyme molecules, i.e., e^{-1} = 37% activity remaining.

plotted in an Arrhenius plot with the idea of seeing if the temperature effect could be adequately described by a sum of exponential functions like:

$$Y_T = \sum_i Y_{io} \exp\left(-E_i/kT\right)$$

where Y_T is the radiation yield at the irradiation temperature T. The parameter E_i, which can be obtained from the slope of the straight line in the Arrhenius plot, may be interpreted as the activation energy of the underlying process. It was found that the results could be adequately fitted by a sum of three straight lines for which the respective values of E_i were: $E_1 = 0$, $E_2 = 1000$ cal/mole, and $E_3 = 3000$–5000 cal/mole (see also Table 6.1).

Table 6.1 *The apparent activation energies for the processes leading to the production of secondary radicals and the loss of enzymatic activity[a]*

Compound	Type of radiation	Type of measurement	E_1	E_2	E_3
			(cal/mole)		
Lysozyme	He^4 Ions	Radicals	0	1000	5000
	He^4 Ions[b]	Radicals	0	1000	4000
	C^{12} Ions	Radicals	0	1000	4000
Trypsin	He^4 Ions	Radicals	0	950	3600
	C^{12} Ions	Radicals	0	950	3300
	C^{12} Ions[b]	Radicals	0	1150	—
	A^{40} Ions	Radicals	0	1300	—
	A^{40} Ions[b]	Radicals	0	800	3100
Trypsin	D^2 Ions	Inactivation	0	1350	4700
	He^4 Ions	Inactivation	0	1350	5200
	B^{11} Ions	Inactivation	0	1100	3400
	C^{12} Ions	Inactivation	0	1150	4200
	Ne^{20} Ions	Inactivation	0	1050	3800
	A^{40} Ions	Inactivation	0	1300	3700

[a] The inactivation data are taken from Brustad's experiments (1964).
[b] These results refer to measurements carried out on samples that have been kept at 295 K for two days between the exposure and the measurements.

Based mainly on these results Augenstein, *et al.* (1964) proposed a new mechanism for enzyme inactivation. These authors cast serious doubts upon the validity of the one ionization theory and suggest that non-ionizing excitations may be more important at room temperature. The inactivation is assumed to be completed when enough radiation energy has been transported from the place where it is absorbed to what they call 'the crucial site' in the enzyme molecule. The important step here is the secondary reactions and the authors introduce a series of processes for the transport of radiation energy in solid proteins. They assume that intermediate species like charges (electrons or electron holes) and excitons can migrate in proteins. No mechanism is suggested for the charge migration except that one of the models is identical to Gordy's hypothesis that electrons can migrate along the protein backbone across the asymmetric carbon atom (Patten and Gordy, 1961). Since our knowledge about the migration of charges and excitons in protons is still very limited, no attempt will be made here to discuss the likelihood of the proposed processes. It should, however, be pointed out that it will be extremely difficult to test experimentally the proposed mechanism. Furthermore, Augenstein, *et al.* seem to ignore the part played by free radicals in transfer of radiation energy and inactivation.

C. THE FREE RADICAL MECHANISM

In the preceding sections we have discussed the types of secondary protein radicals as well as the mechanisms proposed for their formation. It is now of general interest to study the relation between these radicals and the observable biological damage. It is generally accepted that in the case of aqueous solutions the chemical damage is produced largely by the radiation-induced free radicals. This has certainly prompted the assumption that the radiation damage on solid biological systems is also caused fully or partly by the free radicals.† However, so far we have relatively little experimental evidence for this assumption. In the following we will try to work out a free radical mechanism for the radiation inactivation of solid enzymes, and subsequently present some recent experiments which seem to support this hypothesis.

In a recent paper, Braams (1963) tried to outline in more detail a free radical mechanism for radiation damage in the solid state. He assumed that the first step represents a dissociation of the macromolecule into a large and a small radical fragment;

$$MR_i \rightarrow M^{\cdot} + R_i .$$

$M^{\cdot}$ is assumed to be the large, relatively stable, protein radical. $R_i^{\cdot}$ is a small diffusible radical fragment, very often a hydrogen atom. In the next phase, it is assumed that $M^{\cdot}$ can react with its environment leading to both cross-linking and/or to modified protein molecules. The fragment $R_i^{\cdot}$ is assumed to be very reactive and can react (by intermolecular reactions) with other protein molecules. If now other substances such as the radioprotective SH compounds are present, the reactive fragment can also react with these substances. Thus, Braams assumes that if all these fragments react

† Braams, 1963; Ehret, *et al.*, 1960; Henriksen, *et al.*, 1963a; Hunt and Williams, 1964; Powers and Kaleta, 1960.

with the added SH compounds the radiation sensitivity of the macromolecule will be reduced by a factor 2, which is of the same order of magnitude
as that found experimentally.

According to Braams' model the protein radicals are formed only by
rupture of chemical bonds and no radical ions formed by the ionization processes seem to be included.   Furthermore, the possibility that the large protein radical M· can also react with the added SH compound has been neglected.   Based on the experiments which demonstrate that a series of reactions
takes place before the secondary protein radicals are formed, as well as on the

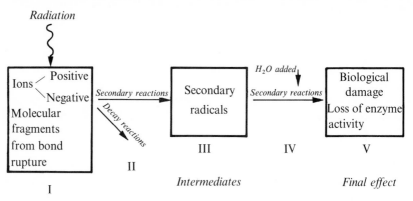

Fig. 6.13   An attempt to visualize a mechanism for radiation damage and repair in the
solid state. It is assumed that the final biological effect, as measured in step V, is the
end result of a sequence of events in which free radicals take part as intermediates.
The main idea is that the early processes in the enzyme inactivation mechanism are
the same as those leading to the secondary protein radicals.

experiments demonstrating the intermolecular transfer of unpaired spins, an
extended free radical mechanism will be proposed here.   This mechanism,
which has certain features in common with that of Braams, is visualized in
Fig. 6.13.   It is assumed that the radiation inactivation of solid enzymes is
the end result of a sequence of events in which free radicals are transient intermediates.   The main idea is that the early processes in the inactivation mechanism are the same as those leading to the secondary protein radicals.   These
radicals (designated as step III in Fig. 6.13) will subsequently be involved in
new reactions, either when the enzymes are still in the solid state or when they
are dissolved in an aqueous solution in order to measure the activity.   According to the model in Fig. 6.13 it is assumed that these reactions lead to the
biological damage.

The radical model here proposed can be tested in experiments where
the production of secondary radicals (step III in Fig. 6.13) is correlated with
the biological damage as measured by the loss of enzymatic activity (step V).

D. *EXPERIMENTAL SUPPORT FOR THE FREE RADICAL MECHANISM*

The first attempts to correlate the production of free radicals with the enzyme inactivation were reported by Hunt, *et al.* (1962) and by Hunt and Williams (1964). They tried to correlate directly the number of radicals formed in ribonuclease with the loss of enzymatic activity. Since they found that the yield of radicals was of the same order of magnitude as the inactivation yield, they concluded that a large fraction of the biological damage can be accounted for by the radicals. However, the most interesting part of their work, with regard to the free radical mechanism, is an experiment on the oxygen effect. It has been mentioned earlier that the radicals formed in proteins very often seem to be sensitive to oxygen. This may result in large qualitative and quantitative changes in the ESR spectra. Very little information

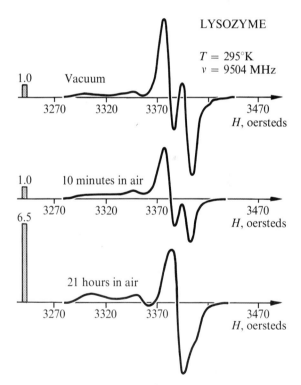

Fig. 6.14   The effect of oxygen on the ESR spectrum of lysozyme. The enzyme was irradiated in vacuum, at room temperature, with 6.5 MeV electrons. All measurements were made at room temperature. After the first measurement the sample was opened to air. The relative spectrometer sensitivity is given by the columns to the left.

exists about the reactions that take place when oxygen is admitted, but the following reaction scheme may be proposed:

$$R\cdot + O_2 \xrightarrow{\ 1\ } ROO\cdot \xrightarrow{\ 2\ } \text{Nonradical species.}$$

It has been assumed that the transient peroxide radical gives rise to a singlet. Drew and Gordy (1963) pointed out that if the second reaction is fast compared to the first one, a decay with no spectral changes will be observed.   On the other hand, if this latter process is slow the ESR pattern will change to a singlet and decay slowly.   For most proteins we can expect something in between these two limits.   In Figs. 6.14 and 6.15 two examples of the oxygen effect are demonstrated.   In the case of lysozyme a large decay in the radical concentration is observed concomitantly with considerable qualitative changes.   It is of interest to note that the doublet resonance, due to the backbone type radicals, is more sensitive to oxygen than the sulfur radicals.   In the case of trypsin (Fig. 6.15), the sample was irradiated in vacuum and kept at room temperature for three days.   This should ensure that most of the reactions in step II have been completed before the sample was opened to air.   It appears that the radical concentration decreases by a factor of 4–5 in the course of a few hours.

    In the experiments by Hunt and co-workers (Hunt, *et al.*, 1962; Hunt and Williams, 1964) on ribonuclease, it was found that oxygen changed

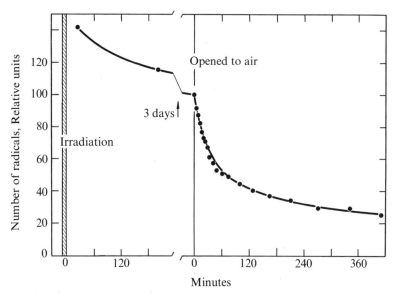

Fig. 6.15   The effect of oxygen on the number of radicals in trypsin. The sample was kept at room temperature, in vacuum, for three days before it was opened to air.

the ESR spectrum as well as the radio-sensitivity as measured by the loss of enzymatic activity.   They assumed that the sulfur radicals lead to the formation of SH groups, and since the yield of SH groups was found to be independent of oxygen, they concluded that the sulfur radicals are unlikely to take part in the oxygen effect.   They assumed that the doublet-type radicals lead to inactivation when they react with oxygen.   Based on this assumption, they calculated an expected inactivation curve (loss of enzymatic activity versus dose) for post-treatment in oxygen, by using the observed dose effect curve for the radical concentration in vacuum.   The good correlation obtained in a certain dose range between the calculated and the experimental inactivation curve seems to support the free radical mechanism.   However, a direct correlation of this kind where one secondary radical is correlated to the inactivation of one macromolecule is, in the opinion of the present author, uncertain and may lead to considerable errors.   The reason is that we still have great problems with the determination of the radical concentration. (See chapter 2, section 2.2).   Furthermore, parameters such as the stability of the radicals, the vacuum in the sample, the bound water, etc., may also cause uncertainties.

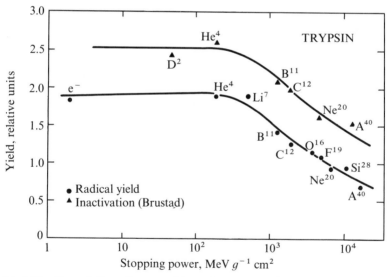

Fig. 6.16   The radiation effect on solid trypsin as measured by the loss of enzyme activity (these data are taken from Brustad, 1964) and by the production of secondary radicals, as a function of the stopping power. The inactivation curve for solid trypsin is exponential with respect to the radiation dose. The parameter used for the inactivation is the reciprocal of the D_{37} dose. In this figure the original data have been recalculated and are given in relative units in order to be plotted on the same scale as the radical data. The flat portion of the curve was given the value 2.5.

In the following, two different experiments will be presented where efforts have been made to overcome the difficulties that are involved in direct correlations.   The main idea with these experiments is to vary the physical conditions for the reactions that take place prior to the formation of the secondary radicals (that means steps I and II in Fig. 6.13).   These variations are expected to result in changes in the yield of secondary radicals and, according to the model in Fig. 6.13, in similar changes in the inactivation yield.   In the first type of experiment the spatial distribution of the energy absorption was changed by using radiations with different stopping powers. The results for the enzyme trypsin are shown in Fig. 6.16.   The enzyme was irradiated in the solid state by 6.5 MeV electrons and a large variety of fast, heavy ions such as helium, lithium, boron, carbon, oxygen, fluorine, neon, silicon, and argon ions.   The yield of radicals, given as the G-value, is plotted as a function of the stopping power of the radiation.   The parameter used to measure the inactivation is the reciprocal of the D_{37} dose.   The inactivation data, which have been taken from Brustad's experiments (1964), have been recalculated and the plateau has been given the value 2.5 in order to be plotted on the same scale as the radical data.   The shape of these two

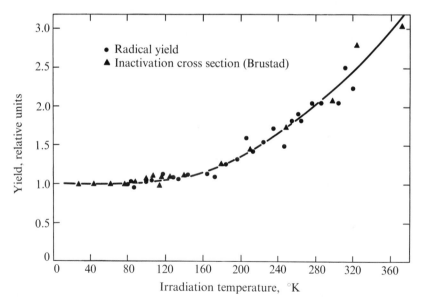

Fig. 6.17   Effect of the irradiation temperature on both the production of secondary radicals and the loss of enzymatic activity for trypsin. The enzyme was irradiated in the solid state, in vacuum, with fast carbon ions. The parameter for the inactivation (the data are taken from Brustad, 1964) is the apparent inactivation cross-section. The average value of the data below 100°K has been set equal to 1.0.

curves is the same.   The yields are constant up to about 200 MeV g^{-1} cm^2. They then decrease and the total variation within the LET range studied here is approximately a factor of 2.4.

In the other type of correlation experiment which has been carried out, the irradiation temperature is varied.   Trypsin was again used and one example is shown in Fig. 6.17.   Solid trypsin was irradiated with fast carbon ions at different temperatures.   The radical data refer to measurements after the samples have been at room temperature for 20 min.   This procedure ensures that most of the secondary reactions (step II) are completed and that only secondary radicals are present in the samples.   In both types of measurements the average value of the data below 100°K has been set equal to 1.0.   The yields are constant up to about 120°K and they then start to increase.   The total difference between 77°K and room temperature is a factor of approximately 2.1 for both types of measurements.

If the yield of secondary radicals is plotted in an Arrhenius plot we obtain the curves shown in Fig. 6.18.   The idea with this plot is to see if also the radical data, like the inactivation results (see above), can be fitted by a sum of straight lines.   It appears that a sum of three straight lines gives an adequate fit to the experimental curves in Fig. 6.18.   Consequently, a quantitative correlation between the production of secondary radicals and the loss of enzymatic activity can be obtained by comparing the apparent activation energies.   The results obtained so far are presented in Table 6.1. Although the radical data show a much larger spread in the apparent activation energies, there seems to be a remarkably good correlation between these two types of measurements.   It is therefore reasonable to assume that the same processes are responsible for both the observed effects.

6.4.3   RADIOPROTECTION IN THE SOLID STATE

It would be of interest to discuss the implication of the free radical hypothesis with respect to the mechanism for the action of radioprotective substances in solid biological systems.   The observation that the ESR centers originally induced in a protein molecule may be subsequently transferred to a small molecular sulfur compound can be described as a protection against the formation of the secondary protein radicals.   According to the model outlined in Fig. 6.13 this would imply that we also have a protection against the biological damage.   It seems therefore possible to ascribe the many protection experiments reported† to a partial interception of the radical reactions in step II (Fig. 6.13).   This would imply that the key to the understanding of the mechanism for protection in the solid state is the secondary

† Braams, 1960; Braams et al., 1958; Brustad, 1961; Butler and Robins, 1962; Norman and Ginoza, 1958; Pihl and Sanner, 1963; Wilson, 1959.

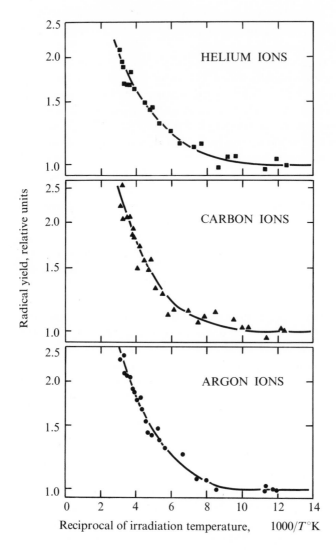

Fig. 6.18 The yield of secondary radicals in solid trypsin as a function of the reciprocal of the irradiation temperature. The solid enzyme was irradiated at different temperatures with helium, carbon, and argon ions. After irradiation the samples were kept at room temperature for 20 min. before the ESR measurements were carried out. The dose was the same for all samples irradiated with one type of ions. The curves were analysed as a sum of straight lines, and the apparent activation energies (given in Table 6.1) were obtained from the slopes of these lines.

radical reactions.   Unfortunately, very little is known about these reactions. One possibility would be a hydrogen transfer reaction:

$$P \cdot + RSH \rightarrow PH + RS \cdot$$

where $P \cdot$ is a large protein radical or a smaller protein fragment (see also Braams, 1963).   Direct support for the hydrogen transfer reaction was recently reported by Sanner (1965) in some experiments on mixtures of trypsin and pyridine coenzymes.   Thus, he found that the reduced coenzymes protected trypsin against inactivation to a greater extent than did the oxydized coenzymes.

It has also been mentioned that an added compound may increase the probability for a direct dissipation of excitation energy (Augenstein, *et al.*, 1964; Sanner, 1965).   However, since we so far have no experimental evidence for such a mechanism, it will not be discussed here.

6.4.4   CONCLUSION

It has been pointed out throughout this discussion that we still have little information about the basic mechanisms for radiation damage and repair in the solid state.   However, since we now have tools which allow us to study intermediate species formed by radiation, it seems possible to go deeper into these mechanisms.   Some of the working models for the inactivation of enzymes in the solid state have been discussed.   In the case of the free radical mechanism some experimental support has been presented.   In the case of the enzyme trypsin, a good correlation between the production of secondary radicals and the loss of enzymatic activity was found.   Additional support for this model is derived from the protection experiments mentioned above.   However, if we look in more detail into this model we realize that there are large gaps in the available information.   For example, we know that a number of the initial ESR centers disappear in the secondary reactions in step II (see Fig. 6.13).   The possibility that the nonradical species thus formed in turn may lead to the inactivation of the molecule should therefore be considered.   Another point where more information is desirable is the stability of the secondary radicals.   The influence of gases such as O_2, NO, H_2, etc., during and after irradiation, on the secondary radicals as well as on the enzyme activity, should be studied in more detail.

A very important point, which has not been discussed in this chapter, is what actually happens to the enzyme molecule when it is inactivated. Thus, we do not know if the enzymes are inactivated as the result of chemical changes in the active site or by physical changes in the tertiary structure of the molecules.   It may well be that the enzymes are inactivated by several different mechanisms and that the secondary radicals studied in the present work can account for only a part of the inactivation.

ACKNOWLEDGEMENTS

I wish to express my gratitude to Professor C. A. Tobias and his group for the hospitality and working facilities offered me at Donner Laboratory.

It is a pleasure to acknowledge the financial support from the U.S. Atomic Energy Commission through the Lawrence Radiation Laboratory, and from the U.S. Public Health Service.

REFERENCES

Akasaka, K., Ohnishi, S. I., Suita, T., and Nitta, I., 1964, *J. chem. Phys.*, **40**, 3110.
Alexander, P., and Toms, D. J., 1958, *Radiat. Res.*, **9**, 509.
Augenstein, L. G., 1963, *Progress in Biophysics and Molecular Biology*, (Oxford: Pergamon Press), Vol. 13, pp. 1–58.
Augenstein, L. G., Brustad, T., and Mason, R., 1964, *Adv. Radiat. Biol.*, **1**, 227–66.
Baxter, S., 1943, *Trans. Faraday Soc.*, **39**, 207.
Blumenfeld, L. A., and Kalmanson, A. E., 1958a, *Biofizika*, **3**, 87; 1958b, *Proc. 2nd Int. Conf. Peaceful Uses of Atomic Energy*, **22**, 524 (Geneva); 1961, *The Initial Effects of Ionizing Radiation*, Ed. R. J. C. Harris (London: Academic Press), p. 59.
Box, H. C., and Freund, H. G., 1964, *J. chem. Phys.*, **40**, 817.
Box, H. C., Freund, H. G., and Lilga, K. T., 1963, *J. chem. Phys.*, **38**, 2100.
Braams, R., 1960, *Radiat. Res.*, **12**, 113; 1963, *Nature*, Lond., **200**, 752.
Braams, R., Hutchinson, F., and Ray, D., 1958, *Nature*, Lond., **182**, 1506.
Brillouin, L., 1962, *Horizons in Biochemistry*, Ed. M. Kasha and B. Pullman (London: Academic Press), pp. 295–318.
Brookhaven Symposia in Biology, 1960, **13**, Protein Structure and Function.
Brustad, T., 1961, *Radiat. Res.*, **15**, 139; 1964, *Biological Effects of Neutron Irradiations* (Vienna: Int. Atomic Energy Agency).
Butler, J. A. V., and Robins, A. B., 1962, *Radiat. Res.*, **17**, 63.
Cardew, M. H., and Eley, D. D., 1959, *Discuss. Faraday Soc.*, **27**, 115.
Corey, R. B., and Pauling, L., 1953, *Proc. R. Soc. B*, **141**, 10.
Davis, K. M. C., Eley, D. D., and Smart, R. S., 1960, *Nature*, Lond., **188**, 724.
Del Re, G., Pullman, B., and Yonezawa, I., 1963, *Biochim. biophys. Acta*, **75**, 153.
Dolphin, G. W., and Hutchinson, F., 1960, *Radiat. Res.*, **13**, 403.

Drew, R. C., and Gordy, W., 1963, *Radiat. Res.*, **18**, 552.

Ehret, C. F., Smaller, B., Powers, E. L., and Webb, R. B., 1960, *Science, N.Y.*, **132**, 1768.

Eley, D. D., 1962, *Horizons in Biochemistry*, Ed. M. Kasha and B. Pullman (London: Academic Press), pp. 341–80.

Evans, M. G., and Gergely, J., 1949, *Biochim. biophys. Acta*, **3**, 188.

Garrett, C. G. B., 1959, *Semiconductors*, Ed. N. B. Hannay (New York: Reinhold Publ. Corp.).

Gordy, W., Ard., W. B., and Shields, H., 1955, *Proc. natn. Acad. Sci., U.S.A.*, **41**, 983.

Gordy, W., and Miyagawa, I., 1960, *Radiat. Res.*, **12**, 211.

Gordy, W., and Shields, H., 1958, *Radiat. Res.*, **9**, 611; 1960, *Proc. natn. Acad. Sci., U.S.A.*, **46**, 1124.

Green, D. W., Ingram, V. M., and Perutz, M. F., 1954, *Proc. R. Soc.* A, **225**, 287.

Henriksen, T., 1962, *J. chem. Phys.*, **37**, 2189; 1963, *Electron Spin Resonance Studies on the Formation and Properties of Free Radicals in Irradiated Sulfur-Containing Substances* (Oslo: University Press).

Henriksen, T., and Pihl, A., 1961, *Int. J. Radiat. Biol.*, **3**, 351.

Henriksen, T., Sanner, T., and Pihl, A., 1963a, *Radiat. Res.*, **18**, 147; 1963b, ibid., **18**, 163.

Hirs, C. H. W., Moore, S., and Stein, W. H., 1960, *J. biol. Chem.*, **235**, 633.

Hunt, J. W., Till, J. E., and Williams, J. F., 1962, *Radiat. Res.*, **17**, 703.

Hunt, J. W., and Williams, J. F., 1964, *Radiat. Res.*, **23**, 26.

Jordan, P., 1938, *Naturwissenschaften*, **42**, 693.

Katayama, M., and Gordy, W., 1961, *J. chem. Phys.*, **35**, 117.

Kendrew, J. C., Bodo, G., Dintzis, H. M., Parrish, R. G., Wychoff, H., and Phillips, D. C., 1958, *Nature*, Lond., **181**, 662.

Kendrew, J. C., Dickerson, R. E., Strandberg, B. E., Hart, R. G., Davis, D. R., Phillips, D. C., and Shore, V. C., 1960, *Nature*, Lond., **185**, 422.

King, G., and Medley, J. A., 1949, *J. Colloid Sci.*, **4**, 1.

Kneubühl, F. K., 1960, *J. chem. Phys.*, **33**, 1074.

Kurita, Y., and Gordy, W., 1961, *J. chem. Phys.*, **34**, 282.

Lea, D. E., 1947, *Actions of Radiations on Living Cells* (Cambridge: University Press).

Libby, D., Ormerod, M. G., Charlesby, A., and Alexander, P., 1961, *Nature*, Lond., **190**, 998.

Lin, W. C., and McDowell, C. A., 1961, *Molec. Phys.*, **4**, 333.

Low, B. W., and Edsall, J. T., 1956, *Currents in Biochemical Research*, Ed. D. E. Green (New York: Interscience Pub. Inc.), pp. 378–433.

McConnell, H. M., and Strathdee, J., 1959, *Molec. Phys.*, **2**, 129.

Miyagawa, I., Kurita, Y., and Gordy, W., 1960, *J. chem. Phys.*, **33**, 1599.

Muirhead, H., and Perutz, M. F., 1963, *Nature*, Lond., **199**, 633.

Müller, A., 1963, *Int. J. Radiat. Biol.*, **6**, 137.

Norman, A., and Ginoza, W., 1958, *Radiat. Res.*, **9**, 77.

Ore, A., 1957, *Radiat. Res.*, **6**, 27.

Ormerod, M. G., and Alexander, P., 1962, *Nature*, Lond., **193**, 290; 1963, *Radiat. Res.*, **18**, 495.

Patten, F., and Gordy, W., 1961, *Proc. natn. Acad. Sci. U.S.A.*, **46**, 1137; 1964, *Radiat. Res.*, **22**, 29.

Pauling, L., and Corey, R. B., 1951a, *Proc. natn. Acad. Sci. U.S.A.*, **37**, 235; 1951b, ibid., **37**, 729.

Pauling, L., Corey, R. B., and Branson, H. R., 1951, *Proc. natn. Acad. Sci., U.S.A.*, **37**, 205.

Peersen, E., and Ore, A., 1964, *Physica Norvegica*, **1**, 205.

Perutz, M. F., Rossman, M. G., Cullis, A. F., Muirhead, H., Will, G., and North, A. C. T., 1960, *Nature*, Lond., **185**, 416.

Pihl, A., and Sanner, T., 1963, *Biochim. biophys. Acta*, **78**, 537; 1964, *First Int. Symp. on Radiosensitizers and Radioprotective Drugs* (Milano: in press).

Pollard, E. C., Guild, W. R., Hutchinson, F., and Setlow, R. B., 1955, *Prog. Biophys. biophys. Chem.*, **5**, 72.

Pollard, E. C., Powell, W., and Reame, S., 1952, *Proc. natn. Acad. Sci., U.S.A.*, **38**, 173.

Pollard, E. C., and Whitmore, G. F., 1957, *Science, N.Y.*, **122**, 335.

Powers, E. L., and Kaleta, B. F., 1960, *Science, N.Y.*, **132**, 959.

Pryce, M. H. L., 1950, *Proc. phys. Soc.* A, **63**, 25.

Pulatova, M. K., Rogulenkova, V. N., and Kayushin, L. P., 1961, *Biofizika*, **6**, 548.

Pullman, B., and Pullman, A., 1963, *Quantum Biochemistry* (New York: Wiley Interscience).

Riehl, H., 1957, *Kolloidzeitschrift*, **151**, 66.

Rosenberg, B., 1962, *J. chem. Phys.*, **36**, 816.

Sanger, F., 1956, *Currents in Biochemical Research*, Ed. D. E. Green (New York: Interscience Pub. Inc.), pp. 434–59.

Sanger, F., and Thompson, E. O. P., 1953a, *Biochem. J.*, **53**, 353; 1953b, ibid., **53**, 366.

Sanger, F., and Tuppy, H., 1951a, *Biochem. J.*, **49**, 463; 1951b, ibid., **49**, 481.

Sanner, T., *Radiat. Res.*, 1965, **26**, 95.

Setlow, R., 1952, *Proc. natn. Acad. Sci., U.S.A.*, **38**, 166.

Söyrm, F., 1962, *Advances in Enzymology*, Ed. F. F. Nord (New York: Interscience Pub. Inc.), Vol. 24, p. 415.

Suard, M., Berthier, G., and Pullman, B., 1961, *Biochim. biophys. Acta*, **52**, 254.

Szent-Györgyi, 1941a, *Nature*, Lond., **148**, 157; 1941b, *Science, N.Y.*, **93**, 609.

Timoféeff-Ressovsky, N. W., and Zimmer, K. G., 1947, *Biophysik I. Das Trefferprinzip in der Biologie* (Leipzig: S. Hirzel).

Wilson, D. L., 1959, *Int. J. Radiat. Biol.*, **1**, 360.

Zimmer, K. G., 1961, *Studies on Quantitative Radiation Biology* (Edinburgh and London: Oliver and Boyd).

CHAPTER SEVEN

BIOLOGICAL FREE RADICALS AND THE MELANINS

M. S. Blois, Jr.

Department of Dermatology, School of Medicine, Stanford University, Stanford, California, U.S.A.

7.1 INTRODUCTION

Melanins are one of the relatively few substances of biological origin and of medical interest, having properties which may be appropriately described by the term 'solid state'. The term 'melanin' itself is a purely descriptive one (Gr. *melas*—black) which conveys no chemical information and merely denotes a black or brown pigment of biological origin. Such pigments are widely distributed throughout the living world, and the comparative biochemical question as to whether different species have different kinds of melanin is under active investigation. Since no sample of melanin has been completely and unambiguously characterized chemically (Swan, 1963) it is perhaps safest to assume for the present that there may be several varieties of natural melanins and to emphasize that even when the singular, 'melanin', is used, that it necessarily refers to a class of substances.

While melanin is apparently found at all phylogenetic levels from the fungi to man, in the more complex organisms it occurs only in specialized cells and tissues. In man it is present in skin and hair, the retinal pigment epithelium and irides of the eye, the adrenal medulla, the pineal body, and probably, the substantia nigra of the brain. Even within a single species, it is not certain that the melanin found in one tissue is identical with that synthesized in another, and there is, indeed, suggestion that it may not be. It is interesting that the tissues enumerated above are all of ectodermal origin, and the striking similarity between the melanogenesis of melanocytes and certain biochemical pathways in neural tissue will be considered below.

Present knowledge of natural melanins is derived in large part from studies on the pigment taken from the ink sac of the squid or from melanoma tissue—a tissue resulting from growth and accumulation of the neoplastic melanocyte. Recent studies by Nicolaus and his group (1964) have been extended to a variety of melanic pigments of plant and insect origin, and chemical differences in the pigment appear to have a phylogenetic basis.

7.2 SITE OF MELANIN SYNTHESIS

In higher forms, including man, it appears that melanin is formed in a single specialized cell, the melanocyte, which itself has been shown to be of neural crest origin (for amphibia by Du Shane (1938) and for higher phyla by others) and during embryologic development migrates to its final anatomic site. Electron microscopy has in the past few years disclosed a unique organelle within the melanocyte, known as the *melanosome* in which melanin synthesis occurs. Figure 7.1 indicates schematically the general morphology of the melanosome during several states of melanization. In its early stages, the melanosome may be considered to consist largely of a protein membraneous matrix upon which the melanin polymer is destined to be formed. A portion at least of this protein provides the enzyme activity necessary for the biosynthesis of melanin. It may be supposed that after the synthesis of this

245

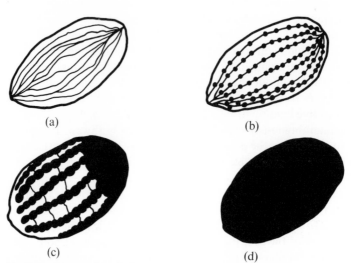

(a)   (b)

(c)   (d)

Fig. 7.1 Stages of melanization of the melanosome. (Schematic, after Moyer: *Ann. N.Y. Acad. Sci.* 1963 **100**: 603).

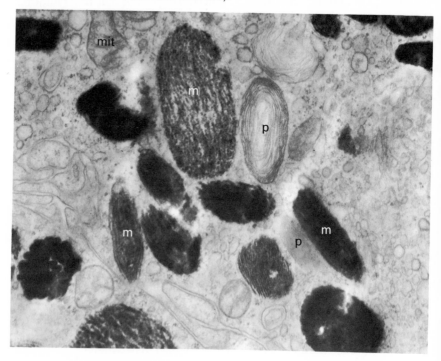

Fig. 7.2   Electron micrograph of a portion of a retinal melanocyte (human fetus of menstrual age 14 weeks) showing several stages of melanization. (Courtesy of A. Breathnach.)

matrix, the melanin precursors then diffuse into the melanosome and are incorporated into polymer.   As the polymer is formed, the protein matrix is eventually covered up until finally no catalytic sites are available for the conversion of further precursor and melanization is complete.   The comparable states of melanization will be seen readily in the electron micrograph of Fig. 7.2.   This fully melanized organelle thus constitutes a small particle, about a micron or less in diameter, of melanin polymer admixed with protein.   This may be extruded by the melanocyte as a melanin granule into the epithelial cells of the epidermis, into a developing hair shaft, or into the lumen of the ink sac of the squid.   The sample of natural melanin which is available for study, then, is this insoluble supramolecular particle of melanoprotein.

7.3 PHYSICO-CHEMICAL PROPERTIES

X-ray diffraction studies of natural melanins have revealed no evidence of periodicity or crystallinity.   Because these granules are not readily soluble, it has not yet been possible to form fibres in the hope of inducing orientation. If these granules are mixed with KBr and pressed into pellets for absorption spectroscopy, it is found that there are no absorption bands in the ultraviolet, or near-infrared (Figs. 7.3 and 7.4).   When the infrared is reached, there are a series of broad absorption bands (Fig. 7.5) which are quite similar amongst substances which are known to differ in considerable degree.

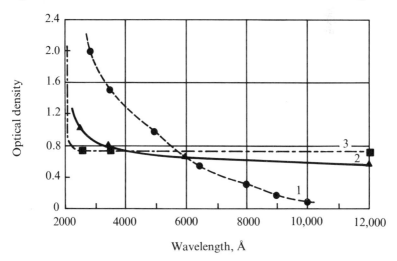

Fig. 7.3   Ultraviolet and visible absorption spectra of (1) 0.1 mg squid melanin dispersed in a 300 mg KBr pellet, compared with (2) 0.3 mg charcoal and (3) 0.1 mg graphite prepared similarly.

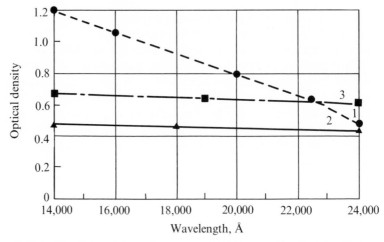

Fig. 7.4   Near infrared absorption spectra of (1) 2 mg squid melanin in a 300 mg KBr pellet. (2) and (3) refer to the samples as in Fig. 7.3.

For example, natural squid melanin and the synthetic polymer prepared by the auto-oxidation of catechol are seen to be quite alike although they are obviously chemically quite different.   These similarities must therefore reside in electronic properties which are shared by these materials but which do not reflect closely the elemental composition or details of chemical structure.

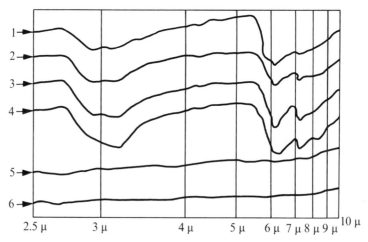

Fig. 7.5   Infrared absorption spectra of (1) squid melanin, (2) catechol melanin—autoxidized, (3) L-DOPA melanin-autoxidized, (4) hydroquinone polymer—autoxidized, (5) graphite, and (6) charcoal. All samples prepared in KBr pellets.

Since these melanin granules are supramolecular, it follows that they can at best form colloidal systems under biological conditions. For true solutions to be formed it would first be necessary for the hydrolysis of primary bonds to occur, and the complete hydrolysis and solubilization of melanins has not yet been achieved, though a certain amount of low molecular weight material becomes dispersed when natural melanins are placed in such solvents as dimethylformamide or dimethylsulfoxide. Because of the difficulty of getting melanin into true solution, its study by chemical means must be quite indirect. Destructive chemical methods, as used in elemental analysis, had been applied to melanins before the turn of the century, but the only conclusion reached was that it was a nitrogen-containing polymer.

The involvement of enzymes in melanin synthesis was discovered quite early. In 1895 Bourquelot and Bertrand reported the isolation of an enzyme from mushrooms which converted tyrosine to melanin. This enzyme was named tyrosinase and has subsequently been shown to occur in all phyla. From 1925 onward, this transformation was studied by Raper (1928), and the last step of the synthesis was later supplied by Mason (1948). This Raper–Mason pathway of melanin synthesis is shown in Fig. 7.6. Some of the intermediates in the Raper–Mason synthesis have never been isolated,

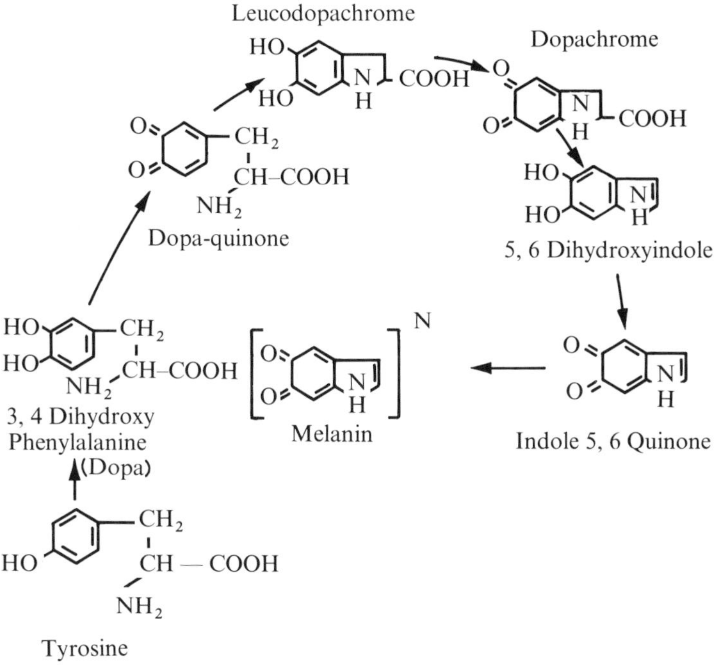

Fig. 7.6   The Raper–Mason pathway of melanin biosynthesis.

and their fleeting existence has been inferred from the results of optical absorption spectroscopy.   This synthetic scheme itself gives no indication as to the chemical structure of the pigment material.   A number of possible structures have been proposed from time to time; several of these are shown in Fig. 7.7.   It has been generally assumed that melanin was extensively conjugated in order to account for the deep, black color, but until quite recently no chemical determinations of structure had been made.   By 1954 the general concept of the melanins seemed to be that these pigments consisted of a high molecular weight, conjugated polymer, of indolequinone. No direct experiments had given information as to the bonding arrangements by which the monomeric units were held together.

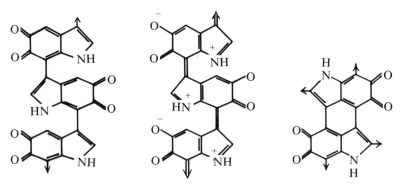

Fig. 7.7   Hypothetical structures for melanin, based upon the condensation of the indole 5, 6 quinone of the Raper–Mason synthesis.

In 1954 a paper appeared by Commoner, Townsend, and Pake reporting on the observation of an electron spin resonance (ESR) in natural melanin.   They proposed that the paramagnetism was due to free radicals trapped in the pigment material which in their case was the melanin of frog eggs.   The plausibility of their hypothesis was supported by the findings of Fraenkel, *et al.* (1954) who showed by means of electron spin resonance that trapped free radicals did occur in polymethacrylate.

In our early studies of semiquinone free radicals (Adams, *et al.*, 1958) we had noticed that as the oxidation of the quinol starting materials came to an end, the solutions were dark and contained an insoluble material which proved to have a permanent paramagnetism.   The auto-oxidation of phenolic compounds inevitably results in the production of melanin-like, high molecular weight, insoluble, polymeric materials.   The electron spin resonance of these polymers is generally characterized by a single, usually structureless, absorption line, a g-value near 2, and a paramagnetism that is permanent.   In later studies on semiquinone free radicals, it appeared that there was a systematic correlation of g-value with the molecular structure of the radical (Blois, *et al.*, 1961) and that, in general, those molecules having a greater delocalization of the odd electron had lower g-values. The examination of natural melanins, however, showed that the g-values observed corresponded more closely to those of monomers or dimers. The concept that melanins were extensively conjugated was thus not borne out by the measurements on the free radical g-values. As far as the polymer structure of melanin was concerned there remained two possibilities: if melanin were highly conjugated, the electron spin resonance spectra might show no hyperfine structure (the number of interacting paramagnetic nuclei would be great, and the spectrum so complex as to be unresolved) and the g-value should be low; however, if melanin were not highly conjugated, one might expect to see the hyperfine structure due to the indolequinone (if as had been supposed, there were only one monomeric species) and to observe a free radical g-value corresponding to that of this monomer. Our results were inconsistent with either, and the Raper scheme, insofar as it implied a single monomer type, seemed an inadequate representation for melanin synthesis. We proposed that in any case the g-value results suggested that the odd electron was probably localized to the monomer or perhaps to a dimer (Vivo-Acrivos and Blois, 1958).

In 1960, Longuet-Higgins proposed a semiconductor model for melanin (based upon structures similar to Fig. 7.7) in which the odd electrons were supposed to be loosely bound to protons along the chain of the polymer. This explanation (that melanin was an intrinsic semiconductor) seemed unlikely because we had observed that the intensity of the melanin resonance did not appear to change as the temperature was lowered to that of liquid nitrogen. Mason, *et al.* (1960) reported in the same year on their electron spin resonance studies of natural melanins and included the observation on the changes in the resonance signal produced by the illumination of the pigment with ultraviolet light. In 1963 Cope, *et al.*, reported on the production of ESR signals in the melanin of eye granules when they were illuminated by visible light under physiological conditions, and they proposed that melanin may play a functional role in the visual process.

Meanwhile, new chemical data obtained by direct methods, and relating to the structure of melanin, was becoming available as the result of the work of Nicolaus and his group at Naples. His approach to the chemistry of melanin had been to employ strong oxidative degradation with such agents as potassium permanganate or hydrogen peroxide or, alternatively, the alkali fusion of natural melanins, and to identify by chromatography the degradation product of these melanins. By working backward from these separated and identified products, it was possible to determine the types of polymeric structure that could yield such products upon degradation. His

conclusions were the following (Nicolaus, 1962): for the case of sepia melanin there are probably several distinct but closely related monomers which
may number as many as 10; there are several bond types responsible for the
bonding of these monomers including carbon–carbon, peroxide, ether, carbon–nitrogen; each of the monomers was polyfunctional so that the melanin
chain could be branched at any monomer position and could also form a
three-dimensional structure; and that melanin probably consisted of a random structure. These features are shown in Fig. 7.8. It will be noticed

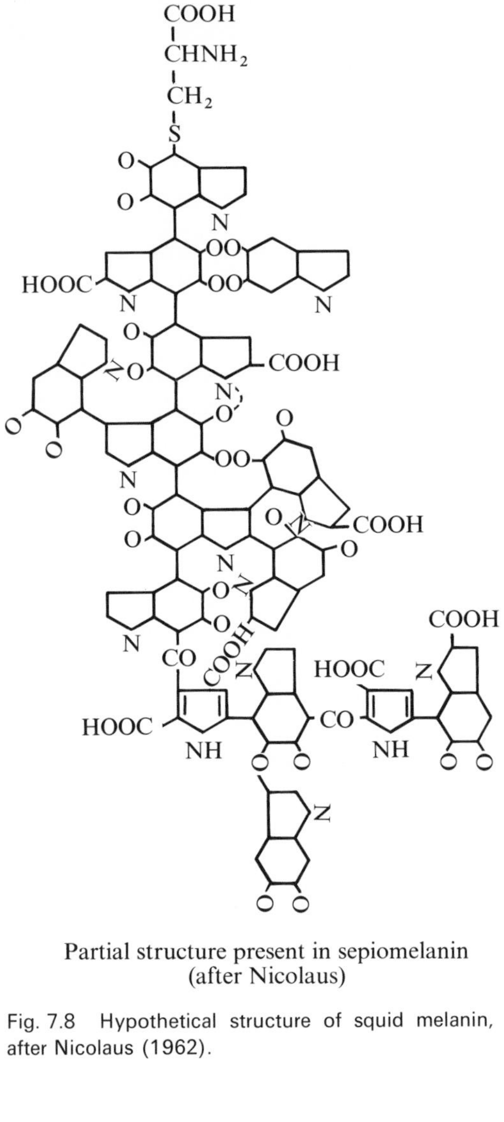

Partial structure present in sepiomelanin
(after Nicolaus)

Fig. 7.8 Hypothetical structure of squid melanin,
after Nicolaus (1962).

that in Nicolaus' proposed structure for melanin there is no conjugation, and that an unpaired electron produced on one monomeric unit would be constrained to remain there.   With this proposed model for melanin structure before us, electron spin resonance studies were then resumed with purified squid melanin.   The following observations were made (Blois, *et al.*, 1964):

(*a*) The electron spin density vs. temperature curve, down to $4°K$ was proportional to the reciprocal of the temperature.   That is, Curie's law was obeyed over this temperature range.

(*b*) Chemical treatment of the melanin:

  (i) Boiling in concentrated sulfuric acid for one hour left the resonance signal unchanged.

  (ii) Treatment with concentrated hydrochloric acid, or alcoholic potassium hydroxide left the absorption unchanged.

  (iii) Treatment with ascorbic acid produced a lightening in color (by virtue of a reversible reduction) but left the ESR signal unchanged.

(*c*) When the dry melanin was heated in air to $200°C$, there was no change in the absorption signal except for a slow loss of intensity as the sample was slowly burned away.

(*d*) Treatment with copper ion (or ferric ion).   The titration of an aqueous suspension of melanin with cupric ion gave a result shown in Fig. 7.9. It will be noted that at first the addition of continuing amounts of cupric ion has little effect upon the spin density but that as a critical value is reached a rapid decrease in spin density then sets in until the signal has entirely vanished.   When the ESR signal had been completely eliminated it was noted that the melanin had not been changed in color.   Thus the color and the paramagnetism of melanin are completely independent.

From the above experimental results we may conclude the following: the fact that the spin density is proportional to $1/T$ essentially rules out a model in which electrons thermally excited into a conduction band are responsible for the paramagnetism of the material.   An attempted explanation of the paramagnetism on the basis of an overlapping triplet-singlet model would require extensive conjugation, and one would expect the spin density to be affected by reducing agents which was contrary to the observations.   In addition, the g-value that we find for melanin is against extensive conjugation as is the hypothetical structure of Nicolaus which is derived from purely chemical studies.   An attempt to explain the paramagnetism on the basis of a charge transfer complex would lead to the result that the spin density should depend upon some activation energy and thus be proportional in an exponential manner to the temperature.   This again is not observed down to liquid helium temperatures.

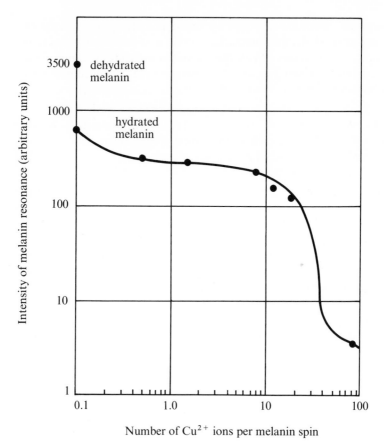

Fig. 7.9   Curve showing the decrease in the spin density of squid melanin upon the addition of Cu^{2+} ions.

Finally, the possibility that the paramagnetism of natural melanins may be due to transition element ions may be ruled out indirectly.   If one starts with metal free quinols and produces polymers autoxidatively, one can be assured there are no metal ions present; yet the polymers are paramagnetic and have the same ESR spectra as natural melanins.   We conclude therefore that the paramagnetism of melanin is probably due to trapped free radicals of the semiquinone type.   This conclusion is consistent with the hypothesis of Nicolaus regarding the structure of melanin.

7.4   BIOSYNTHESIS OF MELANIN

What do these chemical and ESR results imply about the *biosynthesis* of melanin?   The original Raper–Mason scheme, Fig. 7.6, indicates a linear reaction sequence leading from a given starting material to a fixed product. Nicolaus has proposed that this should be modified as indicated in Fig. 7.10 in which several intermediate compounds may go directly to the final product.   Since each of the compounds shown in the Raper–Mason scheme are diamagnetic stable quinones or quinols, and the net reaction is one of successive oxidation and reduction, between each of these compounds one

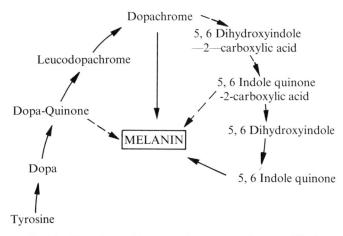

Fig. 7.10 Modified Raper–Mason pathway according to Nicolaus, showing condensation of intermediates with the polymer.

should expect a semiquinone, free radical intermediate to occur.   It may therefore be possible for any of these free radical intermediates to bond directly to the growing polymer.   This concept is shown in Fig. 7.11.

We may suppose, therefore, that melanin biosynthesis probably involves a free radical polymerization reaction.   The evidence supporting this view includes the following:

(a) The *in vitro* polymerization of DOPA and other precursors of melanin has been directly shown to involve free radical mechanisms by Wertz, *et al.* (1961).

(b) The random structure of melanin proposed by Nicolaus suggests a free radical synthesis rather than a conventional enzymatic one.

(c) One finds trapped free radicals in all natural melanins, synthetic melanins, and synthetic polymers which are prepared by a free radical polymerization.

How might one demonstrate this mechanism directly?   The electron spin resonance observation of melanogenesis *in vivo* would be extremely difficult because of the very slow rate at which this occurs and the small amounts of material present in living systems.   The indirect approach, to show that melanin synthesis, at least in part, may be non-enzymatic, might be an easier one.   One characteristic of an enzymatic synthetic pathway is the specificity of substrates.   One may therefore study melanin synthesis in a living system by supplying natural and non-natural melanin precursors which had been radioactively labelled, and then follow the course of the reaction by measuring the radioactivity incorporated into the pigment itself.   Figure 7.11 itself suggests such a possibility, that the aromatic free radicals may condense directly onto the polymer.

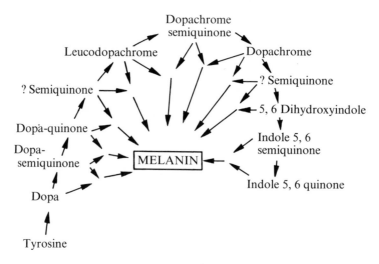

Fig. 7.11   Hypothetical scheme for melanin-synthesis assuming free radical addition reactions between the semiquinone intermediates and the diamagnetic forms.

We therefore chose a biological system in which melanin synthesis was proceeding rapidly, in the form of a transplantable mouse melanoma, which had occurred spontaneously in the animal colony of the Radiology Department at Stanford.   Figure 7.12 shows the biochemical pathway leading from phenylalanine and tyrosine on to melanin and shows the branch leading off to epinephrine synthesis.   The experimental approach taken was the following: one of the melanin precursors along this pathway was labelled with radioactive carbon and this was administered intraperitoneally to a series of mice.   At a fixed time after administration the animals were killed. Samples of tissues were taken and homogenized and known amounts of these tissues were then counted.   By this means the distribution of the administered radioactivity could be determined for each of the different tissues.

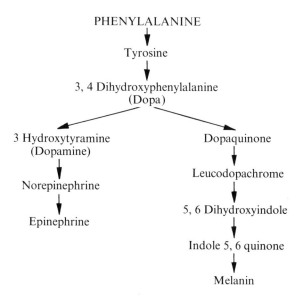

PHENYLALANINE

Tyrosine

3, 4 Dihydroxyphenylalanine
(Dopa)

3 Hydroxytyramine
(Dopamine)   Dopaquinone

Norepinephrine   Leucodopachrome

Epinephrine   5, 6 Dihydroxyindole

Indole 5, 6 quinone

Melanin

Fig. 7.12 The pathways of phenylalanine metabolism, leading to melanin and epinephrine.

Figure 7.13 shows the tissue distribution after the administration of carbon-14 labelled phenylalanine. While this amino acid lies on the pathway of melanin synthesis, it is also incorporated into proteins and can enter other biochemical pathways. It therefore might be expected that there would be nothing particularly specific about the tissue distribution of this material, and the figure shows that, indeed, this is the case. Figure 7.14 shows a similar distribution after the administration of carbon-14 labelled tyrosine.

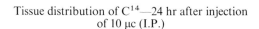

Tissue distribution of C^{14}—24 hr after injection
of 10 μc (I.P.)

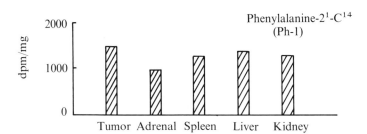

Phenylalanine-2^1-C^{14}
(Ph-1)

2000

dpm/mg

1000

0

Tumor Adrenal Spleen Liver Kidney

Fig. 7.13 The tissue distribution of radioactivity following the I. P. administration of C^{14} labelled phenylalanine to a melanoma-bearing mouse.

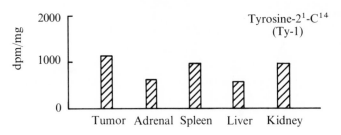

Fig. 7.14   As in Fig. 7.13, except C¹⁴ tyrosine was used.

Again, this amino acid is so widely used biochemically that its appearance in all tissues at comparable levels was not unexpected.   When carbon-14 DOPA was taken, the result obtained is that shown in Fig. 7.15.   Here the distribution shows a quite selective effect, with the radioactivity being concentrated primarily in the tumor tissue and in the adrenals.   Both of these would be expected from examination of the metabolic pathways in Fig. 7.12.

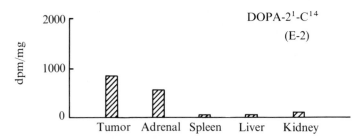

Fig. 7.15   As in Fig. 7.13, except C¹⁴ DOPA was used.

The data suggests that under our experimental conditions DOPA tends to be metabolized in the forward direction (i.e., onward to melanin or epinephrine) rather than backward to tyrosine.   If one then chooses a precursor beyond DOPA, for example dopamine, the results shown in Fig. 7.16 may be obtained.   Again, this conforms to the prediction of the metabolic pathway and shows too that the dopamine is metabolized onward primarily to epinephrine rather than undergoing the reverse reaction to DOPA and down the pathway to melanin.

It could easily be shown that the radioactivity in the melanoma tissue was largely in the melanin pigment. This pigment was extracted from the homogenate, acid-washed and purified, and shown to contain most of the tumor radioactivity. We are not aware of any evidence indicating that melanin pigment itself is metabolized or turned over. In those tissues in which synthesis occurs at significant rates, as in the skin or hair, the pigment is gotten rid of by exfoliation. In other tissue, such as the retinal pigment layer of the eye in which there is no means of eliminating the fully formed pigment, the evidence indicates that pigment synthesis occurs in the fetal stage, followed by a later period of inactivity.

Tissue distributions of C^{14}—24 hr after injection
of 10 μc (I.P.)

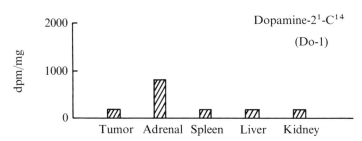

Fig. 7.16   As in Fig. 7.13, except C^{14} dopamine was used.

Radioactivity in the adrenals of these mice, however, is transient because the tagged epinephrine is metabolized. Figure 7.17 shows the results of an experiment in which labelled DOPA was administered to a series of melanoma-bearing mice at the same time, with the animals being serially sacrificed at the indicated later times. The adrenal radioactivity at the time the animals were autopsied is shown, and the curve indicates a turn-over of the labelled epinephrine with a biological half life of some 20 days. The behavior of DOPA does not, of course, distinguish between enzymatic or non-enzymatic synthesis since it is a natural substrate of melanin. To so distinguish it would be necessary to use non-natural melanin precursors and see whether these materials would be incorporated into the melanin pigment. When hydroquinone or catechol was administered the results indicated that there was no specificity as far as uptake is concerned; but the analysis of the pigment shows that radioactivity was present in the purified melanin in each case. These non-natural compounds are thus incorporated into the pigment which would not be expected if the synthesis were totally enzymatic.

What is the biological function of melanin? As far as it is known the answer seems to be that it is protective in one or more of a number of ways. In lower forms, melanin plays an essential role in mimicry, that is, in mechanisms of protective coloration as a means of survival; and in the ink sac of the squid, its employment appears to fall into this general category.   In man, it has a demonstrable effect in protecting him from solar ultraviolet radiation, although it is not the only means for affording this kind of protection.   It has been speculated that this protection extends beyond its mere opaqueness,

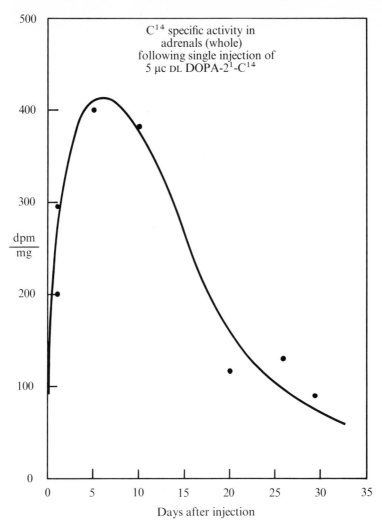

Fig. 7.17   Tissue radioactivity of mouse adrenals at various intervals following administration of C14 DOPA.

and that melanin granules may act as traps for free radicals generated by ultraviolet quanta.   The proposal that melanin may play a functional role in the visual process is an interesting one, but the evidence to date appears insufficient to prove the hypothesis.

7.5 CONCLUSION

The current concept of melanin, then, based upon recent physical and chemical studies is essentially the following: melanin is a unique biopolymer, random or highly irregular in structure, extending in three dimensions and forming large, insoluble, solid, non-hydrolyzable particles.   It is probably not metabolized but appears to form a permanent insoluble granule which must be excreted intact or else remains within the organism.   The pigment is synthesized by a mechanism that may well employ free radical mechanisms in part, and there is evidence suggesting that melanin synthesis may be relatively non-specific with respect to the type of substrate which may be incorporated.   Its striking feature is that it contrasts so sharply with other biopolymers such as proteins or nucleic acid, from which it differs so widely, chemically and physically, and, probably, in mode of synthesis.

ACKNOWLEDGEMENTS

Dr. A. B. Zahlan and Dr. J. E. Maling performed many of the ESR observations described herein.   The assistance of Mrs. Lina Taskovich and Mrs. Linda Jardine with the labelled melanin work is gratefully acknowledged. The experimental work was supported in part by the United States Public Health Service under Grants GM 10847 and CA 08064.

NOTE ADDED IN PROOF

Since the preparation of this chapter, newer experimental data have become available.   Nicolaus and co-workers have shown (*Tetrahedron*, **20**, 1163, 1964) that the plant melanins appear to be of the catechol type, while those of higher phyla are of the indole type.   In a study of the biosynthesis of melanin in the mouse melanoma, Hempel (*Structure and Control of the Melanocyte*, pp. 162–75, Ed. Della Porta and Muhlbock, Springer Verlag, New York, 1966) employed DOPA which had been labelled at various known positions and administered it to the mice.   The amount of radioactivity carried over into the melanin of the melanoma provided information as to whether there were any ring positions of the DOPA which were consistently involved in polymer formation.   It was concluded that no bonding position was consistently involved or excluded in melanin synthesis and that a number of different bonding configurations must occur.   This is in substantial agreement with Nicolaus's hypothesis regarding the non-uniformity of melanin structure.

Physical studies have yielded little additional information; continuing efforts with X-ray diffraction (upon unoriented melanin powders) have reaffirmed the amorphous nature of the melanin polymer though the diffuse rings seen appear to differ in spacing for the catechol and indole melanins (Thathachari, unpublished).   Electron microscopy has continued further to reveal the natural history of the pigment cell and the melanosome but has not yet contributed to the central problem of melanin structure.

REFERENCES

Adams, M., Blois, M. S. Jr., and Sands, R. H., 1958, *J. chem. Phys.*, **28**, 774.

Blois, M. S. Jr., Brown, H. W., and Maling, J. E., 1961, *Free Radicals in Biological Systems*, Ed. M. S. Blois, Jr., *et al.* (New York: Academic Press), Ch. 8.

Blois, M. S. Jr., Zahlan, A. B., and Maling, J. E., 1964, *Biophys. J.*, **4**, 471.

Bourquelot, E., and Bertrand, G., 1895, *C. r. Séanc. Sol. Biol.*, **47**, 582.

Commoner, B., Townsend, J., and Pake, G. E., 1954, *Nature*, Lond., **174**, 689.

Cope, F. W., Sever, R. J., and Polis, B. D., 1963, *Arch. Biochem. Biophys.*, **100**, 171.

Fraenkel, G. K., Hirshon, J. M., and Walling, C. J., 1954, *J. Am. chem. Soc.*, **76**, 3606.

Longuet-Higgins, H. C., 1960, *Archs Biochem. Biophys.*, **86**, 231.

Mason, H. S., 1948, *J. biol. Chem.*, **172**, 83.

Mason, H. S., Ingram, D. J. H., and Allen, B., 1960, *Archs Biochem. Biophys.*, **86**, 225.

Nicolaus, R. A., 1962, *Rass. Med. sper., Anno IX, Suppl.* No. 1.

Nicolaus, R. A., Piatelli, M., and Fattorusso, E., 1964, *Tetrahedron*, **20**, 1163.

Raper, H. S., 1928, *Physiol. Rev.*, **8**, 245.

Du Shane, G. S., 1938, *J. exp. Zool.*, **78**, 485.

Swan, G. A., 1963, *Ann. N. Y. Acad. Sci.*, **100**, 1005.

Vivo-Acrivos, J., and Blois, M. S. Jr., 1958, Paper presented at the Sheffield Meeting of the Faraday Society.

Wertz, J. E., Reitz, D. C., and Dravnieks, F., 1961, *Free Radicals in Biological Systems*, Ed. M. S. Blois, Jr., *et al.* (New York: Academic Press), Ch. 13.

CHAPTER EIGHT

SOME MEDICAL APPLICATIONS OF ELECTRON SPIN RESONANCE SPECTROSCOPY

S. J. Wyard

*Physics Department, Guy's Hospital Medical
School, London, England*

8.1 INTRODUCTION

This chapter will be mostly about electron spin resonance spectroscopy of *unirradiated* biological tissues, first observed by Commoner, *et al.* (1954). In these authors' pioneering experiments tissues were taken from a number of plants, insects, and animals and were lyophilized (freeze-dried) before being placed in the spectrometer. The spectra which were obtained were all alike, consisting of single lines, about 6 Oe wide, and with g-values close to the free electron value (see Fig. 8.1). This indicated that the spectra were due to free radicals, and not to paramagnetic metal ions, but gave no information about the nature of the free radicals. The free radical content, estimated from the spectra, varied between 10^{16} and 10^{18} radicals per gram dry weight.

In some tissues the spectra were due to melanin† and these radicals were resistant to heat and to refluxing in hydrochloric acid. In other tissues the free radicals appeared to be associated with protein components, as shown by fractionation experiments, and were easily destroyed by heating the tissues before lyophilization. Experiments with yeast and with seeds showed that in these materials an increase in metabolic activity was accompanied by an increase in free radical content. In animal tissues also, high metabolic activity, as is present in the liver or kidney, was accompanied by a high free radical content. In green leaves most of the radicals were shown to be due to the action of light. Finally, it was observed that the free radical content of mouse liver hepatoma was only two-thirds that of normal mouse liver.

Prior to these experiments Michaelis (1946) had stated: 'It will now be shown that all oxidations of organic molecules, although they are bivalent, proceed in two successive univalent steps, the intermediate being a free radical, . . .'. Commoner, *et al.* therefore proposed that the ESR spectra they observed which were heat-labile, associated with proteins and dependent on metabolic activity, were due to a small steady-state concentration of free radicals from oxidation-reduction processes.

The experiments of Commoner, *et al.* pointed the way to a number of ESR investigations of biological materials, some with possible medical applications. Before discussing these it will be necessary to consider techniques of measurement and interpretation of the spectra, because the free radical concentration is sufficiently low that sensitivity is a problem, and because the nature of the sample makes the interpretation of the spectra more difficult than for those discussed in the earlier chapters of this book.

8.2 TECHNIQUES OF MEASUREMENT

8.2.1 INTRODUCTION

The problem of sensitivity is due to the low concentration of free radicals coupled with the fact that the presence of water severely restricts the volume

† ESR of melanin is fully discussed in chapter 7.

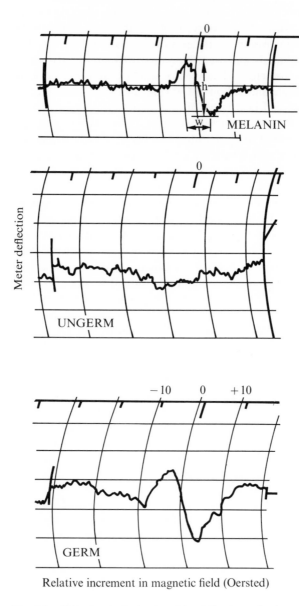

Relative increment in magnetic field (Oersted)

Fig. 8.1   ESR of melanin (top) and lyophilized germinating digitalis seeds (bottom). From Commoner, *et al.* (1954). (In this figure, and all the succeeding ones in this chapter, the first derivative of the absorption spectrum is plotted against the magnetic field strength. See chapter 1 for details of ESR spectra.)

of tissue which can be used, because of the high dielectric loss of water at microwave frequencies.   A few biological tissues are sufficiently dry that this restriction does not apply.   Shields, *et al.* (1956) obtained spectra from certain plant materials (cones, needles, leaves, and stems) taken straight from the plant or picked up from the ground, and placed directly in the spectrometer.   Ants, studied by Krebs and Benson (1965), and bone are other materials which are sufficiently dry to be used in this way.   But the number of such tissues is limited, and in most cases the water content is sufficiently high (e.g., 75% for liver) that special techniques have to be adopted.

Commoner, *et al.* (1954), working at a time when spectrometers were less sensitive than they are now, removed the water from the tissues by lyophilization, and thus increased the sensitivity by a factor which may be estimated as of the order of 100, when comparing free radical concentrations per gram wet weight of tissue.   This technique, which we shall call the *freeze-dry technique*, solved the problem of sensitivity but introduced a new problem; because the question naturally arises as to whether some or all of the free radicals observed are artefacts due to the freeze-drying process.   For this reason most workers nowadays use one of two other techniques.

Commoner, *et al.* (1956), using an improved spectrometer and a specially designed sample holder, obtained sufficient sensitivity to record spectra from a number of wet tissues.   This technique is generally known as the *surviving-tissue technique.*

A third technique, first used by Truby and Goldzieher (1958), consists in rapidly freezing fresh tissue down to a very low temperature (e.g., 77°K) and recording spectra at this temperature.   This will be called the *rapid-freeze technique.*

8.2.2   THE FREEZE-DRY TECHNIQUE

Since the sensitivity is adequate the use of the spectrometer is straightforward. A typical spectrum is shown in Fig. 8.1.   The main difficulty with this technique is the uncertainty about the nature and origin of the free radicals present in the lyophilized material.   Commoner, *et al.* (1954) proposed that the spectra found in lyophilized tissues, apart from special cases such as those due to melanin and those formed by light, were due to a steady-state concentration of semiquinone free radicals from oxidation-reduction processes; but it is not clear that such radicals would survive the freeze-drying process.   It is also conceivable, as mentioned earlier, that some or all of the radicals observed are artefacts produced by freeze-drying.   It has been shown, for example, that rapid freezing of polymers of high molecular weight breaks some of the bonds, giving ESR spectra (Berlin and Penskaia, 1956);

and it has been reported that freeze-drying whole human blood produces free radicals, probably due to breaking the porphyrin ring structure, as observed in the ESR spectrum (Varian Associates, 1957).

Further doubt on the nature of the free radicals in lyophilized tissues comes from an oxygen effect, discovered by Miyagawa, *et al.* (1958). These workers found that animal tissues, lyophilized and observed in vacuum, gave little or no ESR spectra, but after admission of air or oxygen a sizeable signal appeared. Removing the air or oxygen caused the spectra to largely disappear, to reappear again on re-admission of the gas. The spectra had a small asymmetry due to g-value anisotropy of the type expected for an unpaired electron localized on an oxygen molecule. The spectra appeared to be due to molecular oxygen weakly bonded to some site in the lyophilized sample.

Comparison of the two sets of experiments is made difficult because Miyagawa, *et al.* recorded their spectra at 23 GHz, and gave no values for radical concentrations, while Commoner, *et al.* recorded at 9 GHz where the effects of g-value anisotropy are much smaller. Allowing for the difference in frequency the two sets of spectra are very similar; also the order of relative intensity (liver > kidney > heart) was the same for those tissues which were observed in both cases. Presumably the samples studied by Commoner, *et al.* were exposed to air after lyophilization (this point is not made clear), and the same radicals were observed in both sets of experiments.

The oxygen effect was further investigated by Morozova and Bliumenfel'd (1960), who used liver and spleen from rats. They also obtained spectra with g-value anisotropy, but a much smaller oxygen effect. In fact, if the tissues were lyophilized without preliminary freezing, the oxygen effect was almost or completely absent. They suggested that the apparent absence of a spectrum *in vacuo* reported by Miyagawa, *et al.* might be due to the use of rapid freezing before lyophilization, coupled with an insensitive spectrometer. The concentration of free radicals found in rat liver by Morozova and Bliumenfel'd was 1–2.5×10^{17} spins per gram dry weight, similar to the value of 2×10^{17} spins per gram dry weight estimated by Commoner, *et al.* (1954) for lyophilized mouse liver.

A somewhat different oxygen effect was observed by Lion, *et al.* (1961) who worked with bacteria. *Eschericia coli* cells lyophilized and observed *in vacuo* gave little or no ESR spectrum, but on admission of oxygen a spectrum appeared within a few hours. Unlike the experiments with animal tissues, the spectrum from bacteria remained stable after removal of oxygen by re-evacuation. The concentration of free radicals was about 2×10^{16} spins per gram dry weight, i.e., about ten times smaller than in the animal tissues. Similar results were obtained by Dimmick, *et al.* (1961) with other bacteria, *Serratia marcescens*, *Sarcina lutea*, and *Micrococcus radiodurans*, although here the size of the signal only increased two or three times on admission of oxygen, and the maximum concentration of radicals was approximately 10^{15} spins per gram dry weight.   The signal did not decrease upon re-evacuation of the sample.

A fresh approach to the problem of identifying the free radicals in lyophilized tissues was made recently by Kalmanson, et al. (1965).   These authors compared lyophilized tissues with model systems consisting of various quinones, phenols, and heteroaromatic compounds which can form semiquinone free radicals in solution, absorbed on cellulose and proteins. The ESR spectrum was the same in each case.   Furthermore, if evacuated samples were exposed to moist oxygen, the signal increased by about five times to a maximum, and subsequently decreased.   It is of interest that, irrespective of the moisture content of the oxygen, the maximum signal always occurred when the water content of the sample was about 5%, corresponding to the normal 'bound water'.   Replacing oxygen by argon in slightly moistened samples reduced the free radical concentration by a factor of 2–3; subsequent replacement of oxygen restored the concentration almost to its previous level.   The kinetics of the growth and decay of the concentration of radicals was practically identical in lyophilized tissue and in the model systems.   The authors conclude, in agreement with the proposal of Commoner, et al. that the free radicals in lyophilized tissues are derived from enzyme co-factors such as flavins, naphthoquinones, ascorbic acid, ubiquinones, phenols, and flavones of plants, which are present in a semi-oxidized form.   One finding, which was contrary to the results of Commoner, et al. (1954), was that boiling tissues for several hours before lyophilization did not remove the ESR signal.

It is clear that there are enough uncertainties associated with the freeze-dry technique for other techniques to be desirable.

8.2.3   THE SURVIVING-TISSUE TECHNIQUE

In this technique, introduced by Commoner, et al. (1956), the organs to be studied are removed from the animals as rapidly as possible and stored on cracked ice.   Frozen samples have been stored on dry ice for 3–4 weeks without any change in the radical concentration.   Tissue slices, about 0.5 mm thick, are cut when required, and about 50 mg (wet weight) is suspended in either a 5% glucose or in a saline solution contained in a flat ESR cell.   The spectrum is recorded on a high sensitivity 9 GHz spectrometer, usually at room temperature.

The chief difficulty with this technique is in obtaining an adequate signal-to-noise ratio, and there has been considerable discussion on the optimum design of the ESR cavity and associated cell (Commoner, et al., 1956;

Commoner and Ternberg, 1961; Cook and Mallard, 1963; Stoodley, 1963a, b; Wilmshurst, 1963; Commoner, 1965; Horsfield, 1966). It was shown by Stoodley that for spectrometers operating in the microwave region (3 GHz and upwards) optimum sensitivity with aqueous samples is obtained by using a rectangular H_{012} cavity (one wavelength long), and a flat cell extending across the cavity with a thickness 0.31 mm and a volume of 0.072 ml at 9 GHz. Calculations similar to Stoodley's are given in chapter 5, section 5.3.   With a longer cavity the optimum sample thickness increases slightly (but is still less than 1 mm for a cavity 15 wavelengths long), but the sensitivity decreases monotonically as the cavity length increases.   However, several workers with biological tissues have used cells 1 mm thick in cavities several wavelengths long, and claim that the advantages of more space in the cell and less critical positioning of the cell in the cavity more than compensate for the loss of sensitivity.   Stoodley also showed that, having chosen the optimum size for cell and cavity, the sensitivity increases with frequency over the microwave region.   The variation in sensitivity is small, and between the practical limits of 3 and 37.5 GHz the increase is only by a factor of 4.3. Moreover, at the higher frequencies the cell becomes very thin, and would be difficult to use with biological tissues.

    With the optimum size of cavity and cell the sensitivity for an aqueous sample at 9 GHz, under standard conditions of 1 mW power and 1 sec time constant, may be calculated as $4 \times 10^{13} \Delta H$ spins per ml ($6 \times 10^{-8} \Delta H$ M). This assumes a sensitivity of $5 \times 10^{11} \Delta H$ spins for a point sample (see chapter 1, section 1.4) and allows for the reduction in sensitivity due to the finite size of the sample and due to the dielectric loss of water. ΔH is about 10 Oe for biological tissue, so the minimum detectable concentration is 4×10^{14} radicals per ml.   Since the free radical concentration in many surviving tissues is of the order of 6×10^{14} radicals per ml (and is considerably less in some tissues) there is a problem of sensitivity.   However, the power level can be raised, since the radicals do not saturate very easily in solution; and it is also possible to increase the time constant.   With a sufficiently stable spectrometer the time constant may be increased to 100 sec (Horsfield, 1966); some workers have kept the time constant short and summed a number of repeated sweeps of the spectrum on a multi-channel analyser (Vithayathil, et al., 1965; Mallard and Kent, 1966).   In this way the sensitivity may be increased by two orders of magnitude, which will be adequate for all tissues, provided the sensitivity is not impaired by other factors such as instability of the spectrometer, or paramagnetic impurities in the cell or cavity.

    Stoodley's analysis does not apply to spectrometers operating at much lower frequencies, where the cell and cavity used are quite different.   At 280 MHz, Hill and Wyard (1967) obtained a sensitivity of $1.5 \times 10^{14} \Delta H$ radicals per ml in an aqueous sample of 10 ml volume (i.e., four times lower than the sensitivity at 9 GHz).   Because less attention has so far been paid to low

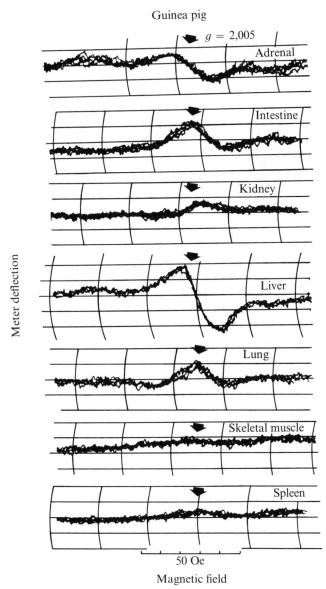

Fig. 8.2   ESR of surviving guinea-pig tissues. Each signal represents superimposed tracings of 3–6 successive runs. From Commoner and Ternberg (1961).

frequency spectrometers it is possible that their sensitivity for aqueous samples may be improved to equal that of the high frequency spectrometers. One possible advantage of working at low frequencies is that it would be easy to oxygenate the solution while recording. This cannot be done in the narrow cells used at high frequencies, so all measurements made so far on surviving tissues have been under essentially anaerobic conditions.

Spectra obtained from surviving tissues are usually single lines with a g-value very close to 2, as shown in Fig. 8.2. The peak-to-peak width is 14 Oe (Mallard and Kent, 1966). In these samples dipolar broadening from the protons in the water molecules would contribute from 6 to 10 Oe to the line width (Wyard, 1965). Allowing for this broadening the spectra are very similar to those in lyophilized tissues, and probably come from the same radicals. However, the concentrations are much lower in surviving tissues; thus for mouse liver the freeze-dry technique gave 4.5×10^{16} radicals per gram wet weight (Commoner, et al., 1954) while the surviving tissue technique gave 2.7×10^{15} radicals per gram wet weight (Commoner and Ternberg, 1961), or nearly 20 times lower.

ESR spectra from surviving tissues are indistinguishable from those given by free radicals in redox enzyme systems, such as succinic dehydrogenase, β-hydroxybutyrate dehydrogenase, and cytochrome reductase, or in mitochondrial particles which contain such systems; moreover the relative intensity of the ESR spectra correlates with the known distribution of mitochondria in mammalian tissues (Commoner and Ternberg, 1961). Thus there is little doubt that the spectra are due to semiquinone free radicals associated with redox enzyme systems. There are certain differences between the temperature dependence of the ESR intensity of surviving tissues and of mitochondrial particles or enzymes isolated from them. However, the ESR intensity is proportional to the steady state concentration of those enzyme co-factors which are in the semi-oxidized free radical form, and this depends on a number of parameters which are likely to differ between intact tissue and isolated systems. The difference in intensity between surviving tissues and lyophilized samples may similarly be due to the freeze-drying process putting more of the enzyme co-factors into the free radical form.

8.2.4   THE RAPID-FREEZE TECHNIQUE

The spectrometer sensitivity is adequate with this technique, being of the same order as for dry samples. In fact, if measurements are made at $77°$K, there is a gain in sensitivity of a factor of four, due to the Boltzmann factor, although this may be offset by a smaller sample volume due to the Dewar arrangements. However, Truby and Goldzieher (1958) were able to use samples of 1.7 g.

The spectrum includes a line due to free radicals with a g-factor very lose to 2 and a peak to peak line width at 9 GHz of 14 Oe for animal issues (Kerkut, et al., 1961). This is the same as for surviving tissues, and a large contribution to the line width is similarly due to the water present in he sample. Very few measurements of radical concentration have been eported for this technique, but Truby and Goldzieher (1958) found that for at liver the concentration of radicals per gram wet weight was five times smaller than for freeze-dried tissue. This is in approximate agreement with he observation of Commoner and Ternberg (1961), who found that the spectrum from surviving guinea-pig kidney increased in intensity by a factor of two as the temperature was lowered from 36 to 0°C, and persisted in the rozen tissue; presumably the intensity would not change on lowering the emperature of the frozen tissue to 77°K. Thus the spectrum seems to be lue to the same free radicals as in the surviving tissue technique, although here may be small differences in the concentrations.

It has been observed that the free radical concentration of excised issue kept at room temperature decays by as much as 50% during the first hour (Kerkut, et al., 1961). At higher temperatures the decay is still more apid. However, it is possible to cool the tissue down to 1-5°C in 1-2 min, and to 77°C within 5 min (Brennan, et al., 1965); and there should be very little radical decay during this time.

The possibility of this technique producing ESR spectra as artefacts should also be borne in mind. Brennan, et al. (1965) have discussed the question of damage to tissues by freezing, and conclude that injuries are minimal and that, in fact, the rapid-freeze technique may provide the best conditions for studying ESR spectra.

As well as the line at $g = 2$ due to free radicals, frozen tissue frequently gives a broad spectrum due to paramagnetic metal ions (Fig. 8.3). Swartz and Molenda (1965) showed that either part of the spectrum could be brought out by adjustment of the level of power incident on the sample. In fact, spectra a and b of Fig. 8.3 were recorded from the same specimen, the power being attenuated by 20 dB in going from a to b. Paramagnetic metal ions are not normally observed in surviving tissues (although Mallard and Kent (1966) reported lines at $g = 2.01$ and possibly $g \sim 4$ in tumors which they attributed to paramagnetic metal ions) and this can be explained by the lower sensitivity of this technique. They have not been observed in freeze-dried material either, apart from whole blood (Varian Associates, 1957), although it is probable that spectra from paramagnetic metal ions would be found in other lyophilized tissues if a search was made for them. Paramagnetic metal ions have been observed in naturally dry tissues: copper and manganese in plant materials (Shields, et al., 1956), manganese, and possibly iron in ants (Krebs and Benson, 1965).

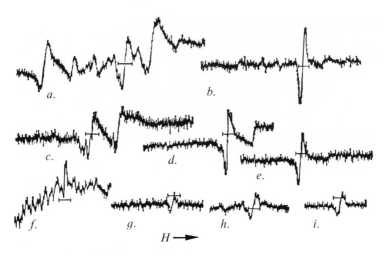

$H \longrightarrow$

Fig. 8.3   ESR of animal tissues at 77°K, showing effect of saturation. From Swartz and Molenda (1965). The markers indicate the position and width of the DPPH (free radical) spectrum. *a*: Liver at 'normal' power; *b*: liver at 20 dB attenuation from 'normal' power; *c*: heart at 'normal' power; *d*: heart at 10 dB attenuation; *e*: heart at 20 dB attenuation; *f*: lung at 'normal' power; *g*: lung at 20 dB attenuation; *h*: liver at 10 dB attenuation; *i*: liver at 20 dB attenuation.

8.2.5   COMPARISON OF THE THREE TECHNIQUES

To summarize the conclusions of the previous sections, the conditions in the surviving-tissue technique are closest to normal, which is presumably the state one is interested in.   The measurements are made however under essentially anaerobic conditions, and it would be interesting to compare the effect of oxygenating the solution, which would be possible with a low frequency spectrometer; although it should be borne in mind that Commoner and Ternberg (1961) found no difference if the sample was saturated by either O_2 or N_2 immediately before recording the spectrum.   The sensitivity is adequate for free radicals in most tissues, but may be too low for some tissues, and for paramagnetic metal ions generally.

The rapid-freeze technique gives considerably greater sensitivity. Although no detailed comparison has yet been made in any one laboratory, it seems that the concentration of radicals is similar to that in surviving tissues.   There are differences, which although small could be important. For example, the free radical concentration is very low, usually undetectable, in surviving tumor tissues; but when the rapid-freeze technique is used a small concentration is clearly present, being, in the case of rat hepatoma, about one-third of the concentration in the corresponding normal tissue (Truby and Goldzieher, 1958). With the freeze-dry technique there is still less difference between tumor and normal tissue, the radical concentration in mouse hepatoma being two-thirds of that in mouse liver (Commoner, et al., 1954). The rapid-freeze technique is suitable for accurate measurements of radical concentrations, since the Q of the cavity is very little affected by small changes in the size, shape, and position of the sample. It is essential for the study of paramagnetic metal ions.

The freeze-dry technique was important historically, but is of less value now, partly because the free radical concentrations obtained differ considerably from those obtained with the other two techniques, and partly because the concentrations depend considerably on the details of the freeze-drying process. Because of its great sensitivity, it may still be useful for a preliminary survey.

8.2.6 INTERPRETATION OF THE SPECTRA

Interpretation is difficult because the conditions of the sample are unfavorable to good resolution. There is no possibility of orienting the radicals in a given direction and, although liquid suspensions can be used (in the surviving-tissue technique), the radicals will usually be bound to large protein molecules which prevents the rapid tumbling required for averaging out any anisotropy in the spectrum. Moreover, there may be a number of different paramagnetic species present in the sample.

The possibility of artefacts must not be overlooked. These include contamination by paramagnetic and ferromagnetic ions (Blois, et al., 1963; Maling, et al., 1963); production of free radicals by mechanical damage (Ulbert, 1962); changes due to freeze-drying (Varian Associates, 1957).

A determination of the concentration of radicals or paramagnetic metal ions responsible for the spectra is straightforward, and the techniques are discussed in some detail in chapters 1 and 3. The possibility of the presence in the sample of other radicals and ions which do not give detectable spectra because the lines are too broad should always be borne in mind.

It is usually possible to distinguish between free radicals and paramagnetic metal ions. The main criterion is that free radicals have spectra with g-values very close to the free spin value of 2.00232. The biggest divergencies, up to 3%, occur when the unpaired electron is located mainly on an oxygen or a sulfur atom. Paramagnetic metal ions, on the other hand, commonly have wide variations in g-value, e.g., from 1.93 to 6 for iron in proteins. However, some metals can give a line close to $g = 2$ which could be mistaken for a free radical, and in such cases a second criterion to use is that of power saturation. Free radicals, because of their weak spin-orbit coupling, have long relaxation times and saturate easily, whereas paramagnetic metal ions tend to have short relaxation times and are difficult to saturate. The difference is very clearly shown in Fig. 8.3.

The importance of saturation has not been recognized in all work on ESR of biological tissues. It is of course essential to avoid saturation when measuring concentrations. When making saturation measurements the key parameter is the amplitude of the microwave magnetic field at the sample, and this depends on such factors as the design of cavity and the microwave frequency as well as on the level of incident power (see chapter 1 for a fuller discussion). Furthermore, the relaxation time, which determines the saturation behavior, depends on the environment of the radical or ion. In general, it is shorter in liquids than in solids, and in solids it is generally shorter at room temperature than at low temperature. If the relaxation time is sufficiently short the ESR line is broadened (as explained in chapter 1) and may become undetectable. For this reason the spectra of some paramagnetic metal ions are only observed at low temperature.

Having distinguished between free radicals and paramagnetic metal ions, the next logical step would be to identify the individual species; but this is seldom possible, especially for the free radicals.

Spectra of paramagnetic metal ions in biological samples are very complex. A useful compilation of spectra, including those of copper, iron (Fe^{2+} and Fe^{3+}), manganese, molybdenum, cobalt (Co^{2+} and Co^{3+}), and vanadium (V^+, V^{3+}, and V^{4+}) appeared in a recent review by Beinert and Palmer (1965). It may be possible to identify paramagnetic metal ions in tissue samples by comparison with such spectra.

The free radical part of the spectrum is usually the same for all tissues, consisting of a single featureless line from which no identification is possible. Careful measurements of the g-value and line width, and observation of the line shape may enable spectra from different samples to be distinguished and correlated with other biological observations. Occasionally hyperfine splitting has been observed.[†] This implies that the spectrum is either isotropic, or that the radical is tumbling with sufficient rapidity for the anisotropic parts of the hyperfine interaction and g-value variation to be averaged out. The condition for this is

$$\tau_c \ll \frac{1}{\delta} \quad \text{(Pake, 1962)}$$

where δ is the anisotropic term expressed in frequency units, and τ_c is the correlation time, which is a measure of the rate of tumbling. τ_c may be

[†] Any doubt as to whether particular lines in the spectrum are due to hyperfine splitting or to g-value variation can be resolved by recording the spectrum again at a different microwave frequency.

approximated by the expression $4\pi\eta a^3/3kT$, where η is the viscosity of the fluid, and a is the radius of the radical. For small radicals (e.g., semi-quinones) in a non-viscous fluid (e.g., water) the condition is met; but it is not met for large molecules such as proteins. In biological tissues, it is likely that most semiquinones will be bound to proteins sufficiently firmly to prevent tumbling, although looser forms of attachment are also possible (Griffith and McConnell, 1966). There is also the possibility of resolved hyperfine splitting due to free rotation of part of a molecule (e.g., a methyl group), even though the rest of the molecule is firmly fixed, as discussed in chapter 4.

Melanin, if present, may be distinguished from other free radicals by its much greater stability. It is unaffected by boiling, a procedure which irreversibly destroys the rest of the free radical spectrum.†

8.3 ESR OF BIOLOGICAL TISSUES

8.3.1 NORMAL TISSUES

ESR spectra of normal tissues will be surveyed first, both for their own interest and also as a standard with which to compare pathological tissues.

Spectra have been reported for a large variety of animal tissues, including adrenal (d, t), blood (e, k, u), bone (a, b, p), brain (e), collagen (b), heart (d, e, g, i, k, l, n, q), intestine (d), kidney (d, e, g, i, j, k, l), lens (g), liver $(c, d, e, f, g, i, j, k, l, m, n, q, r, s, v)$, lung (d, e, g, k, o, q), lymph node (g), muscle (d, e, k), skin (g), spleen (c, d, g, h, k, l, m), and thymus (g). (References are: a: Becker, 1963; b: Becker and Marino, 1966; c: Brennan, et al., 1965; d: Commoner and Ternberg, 1961; e: Commoner, et al., 1954; f: Cook and Mallard, 1963; g: Detmer, et al., 1967; h: Kalmanson, et al., 1965; i: Kerkut, et al., 1961; j: Mallard and Kent, 1964; k: Mallard and Kent, 1966; l: Miyagawa, et al., 1958; m: Morozova and Bliumenfel'd, 1960; n: Nebert and Mason, 1963; o: Rowlands, et al., 1967; p: Swartz, 1965; q: Swartz and Molenda, 1965; r: Ternberg and Commoner, 1963; s: Truby and Goldzieher, 1958; t: Truby and Goldzieher, 1960; u: Varian Associates, 1957; v: Vithayathil, et al., 1965.)

With very few exceptions the surviving-tissue technique gives spectra which are identical for all animal tissues and appear as in Fig. 8.2. Slight variations in g-value (from 2.001 to 2.005) and in line width (13–14 Oe

---

† The disappearance of the non-melanin free radical spectrum following heating of tissue samples to temperatures up to 100°C was reported by Commoner and Ternberg (1961) using the surviving-tissue technique and by Kerkut, et al. (1961) who used the rapid-freeze technique. There is some doubt on the effects of heating the tissues prior to lyophilization, when the freeze-dry technique is used, since Commoner, et al. (1954) suggest that the non-melanin signal disappears, while Kalmanson, et al. (1965) claim that it is only slightly affected.

between points of inflexion) are probably within the experimental errors for lines with such a poor signal-to-noise ratio. The spectra are characteristic of free radicals and the only further information to be obtained from them is the concentration of spins.

Table 8.1 lists the concentrations of free radicals measured in a number of tissues with the surviving-tissue technique. Very few values of concentrations of free radicals based on either of the other two techniques have been published, but as was stated earlier the rapid-freeze technique gives similar values while the freeze-dry technique gives values 10–20 times larger. Although the relative concentrations differ somewhat depending on the technique used, it appears that, if the tissues are arranged in order according to the concentration, this would be the same for all three techniques.

Table 8.1 *Free radical concentrations in normal tissues measured with the surviving-tissue technique (Radicals × 10^{15}/g wet weight)*

Tissue	Guinea-pig	Rat	Mouse	Man
Liver	3.9 ± 0.9 (a)	2.9 ± 1.1 (a) 3 (c) 5.1 ± 0.4 (d)	2.7 ± 0.6 (a)	3(b)
Kidney	1.9 ± 0.6 (a)	1.5 (c) 3.4 ± 0.2 (d)	1.1 ± 0.3 (a)	
Heart	1.5 ± 0.8 (a)	1.4 ± 0.3 (a) 2.8 ± 0.3 (d)	1.1 ± 0.3 (a)	
Spleen		0.6 ± 0.1 (d)		
Lung		0.5 ± 0.1 (d)		
Muscle		0.8 ± 0.2 (d)		
Blood		0.1 (d)		

Authors: (a) Commoner and Ternberg (1961); (b) Ternberg and Commoner (1963); (c) Mallard and Kent (1964); (d) Mallard and Kent (1966).
(*Note.* Differences of a factor of two between the values of Commoner and Ternberg and those of Mallard and Kent are ascribed by the latter authors to a calibration error.)

It was noted by Commoner, *et al.* (1954) that there appeared to be a relationship between the concentration of free radicals in a tissue and its rate of metabolic activity. The experiments of Truby and Goldzieher (1960) showed that the relationship, if it exists, is not a simple one, since neither stimulation of guinea-pig adrenals by adrenocorticotrophin hormone nor suppression by hydrocortisone phosphate had much influence on the intensity of the ESR spectrum of the adrenal tissue.

A closer parallel can be drawn between concentrations of free radicals and concentrations of mitochondria in animal tissues, as Commoner and Ternberg (1961) pointed out. These authors found that ESR spectra were undetectable in liver, kidney, or heart from newborn rats, were small one day after birth, and approached a constant intensity after about 8 days.† This parallels a similar increase in the concentration of mitochondria and the level of succinoxidase activity, observed by Dawkins in rat liver (1959). These parallels, coupled with the similarity of the tissue spectra with those from isolated mitochondria and from redox enzyme systems found in mitochondria led Commoner and Ternberg to the conclusion that the origin of the spectra is in fact the enzymatic redox activity occurring in mitochondrial particles.   Hence it might be said that ESR spectroscopy of free radicals in normal animal tissues is merely a sophisticated way of measuring the mitochondrial population, and has not yet yielded any new biological information.

In addition to the single line at $g = 2.003$, a few other ESR spectra with g-values close to 2 have been reported for normal tissues.   Thus adrenal tissue from guinea-pigs gives two extra lines situated about 40 Oe on either side of the main line (see Fig. 8.2 for the spectrum), although adrenal tissue from rat and from man gives only a single line (Commoner and Ternberg, 1961).   Mallard and Kent (1966) observed an asymmetry in the spectrum from rat liver and also, to a lesser extent, in that from rat kidney.   Brennan, et al. (1965) reported a minor signal at $g = 2.02$ in normal and in regenerating liver from mice.   All these spectra are barely visible above the noise level, and little can be said about them.

Further spectra from normal tissue were obtained by Nebert and Mason (1963) and by Swartz and Molenda (1965), by using the rapid-freeze technique, and recording at high power.   Nebert and Mason recorded good spectra from mouse liver and from cardiac muscle, and from mitochondria and from rough and smooth microsomes taken from mouse liver, which extended from $g = 1.90$ to 2.50, and in some cases to 4.3 (see Figs. 8.4 and 8.5).   These spectra included a line at $g = 2.00$ due to free radicals, and the rest of the spectra were due to paramagnetic metal ions, chiefly iron and copper.   The spectrum from cardiac muscle is similar to that from mitochondria; the liver spectrum is a summation of spectra from mitochondria and microsomes.   ESR spectra from mitochondria and from microsomes are discussed in the review by Beinert and Palmer (1965). Swartz and Molenda obtained similar spectra from heart and liver taken from a dog (see Fig. 8.3).

There have been a number of investigations into ESR spectra from bone and its constituents (Swartz, 1965; Becker, 1963; Becker and Marino,

† Brennan, et al. (1965) working with mice and using the rapid-freeze technique, found a similar increase in the intensity of ESR spectra from liver during the first few days of life; although with spleen the intensity was 2–3 times higher in 2 and 3 days old mice than in adult (6 months old) animals.

1966).   The spectra are complex, and when whole bone is used they vary
with the orientation of the bone axis in the magnetic field of the spectrometer.

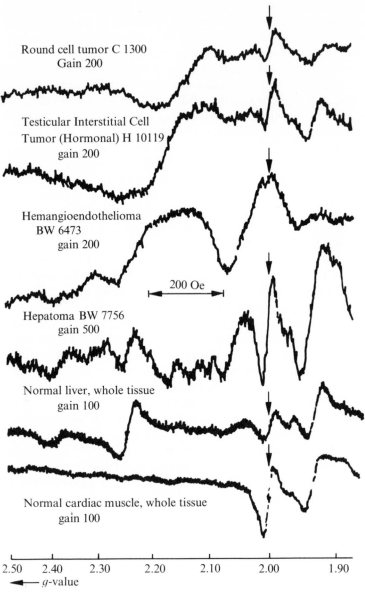

Fig. 8.4   ESR of various mouse tumors, together with normal liver and heart
tissue, recorded at 77°K. Magnetic field increases from left to right, and the
arrow indicates a g-value of 2.00232. From Nebert and Mason (1963).

The spectra have similarities with those from geological apatite, but cannot be attributed entirely to apatite in the bone.

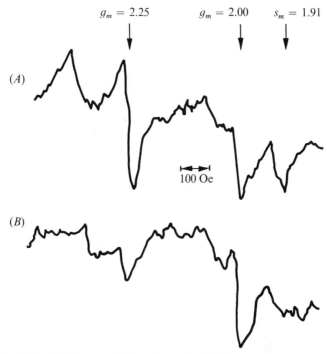

$g_m = 2.25$ $\qquad$ $g_m = 2.00$ $\qquad$ $s_m = 1.91$

(A)

100 Oe

(B)

Fig. 8.5   ESR of normal (A) and neoplastic (B) mouse liver smooth microsomes, recorded at 77°K. From Nebert and Mason (1963).

8.3.2   CANCER

Several investigators have noted significant differences between ESR spectra from cancer tissues and from the corresponding normal tissues.

One common observation is a reduction in the free radical signal at $g = 2.003$, although there is considerable variation in the extent of the reduction.   In their original studies using the freeze-dry technique, Commoner, *et al.* (1954) estimated the free radical concentration in cancer tissue as two-thirds of that in the corresponding normal tissue.   Later, using the surviving-tissue technique, Commoner and Ternberg (1961) reported that neoplastic tissues had relatively low, or wholly undetectable, free radical contents.   This finding was confirmed by Mallard and Kent (1964, 1966), also using the surviving-tissue technique, who found that the free radical signal was absent from cancer tissue (with an upper limit of 10% of normal intensity), with the single exception of a spontaneous kidney carcinoma, for which the free radical intensity was 30% of normal.

Somewhat in contrast with these results, the rapid-freeze technique gives easily observable free radical signals from cancer tissues, even though the intensity is lower than normal. Thus Truby and Goldzieher (1958) found the free radical content in rat hepatoma tissue to be about one-third of that in rat liver. Brennan, *et al.* (1965) also found a reduction, but only to two-thirds normal for infiltrated liver, although to one-quarter for infiltrated spleen. Nebert and Mason (1963) recorded spectra of 29 mouse tumors of different types, all of which included a free radical line. However, these authors did not measure the concentrations.

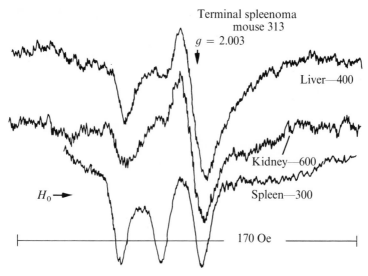

Fig. 8.6   ESR of liver, kidney, and spleen from a mouse in the terminal phase of spleen tumor. Recorded at 77°K. From Brennan, *et al.* (1965).

Whether or not there is a conflict between the results for the two techniques (a point that can only be settled by more careful measurement), there is agreement that the free radical line is less intense; and this seems to reflect the relative absence of mitochondria in many tumors.

The spectra from paramagnetic metal ions also differ for cancer tissues. The 29 spectra recorded by Nebert and Mason show an almost bewildering complexity and variation, and in most cases no attempt was made to compare them with spectra from normal tissues. A few examples, with two normal tissues for comparison, are reproduced in Fig. 8.4. A detailed study was made on one tumor, a hepatoma, for which ESR spectra from mitochondria and from rough and smooth microsomes were compared with those from normal tissue components (see Fig. 8.5 for one such comparison). This comparison established that lines occurring at $g = 1.91$ and 2.25, which are due to a particular iron compound in microsomes, are about three times weaker in hepatoma microsomes than in normal liver microsomes. There was no significant difference in the spectra from mitochondria.

Since it has been suggested that there are similarities between the metabolism of cancer tissue and that of embryonic tissue (one example being the relative lack of mitochondria in either) it would be of interest to compare the spectra of Nebert and Mason with those recorded from fetal tissue.

Brennan, *et al.* (1965, 1966) also used the rapid-freeze technique, but

Neuroblastoma 16 days in transplant

A/JAX ♀ C 1300

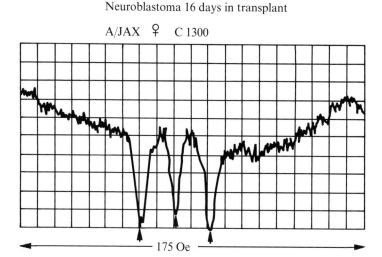

◄─────────────── 175 Oe ───────────────►

Fig. 8.7   ESR of a mouse neuroblastoma, recorded at 77°K. From Brennan, *et al.* (1965).

concentrated on the portion of the spectrum close to $g = 2$. They observed, for the first time with animal tissues, spectra showing hyperfine splitting. The lines are separated by 17.3 ± 0.5 Oe and the g-value is 2.013 for the central line (Figs. 8.6 and 8.7). These spectra were obtained in samples from nodular spleens of mice taken 10–14 days after transplantation of a reticulum-cell sarcoma, and also in a tumor of quite a different origin, a transplantable neuroblastoma. It was verified, by recording the spectra at a different frequency, that the three lines shown in Figs. 8.6 and 8.7 are due to hyperfine splitting; and they probably result from coupling with a nitrogen atom.

Mallard and Kent (1966) also found differences for cancer tissues, in particular a strong line, corresponding to a concentration of 14×10^{15} spins/g wet weight, at $g = 2.016$ in a liver carcinoma induced by butter yellow (dimethyl aminoazobenzene). Metastases of the liver tumor showed this line in even greater concentration, and also a weaker one at $g = 4$. These lines were not detected in normal tissues, nor in the other tumors examined. They were attributed to paramagnetic metal ions, probably iron or molybdenum, and were thought to be due to these metals existing in the tumor in a different valency state, rather than with a different concentration, from that in normal tissues.

Up to this point ESR studies of cancer are of interest as reflecting the differences of metabolism between tumor tissue and normal tissue. An observation of a different kind has recently been made by Vithayathil, et al. (1965).

In this experiment, tumors were induced in the livers of rats by feeding them with a diet containing a carcinogen, either p-dimethyl aminoazobenzene (butter yellow), thioacetamide, or 2-acetylaminofluorene. At intervals of a few days animals were taken from the experimental groups and also from a control group on a normal diet, and ESR spectra of liver samples recorded, using the surviving-tissue technique. One set of spectra is shown in Fig. 8.8. In all the groups on the carcinogenic diet a new ESR line appeared at $g = 2.035$, which had not been observed before in any other tissue. This line, which was in addition to the normal line at $g = 2.005$, appeared a little time after the commencement of the diet, grew to a maximum which was of the same order of intensity as the normal line, and then disappeared again. The time scale for the appearance and disappearance of the new ESR line is proportional to the time required for tumors to appear with the different carcinogens. In each case the new line disappears well before tumors appear, and appears at a very early stage when histological changes are minimal and non-specific, so that this ESR line is the first sign of an approaching tumor. The origin of the new ESR line is not known. Because it is the same for three different carcinogens it seems unlikely to be due to a radical derived from the carcinogen itself, but it may be due to some constituent of the cell.

These recent experiments are sufficiently encouraging to warrant further work on cancer tissues, and suggest that ESR spectroscopy may have three applications: (a) to investigate differences of metabolism between cancer tissues and normal tissues, (b) to provide information on the mechanism of the induction of tumors, (c) to provide an early warning system for the detection of cancer in suspicious but not clearly malignant tissues.

In connection with this last application Hodgkinson and Cole (1965), who recorded spectra from 112 specimens of normal and malignant tissues from the cervix and vagina of 77 patients, reported at the annual meeting of the American College of Obstetricians and Gynaecologists that 'in tissue samples from patients with atypical or presumably precancerous Papanicolaou smears there appears to be an increase in free radical concentration over the normal state as revealed by ESR results'.

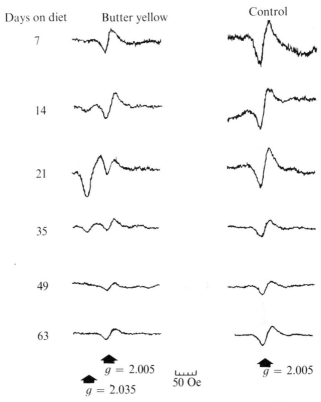

Fig. 8.8   ESR of rat liver, recorded at 15°C. The left-hand spectra are from rats fed on a diet containing butter yellow; the right-hand spectra are from rats on a normal diet. The absolute heights of the different spectra are not comparable. From Vithayathil, *et al.* (1965).

8.3.3   JAUNDICE

The application of ESR to jaundice springs from the empirical observation of Commoner and Ternberg (1961), who were surveying a number of human liver samples obtained by biopsy during various surgical procedures, that samples from cases of jaundice due to obstruction of the extra-hepatic bile ducts gave spectra about three times as intense as those from normal human liver.   Examples of the spectra are shown in Fig. 8.9, where it will be seen

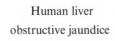

Human liver
obstructive jaundice

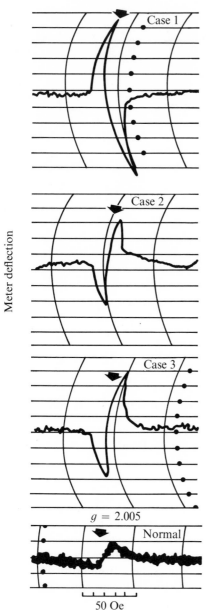

Fig. 8.9   ESR of human liver from three cases of extra-hepatic jaundice, compared with normal human liver. Spectra recorded with surviving-tissue technique. From Commoner and Ternberg (1961).

that the spectra are no different from those of most other biological tissues, except for being more intense.

The initial observation was followed up by the same workers (Ternberg and Commoner, 1963) in a clinical trial covering 65 cases, of which 12 were obstructive jaundice, 8 were non-obstructive jaundice and the other 45 were not jaundice cases and were used as controls.   About 50 mg of tissue was used for the ESR measurements, an amount which is obtainable by needle biopsy.   Spectra were recorded and free radical concentrations determined using the surviving-tissue technique.   For the non-jaundiced patients the concentrations varied between 1.3 and 6.0 $\times$ 10^{15} radicals per gram wet weight, with an average of 3 $\times$ 10^{15}; this is similar to the concentrations found in the livers of laboratory animals.   For the patients with non-obstructive jaundice the concentrations varied between 0 and 7.2 $\times$ 10^{15} radicals per gram wet weight, with an average of 2.9 $\times$ 10^{15}, and were thus very similar to the non-jaundiced patients.   With obstructive jaundice the variation was from 4.8 to 25.8 $\times$ 10^{15} radicals per gram wet weight; with the exception of two overlapping cases the radical concentrations in the livers of patients with obstructive jaundice were higher than in any of the other patients.

In the series reported here an operation was carried out because the cause of jaundice was uncertain, and the diagnosis was confirmed at the operation.   The ESR measurements would have discriminated correctly in the case of 18 patients out of 20, and given a doubtful verdict in the other 2. Since the present methods of clinical diagnosis are sometimes incapable of giving the correct differential diagnosis of jaundice, there would seem to be considerable value in the use of ESR measurements as a laboratory test.

8.4   OTHER MEDICAL APPLICATIONS OF ESR

This section is a brief survey of ESR investigations of other substances, not biological tissues, which may have a medical application.   The results are mostly speculative or else not yet of proven value.

8.4.1   CARCINOGENS

For many years there have been suggestions that certain chemical compounds are carcinogenic because of their ability to exist in a radical form (Kensler, et al., 1942).   ESR spectra of free radicals derived from chemical carcinogens can be obtained in a number of ways (Lipkin, et al., 1953; Kon and Blois, 1958).   Interest in free radicals as possible causes of cancer still persists (Ingram, 1958; Szent-Györgyi, et al., 1960) although there is no direct evidence for this hypothesis.

One carcinogen which has been the subject of a number of investigations by ESR is tobacco smoke.   Lyons, *et al.* (1958) passed tobacco smoke through a tube immersed in liquid oxygen and obtained a pale yellow condensate which gave an ESR spectrum with an intensity corresponding to 10^{15} free radicals per gram.   By warming the condensate to 60°C for about 5 min, refreezing, and recording the spectrum a second time, it was discovered that most of the radicals were relatively unstable; but about a sixth, which were present in a tarry component, were very stable.   Observations in this laboratory (Wyard, 1960) on tar from tobacco smoke showed that the free radicals are present in solid particles, and are probably due to charring. Lyons, *et al.* also reported that the concentration of stable free radicals in soot, which is well known to be another carcinogen, is about one hundred times larger than in cigarette smoke.

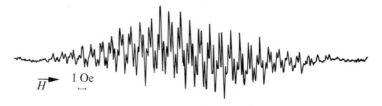

Fig. 8.10   ESR of 3, 4-benzpyrene, heated in vacuum to 197°C. From Forbes and Robinson (1967).

Marsden and Collins (1963) repeated the measurements of Lyons, *et al.* and obtained similar results.   They found that there was a variation in the free radical concentration in smoke from one type of tobacco to another, and that this was paralleled by α-particle activity in the tobacco. They therefore suggested that α-particle radiation in the leaf should be considered as an alternative to pyrolysis as the cause of the free radicals.

Two recent experiments have thrown further interesting light on free radicals in tobacco smoke.   Forbes and Robinson (1967) discovered that certain polynuclear hydrocarbons give very well resolved ESR spectra when heated to temperatures above their melting points.   Figure 8.10 shows one such spectrum, that of 3, 4-benzpyrene, heated in vacuum to 197°C.   Admitting air to the heated compound gives rise to another spectrum; and neither spectrum is identical with the spectra of benzpyrene anion or cation radicals.   Since tobacco smoke condensate includes 3, 4-benzpyrene, which is a well-known carcinogen, and since the carcinogenicity of the condensate is reported to be greater than that of its components, the authors suggest that the increased carcinogenicity might be due to reactive radicals, such as those giving the spectrum of Fig. 8.10, which are produced by heating.

Rowlands, *et al.* (1967) drew cigarette smoke directly into freshly excised lung from rabbits. The lung tissue was quickly homogenized and examined with the rapid-freeze technique, giving the spectrum shown in Fig. 8.11. Figure 8.11 shows a pattern of three lines superimposed on a broader resonance which appears to arise from a different species. The three line pattern is reminiscent of the triplet observed by Brennan, *et al.* in certain cancer tissues, and reproduced in Figs. 8.6 and 8.7.

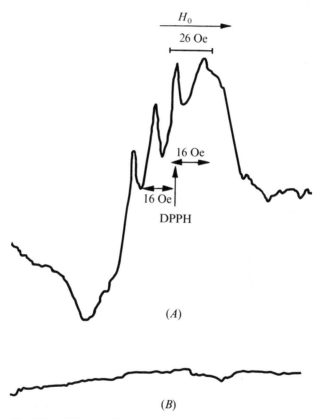

Fig. 8.11   ESR of rabbit lung which has smoked six cigarettes (*A*) compared with normal lung (*B*). Spectra recorded at 77°K. From Rowlands, *et al.* (1967).

The production of free radicals by charring organic materials in general has been extensively investigated (Ingram, 1958). Foodstuffs are no exception, and free radicals are present in high concentration in common foods such as toast (Wyard, 1960). Whether this has any medical significance is quite unknown at present.

8.4.2 TRANQUILIZING DRUGS

Tranquilizing drugs such as chlorpromazine, which are derivatives of phenothiazine, can readily form semiquinone free radicals, which can then be detected and measured by ESR. This fact has been developed into a method of monitoring the level of drug concentration in the blood of patients (Piette, *et al.*, 1964). Although much work had previously been done on drug levels in the urine, little was known about concentrations in the blood, and existing methods of assay were unsuitable in this case. Serum, obtained from blood samples by centrifugation, was placed in a flat quartz cell in the ESR cavity and photolyzed by a 200 watt u.v. lamp *in situ*. Presence of the drug gives rise to the spectrum shown in Fig. 8.12, which is about 5 Oe wide,

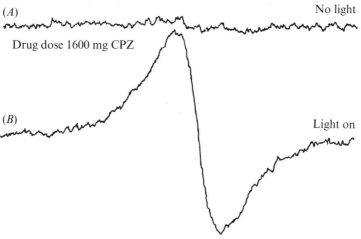

Fig. 8.12   ESR of serum containing tranquilizing drug. From Piette, *et al.* (1964).

with a *g*-value of 2.0053. On extinction of the u.v. lamp the spectrum disappears rapidly. The free radical concentration in the sample can be obtained by double integration of the spectrum, and the method is well suited to monitoring changes in drug level, although it is difficult to obtain the absolute concentration of the drug. It was also discovered that the presence of ascorbic acid in the serum could be simultaneously detected as an ascorbate radical produced by u.v. irradiation. The ascorbate radical spectrum is a doublet of splitting 1.7 Oe and *g*-value 2.0043 (Fig. 8.13), and so can easily be distinguished from the spectrum due to the drug. Since there is an interest in ascorbate levels in psychiatric patients, it is an advantage of the ESR method that it can measure the concentration of this as well as of the drug.

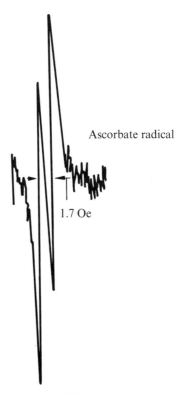

Ascorbate radical

1.7 Oe

Fig. 8.13   ESR of ascorbate radical produced by photolysis of serum. From Piette, *et al.* (1964)

REFERENCES

Becker, R. O., 1963, *Nature*, Lond., **199**, 1304–5.

Becker, R. O., and Marino, A. A., 1966, *Nature*, Lond., **210**, 583–8.

Beinert, H., and Palmer, G., 1965, *Adv. Enzymol.*, **27**, 105–98.

Berlin, A. A., and Penskaia, Ye. A., 1956, *Dokl. Akad. Nauk. SSSR*, **110**, 585–8.

Blois, M. S., Jr., Maling, J. E., and Taskovich, L. T., 1963, *Biophys. J.*, **3**, 275.

Brennan, M. J., Singley, J. A., and Cole, T., 1965, Ford Motor Company Scientific Laboratory, Dearborn, Michigan, U.S.A., Technical Report SL 65–60; 1966, *Proc. Soc. exp. Biol. Med.*, **123**, 715–8.

Commoner, B., 1965, *Instrument News* (Perkin-Elmer Corporation, Norwalk, Connecticut, U.S.A.), **16**, 1–10.

Commoner, B., Heise, J. J., and Townsend, J., 1956, *Proc. natn. Acad. Sci.*, *U.S.A.*, **42**, 710–8.

Commoner, B., and Ternberg, J. L., 1961, *Proc. natn. Acad. Sci., U.S.A.*, **47**, 1374–84.

Commoner, B., Townsend, J., and Pake, G. E., *Nature*, Lond., **174**, 689–91.

Cook, P., and Mallard, J. R., 1963, *Nature*, Lond., **198**, 145–7.

Dawkins, M. J. R., 1959, *Proc. R. Soc.*, B, **150**, 284–97.

Detmer, C. M., Driscoll, D. H., Wallace, J. D., and Neaves, A., 1967, *Nature*, Lond., **214**, 492–3.

Dimmick, R. L., Heckly, R. J., and Hollis, D. P., 1961, *Nature*, Lond., **192**, 776–7.

Forbes, W. F., and Robinson, J. C., 1967, *Nature*, Lond., **214**, 80–1.

Griffith, O. H., and McConnell, H. M., 1966, *Proc. natn. Acad. Sci. U.S.A.*, **55**, 8–11.

Hill, M. J., and Wyard, S. J., 1967, *J. scient. Instrum.*, **44**, 433–6.

Hodgkinson, C. P., and Cole, T., 1965, *J. Am. med. Ass.*, **192**, Adv. 31–2.

Horsfield, A., 1966, *Wld. med. Electronics*, **4**, 4–5.

Ingram, D. J. E., 1958, *Free Radicals as Studied by Electron Spin Resonance* (London: Butterworth Scientific Publications).

Kalmanson, A. E., Trotsenko, V. L., Chumakov, V. M., and Kharitonenkov, I. G., 1965, *Dokl. Akad. Nauk. SSSR*, **161**, 1212–5.

Kensler, C. J., Dexter, S. O., and Rhoads, C. P., 1942, *Cancer Res.*, **2**, 1–10.

Kent, M., and Mallard, J. R., 1964, *Nature*, Lond., **204**, 396–7.

Kerkut, G. A., Edwards, M. L., Leech, K., and Munday, K. A., 1961, *Experentia*, **17**, 497–8.

Kon, H., and Blois, M. S., Jr., 1958, *J. chem. Phys.*, **28**, 743–4.

Krebs, A. T., and Benson, B. W., 1965, *Nature*, Lond., **207**, 1412–3.

Lion, M. B., Kirby-Smith, J. S., and Randolph, M. L., 1961, *Nature*, Lond., **192**, 34–6.

Lipkin, D., Paul, D. E., Townsend, J., and Weissman, S. I., 1953, *Science*, N. Y., **117**, 534–5.

Lyons, M. J., Gibson, J. F., and Ingram, D. J. E., 1958, *Nature*, Lond., **181**, 1003–4.

Maling, J. E., Taskovich, L. T., and Blois, M. S., Jr., 1963, *Biophys. J.*, **3**, 79.

Mallard, J. R., and Kent, M., *Nature*, Lond., **204**, 1192; 1966, *ibid.*, **210**, 588–91.

Marsden, E., and Collins, M. A., 1963, *Nature*, Lond., **198**, 962–4.

Michaelis, L., 1946, Fundamentals of oxidation and reduction. In: *Currents in Biochemical Research*, ed. D. E. Green (New York: Interscience Publishers).

Miyagawa, I., Gordy, W., Watabe, N., and Wilbur, K. M., 1958, *Proc. natn. Acad. Sci. U.S.A.*, **44**, 613–7.

Morozova, G. K., and Bliumenfel'd, L. A., 1960, *Biophysics*, **5**, 273–6.

Nebert, D. W., and Mason, H. S., 1963, *Cancer Res.*, **23**, 833–40.

Pake, G. E., 1962, *Paramagnetic Resonance* (New York: W. A. Benjamin, Inc.).

Piette, L. H., Loeffler, K. O., Green, D. E., and Bulow, G. A., 1964, *Report to U.S. National Institute of Mental Health*, Contract No. PH-43-65-547.

Rowlands, J. R., Cadena, D. G., Jr., and Gross, A. L., 1967, *Nature, Lond.*, **213**, 1256–8.

Shields, H., Ard, W. B., and Gordy, W., 1956, *Nature, Lond.*, **177**, 984–5.

Stoodley, L. G., 1963a, *J. Electron. Control*, **14**, 531–46; 1963b, *Nature, Lond.*, **198**, 1077.

Swartz, H. M., 1965, *Radiat. Res.*, **24**, 579–86.

Swartz, H. M., and Molenda, R. P., 1965, *Science, N.Y.*, **148**, 94–5.

Szent-Györgyi, A., Isenberg, I., and Baird, S. L., Jr., 1960, *Proc. natn. Acad. Sci. U.S.A.*, **46**, 1444–9.

Ternberg, J. L., and Commoner, B., 1963, *J. Am. med. Ass.*, **183**, 339–42.

Truby, F. K., and Goldzieher, J. W., 1958, *Nature, Lond.*, **182**, 1371–2; 1960, ibid., **188**, 1088–90.

Ulbert, K., 1962, *Nature, Lond.*, **195**, 175.

Varian Associates, 1957, *EPR at work*, No. 8, Palo Alto, California, U.S.A.

Vithayathil, A. J., Ternberg, J. L., and Commoner, B., 1965, *Nature, Lond.*, **207**, 1246–9.

Wilmshurst, T. H., 1963, *Nature, Lond.*, **199**, 477–8.

Wyard, S. J., 1960, Electron spin resonance spectroscopy. In: *Tools of Biological Research*, ed. H. J. B. Atkins (Oxford: Blackwell's Scientific Publications); 1965, *Proc. phys. Soc.*, **86**, 587–93.

CHAPTER NINE

THE STUDY OF BIOLOGICAL MOLECULES BY DIELECTRIC METHODS

Edward H. Grant

Department of Physics, Queen Elizabeth College, London, England

9.1 INTRODUCTION

Most molecules of biological interest possess an electric dipole moment which, in general, gives rise to a high dielectric constant and a well defined dispersion region. The behavior of a pure polar liquid is shown in Fig. 9.1 where it is noticed that the dielectric constant (ε') falls from a high value ε_s to ε_∞ as the frequency increases through the dispersion region. When dispersion occurs, there is a phase lag between the motion of the dipoles and the applied field, with a consequent loss of energy. The lower curve in Fig. 9.1 shows the variation of the energy absorption per cycle (ε''), the frequency corresponding to maximum absorption being termed the relaxation frequency, f_s. Corresponding to this parameter is a relaxation wavelength, $\lambda_s = c/f_s$, and a relaxation time, $\tau = \lambda_s/2\pi c$, where c is the velocity of light.

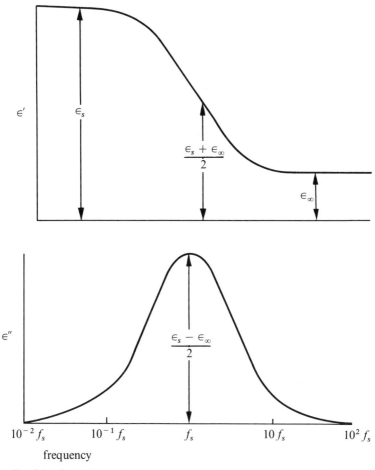

Fig. 9.1   Dispersion and absorption curves for a pure polar liquid (upper and lower curves respectively.)

297

Both ε' and ε'' may be combined in the form of a complex dielectric constant $(\hat{\varepsilon})$ where

$$\hat{\varepsilon} = \varepsilon' - j\varepsilon''. \tag{9.1}$$

As will be explained in more detail later the quantities ε_s, ε_∞, τ, and the dispersion curve shape are all related to various molecular parameters, so that a study of the dielectric behavior of a substance can be used to provide information at a molecular level. At present it should be noted that τ is a measure of the time the dipoles would take to reach a random distribution on removal of a static field which, on a macroscopic level, corresponds to the time taken for the polarization (defined as the electric moment per unit volume of material) to drop to $1/e$ of its initial value.

9.2 DIELECTRIC THEORY

In practice, the investigation of dielectric behavior entails the measurement of ε' and ε'' as a function of frequency and temperature from which the dispersion parameters may be deduced. These, in turn, are interpreted in terms of structure. For a biological material this may be quite a complicated procedure due to the possible presence of several dispersion regions which, in some cases, may overlap. Thus Schwan (1957) has shown for muscle that there are at least three dispersions (α, β, and γ) which occur at Hz, kHz–MHz, and GHz frequencies respectively, and recent work by both Schwan (1965) and Grant (1965a) on protein solutions reveals the existence of another (δ) dispersion occurring between the β and γ regions.

The simplest case is a single dispersion region with a single relaxation time which conforms to the Debye (1929) equations

$$\varepsilon' = \varepsilon_\infty + \frac{\varepsilon_s - \varepsilon_\infty}{1 + (\lambda_s/\lambda)^2} \tag{9.2}$$

$$\varepsilon'' = \frac{\varepsilon_s - \varepsilon_\infty}{1 + (\lambda_s/\lambda)^2} \frac{\lambda_s}{\lambda} \tag{9.3}$$

which are derived from

$$\hat{\varepsilon} = \varepsilon' - j\varepsilon'' = \varepsilon_\infty + \frac{\varepsilon_s - \varepsilon_\infty}{1 + j(\lambda_s/\lambda)}. \tag{9.4}$$

Pure water is an approximation to the above case although a small distribution of relaxation times is also possible. When a spread of relaxation times exists, several distribution functions are available leading to appropriate modification in equations (9.2) and (9.3). For example, Cole and Cole (1941) have deduced the following equation for the case of a distribution of relaxation times

$$\hat{\varepsilon} = \varepsilon' - j\varepsilon'' = \varepsilon_\infty + \frac{\varepsilon_s - \varepsilon_\infty}{1 + \left[j(\lambda_s/\lambda)\right]^{1-\alpha}} \qquad (9.5)$$

from which ε' and ε'' may be obtained.   The parameter α is a measure of the spread of relaxation times and lies between 0 and 1, the former value corresponding to the case of a single relaxation time.   The effect of a positive α on the shape of the ε'' v. log λ curve is to depress the maximum value of ε'' at wavelengths far removed from λ_s on either side of it.

A common way of representing results is to plot ε'' against ε' (a Cole–Cole plot) which will result in a semicircle with its center on the ε' axis if the Debye equations are obeyed.   If, on the other hand, the dielectric behavior approximates more to equation (9.5) a semicircle will be obtained with its

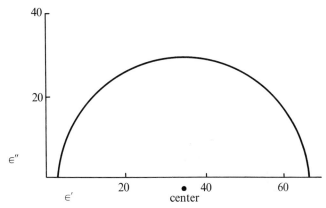

Fig. 9.2   Cole–Cole circle for human serum albumen.

center below the axis.   Another possibility is a skewed arc (Davidson and Cole, 1950).   If two overlapping dispersions are present, the shape of the Cole–Cole plot will be suitably modified.   The Cole–Cole diagram is an invaluable first method of analysis of dielectric results for providing the investigator with the first clue towards the understanding of the nature of the dispersion, or dispersions, present.   However, it should always be followed up by a mathematical analysis to obtain the true picture.   The Cole–Cole plot for an aqueous solution of human serum albumen at microwave frequencies is shown in Fig. 9.2 where it may be noticed that a small distribution of relaxation times is present.

Having now obtained the macroscopic dielectric parameters, the very much more difficult problem of their interpretation in terms of molecular quantities must be discussed.   First of all, let us consider the kind of relation that we should expect to be present between dielectric behavior and molecular structure.   The discussion in the rest of this section and, indeed, in the rest of the chapter will be devoted primarily to liquids since most measurements on biological materials have been concerned with the liquid state.   However, the arguments used are quite general and could equally well be applied to polar solids where the molecules have freedom of rotation as, for example, in the case of ice.

The static dielectric constant (ε_s) is dependent upon the molecular dipole moment (μ) and the type of short-range structure present.   For a simple system such as a polar gas or a very dilute solution of polar molecules in a non-polar solvent the evaluation of the dipole moment μ does not present much difficulty.   In such circumstances the Debye (1929) equation may be used

$$P = \frac{\varepsilon_s - 1}{\varepsilon_s + 2} \frac{M}{d} = \frac{4\pi}{3} N\left(\alpha + \frac{\mu^2}{3kT}\right) \tag{9.6}$$

where P is the molar polarization, M is the molecular weight in grams, d is the density, N is Avogadro's number, and α is the molecular polarizability or moment induced per molecule per unit field.   It can be seen that the polarization can be split up into two parts corresponding to induced dipoles and permanent dipoles, the former being due to atomic and electronic displacement.

Unfortunately, an equation such as (9.6) is unsuitable for biological liquids owing to inadequacies in the assumptions made concerning intermolecular forces.   When formulating equation (9.6) Debye accepted the Clausius–Mossotti expression for the electric field (E_i) acting on a given molecule in a dielectric

$$E_i = \frac{\varepsilon_s + 2}{3} E \tag{9.7}$$

where E is the external applied field.   Onsager (1936) showed that the Clausius–Mossotti value for the applied field should be replaced by

$$E_i = \frac{3\varepsilon_s}{2\varepsilon_s + 1} E \tag{9.8}$$

from which he deduced the following equation for μ in terms of ε_s:

$$\mu^2 = \frac{9kT}{4\pi s} \frac{(\varepsilon_s - n^2)(2\varepsilon_s + n^2)}{\varepsilon_s(n^2 + 2)^2}. \tag{9.9}$$

where n is the refractive index in the far infrared, and s is the number of molecules per ml.   Re-arrangement of equation (9.9) shows that a good approximation to a straight line may be expected if a plot is made of ε_s against $s\mu^2/T$, and this has proved to be the case for many pure polar liquids.

Evidently, Onsager's theory shows that the dominant term in the expression for dielectric constant should be the square of dipole moment of the molecule in the gaseous state (μ), but reference to Table 9.1 should make clear how

Table 9.1   *Dielectric properties of some hydrides*

Substance	Static dielectric constant at 20°C (ε_s)	Vapor dipole moment (μ) (debye)	Hydrogen bond strength (kcal/mole)	Polymerization
HCN	115	2.93	4.6	Linear trimer
H_2O	80	1.84	4.5	?
HF	65	1.94	6.7	Ring structures
H_2S	4	0.95	—	None

wide the departure from this law may be.   For the four liquid hydrides listed, the variation in molecular dipole moment is about a factor of three and the corresponding dielectric constant variation is nearly 30.   Reasons for this variation in ε_s are suggested in the last two columns of the table. Thus, although oxygen and sulfur are in the same group of the Periodic Table, the one striking difference between water and hydrogen sulfide is the lack of polymerization and hydrogen bond formation in the latter.   Hydrogen fluoride has a larger molecular dipole moment than water and exhibits polymerization but in the form of curvilinear aggregates or ring structures which have a small effective dipole moment.   For a completely symmetrical ring structure the dipole moment would be zero, as for benzene.   Hydrogen cyanide in many ways presents the most fascinating case of the four with a dielectric constant of 115 at 20°C increasing to a value as high as 213 at $-15°C$.   This unusual situation is attributable to the existence of linear trimers (Pauling, 1960) with an effective dipole moment of 8.8 debye.†
From the temperature dependence of ε_s the hydrogen bond strength is calculated by Cole (1955) as 4.6 kcal/mole.   It may therefore be concluded that the unmodified Onsager equation breaks down with hydroxylic liquids which precludes its use for biological molecules, where hydrogen bonds play such an important part.

The nature and role of the hydrogen bond will be discussed later in this chapter.   Various attempts have been made to modify Onsager's equation, the most well known being due to Kirkwood (1939):

$$\frac{(\varepsilon_s - 1)(2\varepsilon_s + 1)}{9\varepsilon_s} = \frac{4\pi s}{3}\left(\alpha + \frac{g\mu^2}{3kT}\right). \tag{9.10}$$

† The debye unit is 10^{-18} e.s.u. of electric dipole moment.

The factor g is called the correlation parameter and equals unity for a molecule undergoing free rotation. The departure of g from unity is a measure of the degree of intermolecular attraction and its value must be deduced from a model for the liquid structure. An alternative representation of (9.10) is to write $m \cdot m^*$ in place of $g\mu^2$, where m is the molecular dipole moment in the liquid and m^* is the vector sum of m and the induced moment in the surrounding environment.

The above discussion has been concerned with explaining the main principles involved in the formulation of a dielectric theory. For further information the very readable book by Mansel Davies (1965) should be consulted. More advanced approaches are contained in Böttcher (1952) and Smyth (1954).

It follows in the case of associated liquids, that from a given set of dielectric data it may be possible to envisage several alternative molecular models that fit the facts equally well. Often it is helpful to combine the dielectric data with data obtained from other experimental techniques in order to exclude some interpretations and to reinforce others. The above examples were restricted to small inorganic molecules but, later on in this chapter, the same kind of ideas will be extended to molecules of biological interest. It should not be assumed, however, that a large ε_s necessarily implies the existence of permanent dipoles; other mechanisms of polarization exist which give rise to high dielectric constants but which have nothing to do with dipole rotation. An example of this is the Maxwell–Wagner effect which will be mentioned later.

We must now go on to consider the use of dielectric dispersion measurements and, in particular, the relaxation time, τ_m, or relaxation wavelength, λ_s. As mentioned above, the value of τ_m is a measure of the time that the relaxing unit, which is not necessarily one molecule, takes to rearrange itself. The most simple case is that of a spherical molecule rotating in a continuum, the macroscopic analogy being that of a ball-bearing rotating in oil. For such a case Debye (1929) derived the following expression

$$\tau = 4\pi a^3 \frac{\eta}{kT} \qquad (9.11)$$

in which η is the viscosity of the continuum, a is the radius of the rotating molecule and T is the absolute temperature. Here τ is the molecular relaxation time which is not necessarily the same as the macroscopic relaxation time referred to previously. However, Powles (1953) has shown that τ_m and τ are not very dissimilar, the maximum value of τ_m/τ being 1.5. Equation (9.11) would be expected to hold for large polar molecules in a solvent whose molecules are much smaller, or for a pure polar liquid if the assumed molecular model is a reasonably good approximation to reality.   An example of the former case would be a protein solution.

In practice, it is relatively rare to find relaxation behavior adequately represented by equation (9.11) and it is necessary to correlate relaxation time with some other molecular phenomenon.   For hydrogen bond forming substances it is possible to derive a relationship between the relaxation time and the probability of a bond breaking (Haggis, *et al.*, 1952).   In contrast to this, some liquids may form clusters of molecules and the lifetime of the clusters may be related to the relaxation time (Frank and Wen, 1957).   All three of these possibilities will be considered in the section on water.

Dielectric relaxation may be alternatively assumed to be a process whereby the rotating unit moves between two equilibrium positions separated by a potential barrier.   According to this picture, the relaxation time will be a measure of the number of times per second that such a process will occur and, accordingly, Eyring (Glasstone, *et al.*, 1941) derived the expression

$$\frac{1}{\tau} = \frac{kT}{h} e^{-\Delta F/RT} = A\,e^{-\Delta F/RT} \tag{9.12}$$

where ΔF is the molar free energy of activation and the other symbols have their usual significance.

From thermodynamic considerations

$$\Delta F = \Delta H - T\,\Delta S \tag{9.13}$$

where ΔS is the entropy of activation and ΔH is the enthalpy (or heat) of activation.   Since the variation of A with temperature is much less than the exponential term, a plot of $\ln \tau$ against $1/T$ produces an approximate straight line whose slope provides ΔH and whose intercept gives ΔS.   These two quantities can then be related to structure since ΔH is a measure of bond strength and ΔS is related to local disorder (section 9.4).

In conclusion it should be pointed out that relaxation behavior can occur which has nothing to do with rotating dipoles.   The Maxwell–Wagner (Maxwell, 1892; Wagner, 1913) effect occurs when there is a heterogeneous mixture of components which have different dielectric constants and different conductivities.   When the whole medium is subjected to an electric field, charges take a finite time to build up on the interfaces separating the various components and relaxation is observed.   The relaxation time is given by the expression

$$\tau = \frac{2\varepsilon_1 + \varepsilon_2}{4\pi(2\sigma_1 + \sigma_2)}. \tag{9.14}$$

This equation corresponds to a suspension of particles of dielectric constant

ε_1 and conductivity σ_1 in a continuum whose corresponding parameters are ε_2 and σ_2.

The initial part of this chapter has been devoted to explaining the essentials of dielectric theory and showing how, in general, the dielectric behavior may be related to molecular structure. Detailed discussion has been deliberately postponed until later when specific instances of biological interest will be examined. Furthermore, the types of polarization and relaxation to be mentioned are by no means exhaustive but are selected to illustrate the principles involved.

In the next section, apparatus and techniques of measurement of ε' and ε'' will be explained. The remaining sections of the chapter will be devoted to a description of the dielectric and structural properties of several molecules of biological interest.

9.3   APPARATUS AND TECHNIQUES OF MEASUREMENT

The dielectric constant of a biological material may vary from several millions at frequencies of a few hertz to the square of the refractive index (about three) at optical frequencies. Several dispersion regions may be traversed over this frequency range, the three well known ones being the α, β, and γ occurring at Hz, kHz–MHz, and GHz respectively. Dispersions occurring at frequencies in excess of about 100 GHz are concerned with atomic and electronic polarization only and are beyond the scope of this chapter although of great interest as subjects in their own right. They are studied by optical, infrared, or ultraviolet methods.

For the region of interest (d.c. to 100 GHz) the techniques available can be divided into four categories (Table 9.2) which will be considered in turn.

Table 9.2   *Categories of measuring technique*

Frequency range	d.c.–200 MHz	100 MHz—3 GHz	3 GHz—70 GHz	50 GHz upwards
Technique of measurement	Bridge methods	Coaxial lines	Waveguide techniques	Free space methods

The bridge methods are very simple in principle but require great care in operation if high accuracy is to be achieved. This is because of the presence of interfering second order effects. The impedance presented to the bridge consists of a dielectric cell containing the liquid under test, and the real and imaginary parts are measured in the usual way. The impedance consists of

$$Z = \frac{1}{1/R + jwc} \qquad (9.15)$$

where R is the effective resistance of the condenser and c is the total capacity. If the capacity in air is c_0 then $\varepsilon' = c/c_0$ and $\varepsilon'' \propto 1/R$. $\qquad$ (9.16)

The dielectric constant is given directly but the relationship between R and the dielectric loss requires the evaluation of a conversion factor or 'cell constant' for the dielectric cell. This can be done with a solution of known conductivity such as potassium chloride.

Unfortunately the total capacity measured includes a term due to electrode polarization, another term due to stray capacitance, and an inductive term.

Electrode polarization is important at low frequencies with liquids of high conductivity and all liquids of biological interest fall in this category. Furthermore, the resistive current is very much larger than the capacitive current with biological liquids at low frequencies which makes accurate measurement difficult. Electrode polarization can be detected by measuring the capacity of the condenser containing an electrolyte whose dielectric constant is independent of frequency over the range in question. Any variation of capacity with frequency is then due to electrode polarization and this can be determined and used to correct measurements carried out on a liquid of unknown dielectric properties. It is, of course, necessary to adjust the conductivity of the standard to be the same as that of the liquid under test. Electrode polarization may be minimized by widening the gap between the electrodes or by depositing platinum black upon them. However, this latter procedure may give rise to local heat dissipation in the vicinity of the electrodes and authorities disagree about its desirability. Some workers employ a cell whose electrode spacing may be varied by a micrometer screw gauge so that electrode polarization may be easily corrected for by working at different separations. As a rough indication of the seriousness of electrode polarization, an aqueous solution of 6% serum albumen in an average sized test cell has to be examined at frequencies as high as about 10 kHz before the electrode polarization diminishes to negligible proportions. In addition, as mentioned above, it is necessary to have very high accuracy in the calibration of the reactive components in the bridge, so it is clear that bridge measurements at low frequencies require a great deal of trouble for good results. A suitable bridge has been designed by Schwan and Sittel (1953).

At radio frequencies (1 kHz–1 MHz) the situation becomes much easier and it is usually possible to employ a commercial bridge, but above about 1 MHz the effects of stray capacitance and inductance become important.   It is possible to buy a commercial bridge which will go as high as 250 MHz but the major difficulty of the cell design still remains.   To minimize stray capacitance, the leads to the cell may be dispensed with by screwing it directly on to the bridge mounting.   Inductance may be minimized by careful cell design.   When all these precautions have been taken, experience shows that bridge methods cannot be used at frequencies greater than about 200 MHz.

For details of bridge methods applied to biological materials readers are referred to the works of Rosen (1963) and Schwan and Sittel (1953).

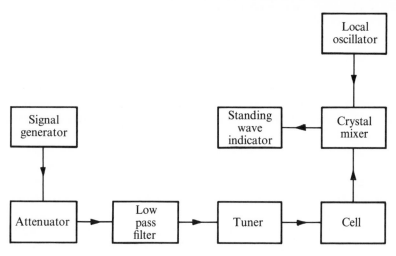

Fig. 9.3   Block diagram of coaxial line apparatus.

In the part of the spectrum between 100 MHz and 3 GHz coaxial lines or twin wires may be used with success.   The techniques of measurement of ε' and ε'' may involve making measurements in the sample, examining reflections from the sample, or plotting a resonance curve.   For liquids of high or medium loss, the second method leads to poor accuracy and so the choice must be between the first and the third.   Space permits the description of only one type of technique and so the first category of method will be chosen since this is the one that has been used by the author (Grant, 1965b; Aaron and Grant, 1963; Buchanan and Grant, 1955).

In essence, the method consists of enclosing the liquid under test in a short-circuited coaxial line and measuring the resulting standing wave with a movable probe that projects from the inner conductor.   The circuit diagram is shown in Fig. 9.3 and the experimental cell in Fig. 9.4.   A more detailed description of these will be given after the theoretical aspects have been considered.

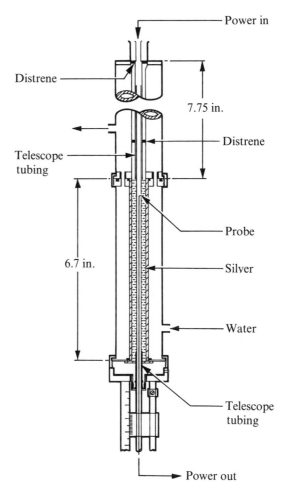

Fig. 9.4   Coaxial line experimental cell.

If the field strength at the short circuit is E_0, the electric vector at a distance x from the short circuit is given by

$$E = E_0(e^{\gamma x} - e^{-\gamma x}) \tag{9.17}$$

leading to

$$|E|^2 \propto \cosh 2\alpha x - \cos 2\beta x. \tag{9.18}$$

The waveform derived from equation (9.18) is shown in Fig. 9.5.

The complex propagation constant (γ) is equal to $\alpha + j\beta$ where α is the attenuation coefficient and β is the phase constant.   It is necessary to measure α and β independently in order to calculate ε' and ε'' from the expressions

$$\varepsilon' = \left(\frac{\lambda}{2\pi}\right)^2 (\beta^2 - \alpha^2) \tag{9.19}$$

$$\varepsilon'' = \left(\frac{\lambda}{2\pi}\right)^2 2\alpha\beta \tag{9.20}$$

where λ is the free space wavelength.

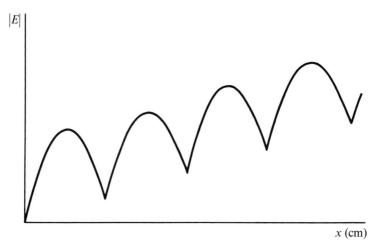

Fig. 9.5   Variation for electric field strength with distance from the short-circuit in a line containing a medium loss liquid.

There are several ways by which α and β can be measured and these have been described in full previously by Buchanan and Grant (1955). In the more recent studies, the two parameters that have been measured are the distances of the minima from the short-circuit and the standing wave ratio. Manipulation of equation (9.18) shows that for small values of α^2/β^2

$$x_{\min} = \frac{n\pi}{\beta}\left(1 - \frac{\alpha^2}{\beta^2}\right) \tag{9.21}$$

where $x_{\min}$ is the coordinate of the minima.

The standing wave ratio $E_{\min}/E_{\max}$ is related to α by the equation

$$E_{\min}/E_{\max} = \frac{\sinh \alpha x_1}{\cosh \alpha x_2} \simeq \sinh \alpha x_1 \tag{9.22}$$

assuming that α^2/β^2 is small and that αx is small.   The coordinates of the minimum and maximum are x_1 and x_2 respectively. For dilute solutions of proteins, peptides, or amino acids both (9.21) and (9.22) are valid. For more concentrated solutions the standing wave ratio and x_{min} are still measured but a computer is used to solve (9.18) for α and β.

The apparatus shown in Fig. 9.3 is standard General Radio equipment except for the experimental cell. This cell (Fig. 9.4) is made of solid silver to minimize ionic conductivity and the inner conductor is made of monel metal moving through cylindrical supports of the same metal at the top and bottom of the cell. The probe projects through the hollow inner conductor, so that the latter acts simultaneously as the inner of the input line and the outer of the output line. The probe is cut down to a fraction of a milli-meter in length so as not to perturb the field. This apparatus can be used to investigate aqueous solutions over the frequency range 150 MHz–3 GHz.

Resonance methods for use with coaxial lines are described by Conner and Smyth (1942) and by Schwan (1954).

At frequencies higher than about 3 GHz waveguides become pre-ferable to coaxial lines, but waveguides only work over a very narrow band and hence more than one set of apparatus is required to cover a modest frequency range. The relaxation wavelength of water is 1.74 cm at 20°C and so several sets of apparatus working at wavelengths near this are re-quired if the γ dispersion is to be studied adequately. Equipment is avail-able commercially at 10 cm, 3 cm, 1.25 cm, 0.8 cm, and 0.4 cm. These are the commonly used wavelengths but it is also possible to work at interme-diate wavelengths and even at wavelengths shorter than 4 mm. For high loss liquids such as water or aqueous solutions, measurements at millimeter wavelength become very difficult to perform and verge on the impossible as 1–2 mm is approached due to the lack of high powered sources and precision waveguide apparatus. Between millimeter wavelengths and the far infra-red lies a small gap which is relatively unexplored as far as polar liquids are concerned. When this region is finally open for investigation, it is possible that new dispersions may be discovered since, for some substances, the extrapolated values from the far infrared do not link up with the values extra-polated from the microwave region. The problem has recently been tackled successfully for water at 300 μ by Geffie and his co-workers (Chamberlain, et al., 1966).

Returning to the question of choice of apparatus and technique, it is clear that at microwave frequencies methods must be used which are speci-fically suited to measuring high loss if biological materials are being con-sidered. Such a method is the Buchanan (1952) method which arranges the apparatus in the form of a bridge. Readers are referred to the original publication for full details but, in essence, the apparatus consists of a dielec-tric cell in one arm of the bridge and a cut-off attenuator in the other arm.

The power is matched in and out of the cell and the specimen is of high loss so that the ratio of the field strengths x cm apart in the specimen is $e^{-\alpha x}$. In the other arm of the bridge, the piston of the attenuator can be moved to vary amplitude without altering the phase. By moving the cell interface and the attenuator piston, the bridge is balanced in two consecutive places down the cell column. The movement of the cell interface gives the wavelength in the liquid and the movement of the attenuator piston provides the attenuation for one wavelength, hence leading to α and β from which ε' and ε'' can be calculated.

Buchanan's method is simple, rapid, and accurate and has been used successfully at 3 cm and 1.25 cm. Attempts are being made to introduce it at 8 mm in spite of the very high loss at this wavelength. For a dilute protein solution at 8 mm, $\alpha = 23$ cm^{-1} at room temperature, i.e., 1 cm of liquid reduces the power by a factor of around 10^{-20}. Obviously, the liquid path must be kept very small and a phase changer used to provide independent phase variation.

Other methods of measuring high loss liquids at microwave frequencies have been used by Poley (1955) and Grant (1959) but much more work has been carried out with low and medium loss liquids using standard reflection techniques. Cavity methods are not usually satisfactory for high loss materials but Vogelhut (1964) has estimated protein bound water using a cavity method at 3 cm wavelength.

Measurements on high loss substances at wavelengths shorter than about 4 mm are exceptionally difficult to perform and free space methods or a combination of free space and guide techniques have to be adopted. Progress has been made by Smyth over the past few years and measurements on water at a wavelength of 3.1 mm have been reported using an interferometric method (Rampolla, *et al.*, 1959).

Before leaving techniques of measurement, it should be pointed out that all methods described measure the total dielectric loss which is made up of dipolar loss and loss due to ionic conductivity. Thus we may write

$$\varepsilon''_M = \varepsilon''_D + \varepsilon''_C \qquad (9.23)$$

where ε''_M is the measured value and the other two terms refer to the dipolar component and the ionic conductivity contribution respectively. The latter term is related to the ionic conductivity by the expression

$$\varepsilon''_C = 60\lambda\sigma \qquad (9.24)$$

where λ is the free space wavelength of measurement and σ is the conductivity in ohm^{-1} cm^{-1} measured at a frequency where there is assumed to be no dipolar loss.

For example, if an amino-acid solution is being investigated at microwave frequencies, ionic conductivity is usually measured on a 1 kHz bridge and assumed not to vary between 1 kHz and the frequency of measurement. Equation (9.23) is then used to obtain ε_D''.

The assumption that σ is constant between radio frequencies and microwave frequencies has been criticized, particularly as there are known cases when this assumption is not valid, an example being the Debye–Falkenhagen effect (Falkenhagen, 1934). Another effect has been noticed by Little and Smith (1955). It seems wise, therefore, to ensure that σ is reduced to as low a proportion as possible and this is achieved by constructing the experimental cell from a metal such as silver. Brass should be avoided when working with biological solutions since many of these form copper complexes.

9.4 THE DIELECTRIC PROPERTIES OF SOME MOLECULES OF BIOLOGICAL INTEREST

In this final section of the chapter it is proposed to discuss some of the work carried out on specific biological molecules. A brief mention will also be made of investigations on cell structures using dielectric methods.

9.4.1 WATER

The smallest molecule of biological interest is water but it is one of the most difficult to study as far as the interpretation of its dielectric properties is concerned. Water has probably been subjected to a more intensive study than any other substance and many theories concerning its structure have been suggested, some of which are mutually exclusive. Such evidence as has been furnished by the dielectric studies has been of qualitative, rather than of quantitative, assistance in the formulation of water structure.

Although the dielectric measurements are difficult to interpret unambiguously, they are relatively easy to perform at wavelengths greater than 1 cm and a great deal of work was carried out in the microwave region 1–10 cm 15 to 20 years ago (see Hasted, 1963, for review). With the exception of Cook (1952) these workers all agreed that the water dispersion was of the Debye type, with the dielectric constant falling from $\varepsilon_s = 80$ to $\varepsilon_\infty \sim 5$ at 20°C. The relaxation wavelength was shown to be strongly dependent on temperature, varying from 3.34 to 0.61 cm as the temperature moves from 0 to 75°C. Later, Grant, et al. (1956), working at longer wavelengths (1–50 cm), suggested that the dielectric behavior of water was more compatible with the Cole–Cole equation (9.5) with $\alpha = 0.02$. They also suggested that $\varepsilon_\infty = 4.5$ which would link up well with the far infrared results and thus obviate the necessity of a subsidiary dispersion region occurring at milli-meter or sub-millimeter wavelengths. Poley (1955) and Grant (1959) measured water at 8 mm wavelength, the former obtaining values suggesting another dispersion region while the latter got values of ε' and ε'' which con-formed to a single dispersion with either one relaxation time or a small spread of relaxation times. Finally, Rampolla, et al. (1959), investigating water at 20°C at 3.1 mm, obtained $\varepsilon' = 8.5$ and $\varepsilon'' = 12.0$. Their results definitely point to the existence of a subsidiary dispersion region at milli-meter or sub-millimeter wavelength but the errors associated with the measurements are high. Summing up, it is evident that although the main features of the water dispersion are understood, there is much disagreement about the second order behavior. Clarification will only appear when it is possible to carry out accurate measurements around one millimeter, al-though careful work around 0°C at the longer millimetric wavelengths would be useful. Lowering the temperature is equivalent to increasing the measuring frequency.

Precise structural interpretation of the dielectric behavior of water is difficult, and this is true of most other methods of investigating water. The value of ε_s is high for the known molecular dipole moment and confirms the associated nature of the liquid and the presence of an open structure main-tained by hydrogen bonds. Haggis, et al. (1952) proposed that water con-sisted of a statistical assembly of five types of water molecules forming 0, 1, 2, 3, or 4 hydrogen bonds per molecule. The static dielectric constant of water was then evaluated using this molecular model and Kirkwood's (1939) theory for associated polar dielectrics, the agreement with experiment being good. In Haggis's theory hydrogen bonds are either formed or broken; there is no provision for a 'bent' hydrogen bond. This latter concept was introduced by Pople (1951) in his theory but the agreement between theory and experiment was less satisfactory than in Haggis's case although the predicted temperature variation was good.

Other theories for water structure postulate the existence of clusters or aggregates and the dielectric behavior is a property of the clusters rather than of individual molecules. This will be considered in more detail below.

The phenomenon of dielectric relaxation may be linked with structure in several ways. In Haggis's theory, the relaxation time is a measure of the probability of the breaking of a hydrogen bond so that a plot of equation (9.12) should provide a straight line with a slope ΔH. The value of ΔH derived from dielectric measurements is about 3.5–4.0 kcal/mole which would confirm the hypothesis that one hydrogen bond is broken or distorted in relaxation. The Debye equation (9.11) appears to hold for water and the value of molecular radius is very nearly equal to half the distance between the oxygen atoms. In view of the disparity between Debye's molecular model and the structure of water, this quantitative agreement is probably coincidental.   On the other hand, it does add weight to the idea that the same molecular mechanism is responsible for both viscosity and dielectric relaxation, particularly as it has been shown that both processes have the same activation energy (Saxton, 1952).   Attempts have been made to show that a proportionality between τ and η/T may also be expected for water if a likely form of structure is assumed (Hill, 1954; Grant, 1957a), and recently the relationship between dielectric relaxation, viscosity, and NMR measurements has been considered (Powles, 1965; Krynicki, 1966).

An entirely different approach is due to Frank and Wen (1957) in their 'flickering cluster' theory.   They proposed that hydrogen bonded water molecules are aggregated in clusters of half life about 10^{-10}–10^{-11} sec and that this corresponds to the observed dielectric relaxation time.   Studies of the absorption bands in water between 1.1 and 1.3 μ have been interpreted in terms of cluster size and suggest that there may be an upper limit of 90 molecules per cluster at 20°C (Buijs and Choppin, 1964).   Pauling (1960) has also produced a theory which requires a cluster formation but in this case the clusters are in the form of pentagonal dodecahedra with 46 molecules at the apices and non-hydrogen bonded molecules at the centers.   Presumably the relaxation time is again a measure of the lifetime of a dodecahedron.

No mention has been made in this chapter of the far infrared dispersion nor of the possible dispersion in the very far infrared.   The latter dispersion is as yet unconfirmed; the former is an example of atomic polarization and may be due to the vibration of the quasi-crystalline lattice.

Summing up this section, the following points emerge clearly.   The dielectric dispersion of water is characterized by a single relaxation time, or small distribution of relaxation times, centered around 0.92×10^{-11} sec at 20°C.   This corresponds to a relaxation wavelength of 1.74 cm at 20°C but which is strongly dependent on temperature.   The dielectric constant falls from 80 to 5.5 ± 1 during this dispersion and a subsidiary dispersion between microwave region and the far infrared is possible but unproven.   In view of Geffie's recent work (Chamberlain, et al., 1966) its presence appears unlikely.

The dielectric properties of water clearly demand an open, highly associated structure with the molecules linked by directed hydrogen bonds.

The previous two paragraphs represent the lowest common denominator of agreement between all workers, but individual hypotheses go much further.   There is clearly great scope for work on this common but fascinating substance.   For a review of the dielectric behavior of water, readers are referred to Hasted (1963).

9.4.2 AMINO ACIDS, PEPTIDES, AND PROTEINS

Aqueous solutions of proteins, peptides, and amino acids are very amenable to study by dielectric methods due to the fact that the solute molecule exists as a dipolar ion in its water environment. Thus, an amino acid which has the general formula

$$H_2N-CH-COOH$$
$$|$$
$$R$$

becomes

$$H_3{}^+N-CH-COO^-$$
$$|$$
$$R$$

in solution with a resulting dipole moment, relaxation time and consequent dielectric behavior. Peptides and proteins have a more complicated charge distribution and the net dipole moment cannot be simply considered as two charges (e) separated by a distance (r). Detailed interpretation of the measurements obtained on these larger molecules is therefore more difficult although at the lower frequencies dielectric relaxation may be explained in terms of the rotation of macroscopic ellipsoids.

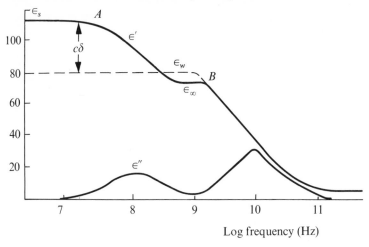

Fig. 9.6   Dispersion curve for an amino-acid solution.

In this section, it is not proposed to explain the detailed molecular structure of amino acids, peptides, and proteins, and readers are advised to consult a book on molecular biology, such as Haggis (1964), for this information.

An aqueous solution of an amino acid will exhibit two dispersion regions A and B corresponding to the two components present (Fig. 9.6).

When a two-component system is being studied, new parameters will be required, an important one being the dielectric increment (δ).   Referring to Fig. 9.6, we see that δ is defined by

$$\varepsilon_s = \varepsilon_w + \delta c \tag{9.25}$$

where ε_w refers to pure water and c is the concentration in moles per litre.   It should be noted that ε_w is not the same as the dielectric constant of the solution (ε_∞) between the two dispersions.   The value of ε_∞ is less than ε_s because at these frequencies the amino acid molecules behave as though they were non-polar and so the dielectric constant of the solution is *smaller* than that of the pure liquid.   The actual change in ε' through the solute dispersion is $\Delta\varepsilon'$ where

$$\Delta\varepsilon' = \varepsilon_s - \varepsilon_\infty. \tag{9.26}$$

Similarly, there will be an incremental dielectric loss $\Delta\varepsilon''$ given by

$$\Delta\varepsilon'' = \varepsilon'' - \varepsilon''_{cw} \tag{9.27}$$

where ε''_{cw} is the dielectric loss of the free water in the solution, i.e., the value for pure water corrected for the volume of the solute molecules.

The characteristics of the amino-acid dispersion can now be discussed in terms of the incremental values.   Amino acids exhibit their dispersion at decimeter wavelengths so that coaxial line apparatus is appropriate for their investigation.   The simplest amino acid is glycine where the R group in the general formula is a hydrogen atom.

Since there is disagreement between the results of the earlier workers, the discussion of the glycine work will be restricted to experiments carried out in the past ten years.   Gent (1954) found from measurements at 300 MHz that $\delta = 22.6$ per mole at 20°C and more recently, Aaron and Grant (1963) obtained $\delta = 22.3$ at the same temperature.   Their measurements were carried out at four frequencies in the range 450–900 MHz and over a temperature range.   They also calculated the activation enthalpy (ΔH) as 4.0 kcal/mole which was interpreted as being due to the rupture or distortion of a hydrogen bond between a glycine molecule and a water molecule.   In solution, the glycine molecule takes up the form of the dipolar ion $H_3{}^+NCH_2COO^-$ and can thus form both N-H–O and O-H–O hydrogen bonds with the water.   Equation (9.11) was plotted and found to give a straight line relationship between τ and η/T with a value of effective molecular radius equal to 2.7 Å.   As mentioned in the previous section, it is unwise to attribute too much significance to the values of effective molecular radius, but the fact that it is of the correct order of magnitude may be taken as evidence that the glycine molecules rotate singly and not in preferred domains.   The dipole moment of glycine in water can be calculated from the increment, using Kirkwood's theory of dielectrics, and values obtained from more recent work agree quite well with the earlier measurements in giving a value of 15.7 debye.   Dividing this by the electronic charge gives the distance of separation between the charge as 3.27 Å which is in good agreement with the value expected from simple structural considerations.   This confirms the correctness of the method and the use of Kirkwood's theory, and allows us to proceed with similar molecules whose configuration in water is unknown.

After glycine the next amino acid in ascending molecular weight is alanine where a methyl group takes the place of the hydrogen atom.   The formula for alanine is therefore

$$H_2N\text{---}CH\text{---}COOH$$
$$|$$
$$CH_3$$

which in solution becomes a dipolar ion.   Alanine exists in two forms depending upon which carbon atom the amino group is attached to.   As drawn above, the molecule is α-alanine, but when the amino group is attached to the carbon of the methyl group (the β carbon atom) the steric configuration is altered and the molecule becomes β-alanine.   In β-alanine the distance between the amino and carboxyl groups is larger than with the α form and hence the dipole moments are different.   For α-alanine at 20°C, $\delta = 25.5$ per mole, the corresponding value for β-alanine being 34.6 per mole.   On the other hand, the relaxation wavelength and the activation enthalpy are the same for both molecules, confirming that these parameters are determined by molecular size and intermolecular bonds rather than by charge distribution considerations.

Dielectric dispersion measurements are now being extended to the other amino acids, and it is hoped to publish some results on these soon. These will supplement the valuable earlier work carried out at low frequencies at one temperature only.

Turning now to peptides, the situation becomes more complex as far as precise structural interpretations are concerned.   As with the amino acids, several peptides have been studied at low frequencies and single temperatures but very little work has been carried out on their dispersions and hence the information available on relaxation times is small.

If a peptide with only two charged groups is considered, the interpretation becomes more straightforward.   For example, diglycine consists of two glycine residues joined through a peptide bond with one water molecule being eliminated.   This becomes ionized in solution with the NH_3^+ and COO^- groups at the ends of the molecule.   Similarly, triglycine, tetraglycine, and the higher peptides can be built up.   Wyman and McMeekin

(1933) measured the first seven glycyl peptides and found that the dielectric increment was proportional to the number of glycine units in the molecule. Conner and Smyth (1942) investigated the relaxation wavelengths of the first five glycyl peptides and showed that they extended from about 22 cm for diglycine to 68 cm for pentaglycine. Aaron and Grant (1964) obtained values for diglycine and triglycine in agreement with Conner and Smyth but went on to measure the activation enthalpies as well. As with the amino acids, the enthalpies calculated were consistent with the idea that one hydrogen bond is broken during dielectric relaxation. Although the behavior of both diglycine and triglycine was reported as being in accordance with a single relaxation time, very recent work suggests that a distribution of relaxation times is present between 0 and 10°C. This has resulted in a slight change in the ΔH values reported previously.

The dielectric properties and molecular parameters of glycine and some of its peptides are shown in Table 9.3.

Table 9.3 *Molecular parameters of glycine and some glycyl peptides at 25°C*

	Molar dielectric increment $\Delta \pm 5\%$	Dipole moment μ(debye) $\pm 3\%$	Charge separation r (Å)	Relaxation wavelength λ_s (cm) $\pm 10\%$	ΔH (kcal/mole) ± 0.5	ΔF (kcal/mole) ± 0.06
Glycine (pH = 6.7)	22.7	15.7	3.27	9.5	3.9	3.44
Diglycine (pH = 5.8)	70.2	27.8	5.8	24.8	3.5	4.0
Triglycine (pH = 5.7)	126.2	37.1	7.73	38.8	3.4	4.25
Alanyl glycine (pH = 5.8)	75.4	28.6	5.95	31.4	3.8	4.1

Dielectric measurements on amino-acid and peptide dispersion are rather sparse and an effort is being made to remedy this state of affairs. With regard to proteins, however, the situation is very different.

A protein solution exhibits two principal dispersion regions due to the protein molecules and water molecules. These are designated the β and γ dispersions respectively.

Work by Schwan (1965) on hemoglobin and Grant (1965a, 1965b, 1966) on two of the albumens has shown the existence of a subsidiary dispersion between the two main regions, and it is proposed to call this the δ dispersion. It will be interesting to see whether this is as fundamental a phenomenon for a protein solution as the other two relaxation regions.   The complete dispersion for bovine serum albumen is shown in Fig. 9.7.

A very thorough investigation of thirteen protein solutions was made by Oncley (1943) at 25°C between about 10 kHz and 40 MHz, which covers the β dispersion completely.   A bridge method was used and the relaxation frequencies (f_s) were found to lie between 100 kHz and 10 MHz for the proteins studied, depending upon the molecular weight.   For insulin $f_s = 10$ MHz and for carboxyhemoglobin f_s was nearer 100 kHz.   For each protein the observed dispersion curve was broken down into two components, each with its own relaxation time.   Oncley argued from this observation that two

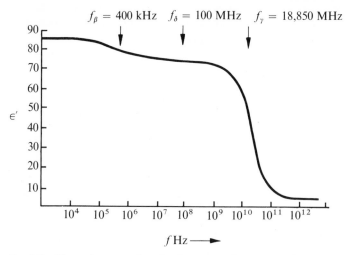

Fig. 9.7   Dispersion curve for a bovine serum albumen solution.

types of rotation were occurring, attributable to the rotation of an ellipsoid of revolution which he assumed the protein molecule to be.   The two observed relaxation times would then correspond to rotation about the major and minor axes of the ellipsoid.   Dispersion curves for ellipsoids of various axial ratios were calculated and compared with the observed curves, thus enabling the shapes of the protein molecules to be deduced.   These studies undoubtedly represent one of the best applications of dielectric measurements in biophysics.

All proteins studied by Oncley were found to be elongated ellipsoids of axial ratio between 1.6 for horse carboxyhemoglobin to 10 for secalin.   A knowledge of the amount of bound water present is required to calculate the axial ratio unambiguously but this may not be critical.   The problem of bound water will be discussed from the dielectric standpoint later on in this section.   The effective dipole moments obtained from Oncley's work were generally in the range 200–700 debye and are not necessarily related to molecular size, in contrast with the simpler molecules.

Although Oncley has assumed that protein molecules are ellipsoids with a permanent dipole moment, other explanations are possible. For example, a completely different approach is the mobile proton theory of Kirkwood and Shumaker (1952). According to their theory, loosely bound protons migrate between the various available sites on the protein molecule, this migration being produced by the external field. This means that the protein molecule has an induced dipole moment in addition to, perhaps, a permanent one as well. In fact, it is possible to interpret the observed dielectric increments of the protein molecules without the necessity of a permanent dipole moment at all. From this molecular picture it would be expected that the induced dipole moment would be dependent upon the pH of the solution since this would determine the availability of the sites for proton migration. In keeping with this, a pH dependence of dielectric increment has been observed for some proteins.

It is not possible in the light of present knowledge to come down firmly in favor of either of these two theories and opinions on the subject are divided. Takashima (1965) has produced evidence that, in the case of egg albumen, the results are incompatible with the original Kirkwood–Shumaker theory but may be explained by a revised theory still involving proton fluctuation. The problem is further discussed by Moser, et al. (1966).

Denaturation studies have been carried out on hemoglobin and serum albumen by Takashima (1960, 1964) using dielectric methods.

So far, we have considered the properties of proteins in their own relaxation region but Buchanan, et al. (1952) have looked at the problem from other standpoints. They measured the dielectric properties of six proteins in the microwave region (1–10 cm) in order to find the effect of the protein molecules on the water (γ) dispersion. The relaxation wavelengths were found to be slightly greater than pure water which is due to the structure promoting effect of the protein molecules. Buchanan, et al. (1952) extrapolated their results to lower frequencies in order to find the dielectric constant at frequencies just below the water dispersion. The difference between this and the value due to pure water was attributed to the protein bound water and to contributions from the protein molecule itself arising from atomic polarization. Assuming a value for the latter contribution, the protein bound water was estimated for the six proteins. In spite of the many assumptions made, this was a useful study and pointed to the existence of the δ dispersion (Fig. 9.7). The values obtained for hydration (bound water) were in the region 0.2–0.4 g/g protein, the precise value depending upon the assumed molecular shape.

The range of measurement employed by Buchanan was extended by

Grant (1957b) who investigated serum albumen in the region 1–50 cm.   The Cole–Cole circle resulting from this work is shown in Fig. 9.2 where a small distribution of relaxation times is noticed.   The bound water calculated from the dielectric decrement was rather lower than the values obtained by Buchanan, *et al.*

More recently, proteins have been studied at decimeter wavelengths, that is, between the main protein and water dispersions.   As mentioned previously, the existence of a small subsidiary (δ) dispersion has been shown and both Schwan and Grant have suggested independently that it may be due to the bound water relaxing.   It should be pointed out, however, that, although the results are compatible with this suggestion, other possibilities cannot be ruled out.   The activation enthalpy associated with the relaxation process appears to be about 11 kcal/mole on a rough estimate, which is about twice as high as the free energy that would be anticipated (equation (9.9)).   This would mean that large positive entropy changes would be involved which, of course, means an increase in the local disorder during the relaxation process.   Considering the problem from the molecular side, one would anticipate a fairly ordered water structure in the neighborhood of the protein molecule.   If the structure is destroyed during dielectric relaxation, an increase in disorder would also be expected.   Hence the bound water hypothesis is tenable from thermodynamic considerations as well as from the purely dielectric point of view.   Some dielectric data for two of the albumens are summarized in Table 9.4.

So far in this chapter we have been concerned with solutions but some work has been carried out on hydrated solids which involves a different type of measurement.   An example of this is Rosen's (1963) work on four different protein powders.   The powders were placed in a desiccator maintained at a known relative humidity and allowed to equilibriate.   The specimen was then transferred to the dielectric cell and its dielectric constant measured by a bridge method, the bridge operating over the frequency range 50 kHz–20 MHz.   The procedure was repeated at various humidities and the dielectric constant measured as a function of adsorbed water.   It was noticed that for each protein a critical hydration (w) exists above which the dielectric constant rises sharply.   This critical hydration corresponds to what we have been calling bound water and therefore the amount present should compare favorably with the estimates obtained at higher frequencies, although it would be unlikely to be exactly the same for both systems.   In fact, Rosen's value of w for bovine serum albumen was 0.25 compared with 0.25 suggested from Grant's (1965b) measurements on the δ dispersion and 0.3 predicted from the microwave measurements of Buchanan, *et al.* (1952). This is satisfactory since the deductions from the solution results involve many assumptions and the experimental error is much higher than in Rosen's

Table 9.4 *Dielectric parameters of the albumens at 25°C*

	Molecular weight	Measured parameters						Deduced parameters		
		β Dispersion		δ Dispersion		γ Dispersion		Hydration	Axial ratio	Dipole moment (debye)
		$\Delta\varepsilon'$	λ_s (m)	$\Delta\varepsilon'$	λ_s†(m)	$\Delta\varepsilon'$	λ_s (cm)			
Egg albumen (pH = 4.75)	45,000	1.9	250	0.25	1	72.20	1.56	0.20	5:1 Prolate spheroid	250
Bovine serum albumen (pH = 4.98)	69,000	1.4	380	0.43	3	72.25	1.57	0.25	5:1 Prolate spheroid	220

$\Delta\varepsilon'$, Change in ε for 1% solution.

† Approximate values

method.   Furthermore, the different methods are probably not measuring precisely the same parameter because a hydrated powder is involved in one case and an aqueous solution in the other.   Apart from accuracy, the hydrated solid kind of measurement has the merit that proteins relatively insoluble in water can be examined.

Takashima (1962) carried out an investigation similar to the above on crystals of bovine serum albumen and egg albumen and arrived at a value of critical hydration in agreement with Rosen.

In this section on proteins it has been possible only to touch on some items such as the dependence of dielectric properties on pH and the effect of denaturation.   Readers are referred to the appropriate references for more information on these important topics.

9.4.3 NUCLEIC ACIDS

Very little dielectric work has been done on nucleic acid solutions and none at all on the purine and pyrimidine bases and their associated nucleotides and nucleosides.   As far as DNA is concerned, the earlier work of Jungner (1950) and Allgen (1950) was performed with low molecular weight DNA and is therefore unrepresentative of the DNA molecule as now understood.   This explains why their results are at variance with those of later workers.

A comprehensive study of DNA has been carried out by Takashima (1963) who investigated several specimens of DNA from different sources, all of which were double stranded with a molecular weight in excess of one million.   A bridge method was used covering the range 30 Hz–5 MHz and aqueous solutions were studied at 15°C.   The results revealed a wide distribution of relaxation times centered around 10^{-4} sec and a static dielectric constant of over a thousand for a solution of only 0.2% concentration.   This leads to a dipole moment of about 15,000 debye which is extremely high, even compared with the protein molecules referred to earlier.   The precise interpretation of these results is being held over pending further investigation.   At present it does not appear that either a permanent dipole or a Kirkwood–Shumaker type of process can be the sole mechanism underlying the observed behavior.

Jerrard and Simmons (1959) found a smaller increment and shorter relaxation time than Takashima, presumably because the molecular weight of their DNA specimen was lower.   Jacobsen (1955) investigated sodium desoxyribonucleate using a bridge method and interpreted the results by postulating that the whole dielectric polarization of the macromolecule arises from the water of hydration.

9.5 QUASI-MACROSCOPIC STRUCTURES OF BIOLOGICAL INTEREST

Although the purpose of this chapter has been to show how dielectric investigations provide information at a molecular level, it would be incomplete without a reference to the work done on biological suspensions. A great deal of information has been obtained concerning membrane structure by measuring their electrical properties, particularly by Schwan (1957) and his associates.

Measurements carried out by Schwan on suspensions of bacteria *Eschericia coli* show the existence of a low conductance surface membrane of thickness between 40 and 100 Å. The dielectric constant of the suspension falls from several tens of thousands to the free water value as the frequency increases from a few Hz to tens of MHz. This is accompanied by two dispersion regions, the α region occurring below 10 kHz and the β dispersion around 1 MHz. Schwan has noticed comparable behavior for blood cells and Cook (1952) has extended this work to microwave frequencies where the dielectric properties of blood are shown to be closely related to their free water content. Another interesting investigation by Schwan and Morowitz (1962) is the structure of the pleuropneumonia-like organism A 5969, where the dielectric measurements revealed the existence of a membrane about 125 Å thick of which 40 Å consists of lipid.

Quite apart from the fact that dielectric measurements are a research tool is the consideration that they are needed for their own sake. This is becoming increasingly important with the introduction of high powered microwave sources for radar and other purposes since a health hazard is involved. The tolerance levels for microwave radiation for a particular tissue depend upon the dielectric constant and loss of the tissue, and these therefore have to be known in detail. Examples of this type of study may be found in the work of Cook (1951) and Schwan (1957).

9.6 CONCLUSION

In this chapter, an attempt has been made to explain the nature of dielectric parameters, how they can be measured and what kind of information at a molecular level can be obtained from their interpretation. The aim has been to describe in detail one particular example of each technique or type of measurement that has been made, while giving references to other examples in the same field.

ACKNOWLEDGEMENTS

Some of what has been described has been based on work carried out at Guy's Hospital Medical School. In this connection it is a pleasure to acknowledge the support of Professor C. B. Allsopp, Mrs. M. W. Sharp, Miss S. E. Young, and the technical assistance of Mr. F. W. Huthwaite.

REFERENCES

Aaron, M. W., and Grant, E. H., 1963, *Trans. Faraday Soc.*, **59**, 85; 1964, *Proc. 13th Colloque Ampere* (Bruges: Elsevier), p. 352.

Allgen, L. G., 1950, *Acta physiol. scand.*, **22**, Suppl., p. 76.

Böttcher, C. J. F., 1952, *Theory of Electric Polarisation* (Bruges: Elsevier).

Buchanan, T. J., 1952, *Proc. Inst. Radio Engrs.*, **99**, pt. III, p. 61.

Buchanan, T. J., and Grant, E. H., 1955, *Br. J. appl. Phys.*, **6**, 64.

Buchanan, T. J., Haggis, G. H., Hasted, J. D., and Robinson, B. G., 1952, *Proc. R. Soc. A*, **213**, 379.

Buijs, K., and Choppin, G. R., 1964, *J. chem. Phys.*, **39**, 2035.

Chamberlain, J. E., Chantry, G. W., Gebbie, H. A., Stone, N. W. B., Taylor, T. B., and Wyllie, G., 1966, *Nature*, Lond., **210**, 790.

Cole, K. S., and Cole, R. H., 1941, *J. chem. Phys.*, **9**, 341.

Cole, R. H., 1955, *J. Am. chem. Soc.*, **77**, 2012.

Conner, W. P., and Smyth, C. P., 1942, *J. Am. chem. Soc.*, **64**, 1870.

Cook, H. F., 1951, *Br. J. appl. Phys.*, **2**, 295; 1952, ibid., **3**, 249.

Davidson, D. W., and Cole, R. H., 1950, *J. chem. Phys.*, **18**, 1417.

Davies, M., 1965, *Some Electrical and Optical Aspects of Molecular Behaviour* (London: Pergamon Press).

Debye, P., 1929, *Polar Molecules* (New York: The Chemical Catalogue Co.).

Falkenhagen, H., 1934, *Electrolytes* (Oxford: University Press).

Frank, H. S., and Wen, W. Y., 1957, *Discuss. Faraday Soc.*, **24**, 133.

Gent, W. L. G., 1954, *Trans. Faraday Soc.*, **50**, 1229.

Glasstone, S., Laidler, K. J., and Eyring, H., 1941, *The Theory of Rate Processes* (New York: McGraw-Hill), Ch. 9.

Grant, E. H., 1957a, *Physics Med. Biol.*, **2**, 17; 1957b, *J. chem. Phys.*, **26**, 1575; 1959, *Br. J. appl. Phys.*, **10**, 87; 1965a, *Ann. N.Y. Acad. Sci.*, **125**, Art. 2, 418; 1965b, *Proc. 13th Colloquium, Protides of the Biological Fluids* (Bruges: Elsevier), p. 409; 1966, *J. molec. Biol.*, **19**, 133.

Grant, E. H., Buchanan, T. J., and Cook, H. F., 1956, *J. chem. Phys.*, **26**, 151.

Haggis, G. H., 1964, *Introduction to Molecular Biology*, Ed. G. H. Haggis (London: Longmans), Ch. 3.

Haggis, G. H., Hasted, J. B., and Buchanan, T. J., 1952, *J. chem. Phys.*, **20**, 1452.

Hasted, J. B., 1963, *Progress in Dielectrics* (London: Heywood and Co.), Vol. 3.

Hill, N. E., 1954, *Proc. phys. Soc. B*, **67**, 149.

Jacobsen, B., 1955, *J. Am. chem. Soc.*, **77**, 2919.

Jerrard, H. G., and Simmons, B. A. W., 1959, *Nature*, Lond., **184**, 1715.

Jungner, I., 1950, *Acta physiol. scand.*, **20**, Suppl, p. 69.

Kirkwood, J. G., 1939, *J. chem. Phys.*, **7**, 911.

Kirkwood, J. G., and Shumaker, J. B., 1952, *Proc. natn. Acad. Sci. U.S.A.*, **38**, 855.

Krynicki, K., 1966, *Physica*, **32**, 167.

Little, V. I., and Smith, V., 1955, *Proc. phys. Soc.* B, **68**, 65.

Maxwell, J. C., 1892, *A Treatise on Electricity and Magnetism* (Oxford: University Press), Vol. 2.

Moser, P., Squire, P. G., and O'Konski, C. T., 1966, *J. phys. Chem.*, Ithaca, **70**, 744.

Oncley, J. L., 1943, *Proteins, Amino-Acids and Peptides*, Ed. E. J. Cohn and J. T. Edsall (New York: Reinhold Publ. Corp.), Ch. 22.

Onsager, L., 1936, *J. Am. chem. Soc.*, **58**, 1486.

Pauling, L., 1960, *The Nature of the Chemical Bond*, 3rd Edn. (Ithaca: Cornell University Press).

Poley, J. Ph., 1955, *Appl. scient. Res.* Section B, **4**, 337.

Pople, J., 1951, *Proc. R. Soc.* A, **205**, 163.

Powles, J. G., 1953, *J. chem. Phys.*, **21**, 633; 1965, *Molecular Relaxation Processes* (The Chemical Society, Aberystwyth: Academic Press).

Rampolla, R. W., Miller, R. C., and Smyth, C. P., 1959, *J. chem. Phys.*, **30**, 566.

Rosen, D., 1963, *Trans. Faraday Soc.*, **59**, 2178.

Saxton, J. A., 1952, *Proc. R. Soc.* A, **213**, 473.

Schwan, H. P., 1954, *Z. Naturf.*, **9a**, 35; 1957, *Adv. biol. med. Phys.*, **5**, 191; 1965, *Ann. N.Y. Acad. Sci.*, **125**, Art. 2, 344.

Schwan, H. P., and Morowitz, H. J., 1962, *Biophys. J.*, Vol. 2, **5**, 395.

Schwan, H. P., and Sittel, K., 1953, *Trans. Am. Inst. elect. Engrs.*, May, 114.

Smyth, C. P., 1954, *Dielectric Behavior and Structure* (New York: McGraw-Hill).

Takashima, S., 1960, *Biochim. biophys. Acta*, **51**, 260; 1962, *J. Polym. Sci.*, **62**, 233; 1963, *J. molec. Biol.*, **7**, 455; 1964, *Biochim. biophys. Acta*, **79**, 531; 1965, *13th Colloquium, Protides of the Biological Fluids* (Bruges: Elsevier).

Vogelhut, P. O., 1964, *Nature*, Lond., **203**, 1169.

Wagner, K., 1913, *Annln. Phys.*, **40**, 817.

Wyman, J., and McMeekin, T. L., 1933, *J. Am. chem. Soc.*, **55**, 908.

CHAPTER TEN

THE APPLICATION OF MÖSSBAUER SPECTROSCOPY TO THE STUDY OF IRON IN HEME PROTEIN

J. E. Maling and M. Weissbluth

Biophysics Laboratory, Stanford University, Stanford, California, U.S.A.

10.1 INTRODUCTION

The resonant absorption of γ-rays by nuclei is generally known as Mössbauer absorption, so named after its discoverer (Mössbauer, 1958, 1959). It is of great interest both as a fundamental physical phenomenon and as a basis for a new spectroscopic technique of very high resolution. Mössbauer spectroscopy discloses certain types of hyperfine interactions, i.e., interactions between nuclei and electrons. It therefore has a wide range of application, including nuclear, solid state, and chemical physics. Several reviews, books, and conference proceedings have been published (Compton and Schoen, 1962; Frauenfelder, 1962; Boyle and Hall, 1962, Mössbauer, 1962; Bearden, 1964; Abragam, 1964; Wertheim, 1964). A bibliography to published literature has been compiled by Muir, *et al.* (1966).

Since hyperfine interactions often reflect certain features of chemical binding, it has been possible to extract useful information on ion–ligand interactions from a study of Mössbauer spectra. In particular, such experiments yield a measure of s-electron density, electric field gradient, and effective magnetic field at the position of the nucleus in which resonant γ-ray absorption occurs. A number of isotopes show this effect, among them is the stable isotope of iron, Fe-57, which occurs naturally with an abundance of 2.2%; as a consequence Mössbauer spectroscopy is applicable to iron compounds. In this chapter, we are concerned with applications to the study of iron binding in hemoglobin, myoglobin, and cytochrome c, which are all members of an important class of biological molecules, the heme proteins. Such a study is of direct biological interest because iron plays a central role in the function of heme proteins. Thus, in the physiological state, iron in hemoglobin and myoglobin binds oxygen reversibly; also, iron in cytochrome c participates in biological oxidation and reduction processes.

Of considerable importance in the interpretation of Mössbauer spectra is the structural information which, in the case of hemoglobin and myoglobin, is well established (Perutz, 1963; Kendrew, 1963). These molecules, as well as cytochrome c, contain heme (iron protoporphyrin IX) which is an approximately planar molecule having a molecular weight of 600; each heme contains one iron atom situated in the center of a square array of four pyrrole nitrogens. Derivatives of heme consist of heme plus certain atoms or molecules bound at one or both out-of-plane (fifth and sixth) positions on the iron. Iron in the center of four pyrrole nitrogens and with both out-of-plane positions occupied forms an ion–ligand complex of essentially octahedral symmetry.

Hemoglobin, the molecule responsible for the transport of oxygen from the lungs to the tissues, contains four subunits, each of which consists of a protein chain attached to a heme through the iron at the fifth position; the total molecular weight is about 67,000. Derivatives of hemoglobin are defined by the oxidation state of the iron and the ligand in the sixth position. In oxyhemoglobin, for example, an oxygen molecule is attached to a divalent

329

iron in the heme.   Myoglobin is closely related in structure and function to hemoglobin.   It consists of a single protein chain attached to one heme; the molecular weight is approximately one-fourth that of hemoglobin.   Myoglobin binds oxygen in the same fashion as hemoglobin and functions as an oxygen storage protein in muscle.

Cytochrome c is a heme protein involved in the respiration of aerobic organisms and tissues.   It has a molecular weight between 12,000 and 13,000 and one heme group per molecule.   At least three bonds link the heme to the protein in cytochrome c (Margoliash, 1966); one is thought to be an iron–protein bond as in hemoglobin, and two are covalent bonds to the porphyrin ring.

It is desirable to characterize as precisely as possible the iron–ligand complex; and Mössbauer spectroscopy, because of its ability to probe the microscopic electronic environment of the iron, is a powerful tool in this respect.   The discussion will develop this aspect in more detail.   It will consist first of a brief discussion of the phenomenon as a basis for spectroscopy and then the application of the technique to heme protein derivatives which vary among themselves as to protein moiety, sixth position ligand, valency, and spin state of the heme iron.

10.2   THE BASIC PHENOMENON: RECOILLESS EMISSION AND ABSORPTION OF γ-RAYS

Mössbauer spectroscopy is completely analogous to optical spectroscopy. In the latter, the ultimate source of radiation consists of excited atoms or molecules which decay to the ground state.   The radiation after being suitably monochromatized by a prism or grating, is incident upon the sample under study.   The intensity of the beam which is transmitted through the sample (absorber), as a function of wavelength (or photon energy) constitutes the basic data of an absorption spectrum.   In Mössbauer spectroscopy the source consists of excited nuclei which, in decaying to their ground state, emit γ-radiation.   With certain nuclei in appropriate surroundings (as described below), the radiation is highly monochromatic.   In fact, the γ-ray line can be so narrow that its energy may be shifted significantly by means of the Doppler effect, that is, by oscillating the source (or absorber) at moderate velocities.   Thus the velocity drive, which provides a Doppler shift to the γ-ray photons, is the analog to the dispersive device in optical spectroscopy. The γ-rays are incident on the sample being investigated; and the transmission as a function of γ-ray energy, which may be expressed in velocity units, becomes the basic data for a Mössbauer absorption spectrum.

To obtain Fe-57 in the proper excited state it is necessary to use the radioactive isotope Co-57 which decays, with a half-life of 270 days, to the

136 keV excited state of Fe-57 (Fig. 10.1); the latter nucleus in reverting to its own ground state emits three γ-rays, one of which has an energy of 14.4 keV. It is this γ-ray which has characteristics suitable for Mössbauer spectroscopy.

For a free atom of mass M the recoil energy due to emission of a photon of energy E_0 is $E_0^2/2Mc^2$ where c is the velocity of light. If the atom is in motion during emission the photon energy will be modified by a term,

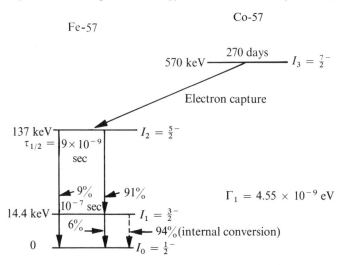

Fig. 10.1   The decay scheme for the radioactive nucleus Co-57. Co-57 decays with a half life of 270 days to the 137 keV state of Fe-57. The excited Fe-57 nucleus decays directly to its ground state emitting a 137 keV photon and to the 14.4 keV first excited state emitting a 123 keV photon. Radiative decay to the ground state from the first excited state provides the Mössbauer emission. The natural line width of the 14.4 keV state is 4.55 × 10^{-9} eV; the nuclear spin is $\frac{3}{2}$. The spin of the ground state is $\frac{1}{2}$. The superscript minus sign after the nuclear spin indicates that the nuclear state has odd parity.

$E_0|\mathbf{v}/c|\cos\theta$, where $\mathbf{v}$ is the velocity of the atom and θ is the angle between $\mathbf{v}$ and the momentum vector of the photon.   The energy of the photons emitted by such atoms is given by

(emission) $E_\gamma = E_0 - E_0^2/2Mc^2 + E_0\,|\mathbf{v}/c|\cos\theta$ (10.1)

where E_0 is the photon energy in the rest frame of the nucleus.   The photon energy for resonant absorption by a similar nucleus moving with velocity $\mathbf{v}'$ and direction θ' is

(absorption) $E_\gamma' = E_0 + E_0^2/2Mc^2 + E_0\,|\mathbf{v}'/c|\cos\theta'$ (10.2)

The energy of γ-rays emitted from a system of free atoms moving with thermal velocities would be centered at $E_0 - E_0^2/2Mc^2$ while the resonant absorption cross-section would be centered at $E_0 + E_0^2/2Mc^2$. Thus resonant absorption would be expected to occur for the fraction of events represented by the overlap in energy of the emission and absorption lines. The width of this overlap region is of the order of thermal energy: about 10^{-2} eV at room temperature.

In a solid, the situation is altered considerably from the case of the free atom. Mössbauer (1958, 1959) discovered that a certain fraction of the γ-rays emitted by excited Ir-191 nuclei in a solid do not obey equation (10.1). Instead they had an energy equal to E_0 and a line width close to the natural line width, $\Gamma = \hbar/\tau_m$ where τ_m is the mean life of the excited state. Corresponding effects were observed in absorption. The significant fact is that the emitting (or absorbing) atom is bound to other atoms in a solid. There then exists a certain probability that the recoil momentum associated with the emission (or absorption) of a photon will be taken up by the lattice rather than by the individual atom. When this occurs, the recoil energy $E_0^2/2Mc^2$ becomes vanishingly small because M is now essentially the mass of the crystal rather than the mass of a single atom. In addition, the lattice has a discrete set of vibrational excitations. This means that the last term in (10.1) or (10.2) is replaced by a quantity which describes the number of phonons that have been interchanged between the lattice and the γ-ray photons. Here too there is a non-vanishing probability that no phonons are exchanged. When these conditions prevail the emission (or absorption) is described as 'recoilless' or 'recoil-free' and emitted (or absorbed) photons match very closely the energy and level widths of the nuclear transition. It is this feature which characterizes the Mössbauer effect.

In Fe-57, the 14.4 keV level has a mean life of 1.0×10^{-7} sec or a level width of 4.5×10^{-9} eV so that when Co-57 is embedded in a non-magnetic solid the 14.4 keV photons have a spectral homogeneity of three parts in 10^{13}. As a consequence, hyperfine interactions as small as 10^{-8} eV become accessible to observation by Mössbauer techniques.

The probability of a recoilless event (emission or absorption) depends on certain properties of the solid as well as the energy and mean life of the nuclear excited state. The solid need not be crystalline; Mössbauer effects have been observed in amorphous materials and even in liquids of high viscosity. If f is the probability of a recoilless event, also known as the Debye–Waller factor, it is shown (Freuenfelder, 1962) that

$$f = \exp\left(-\frac{4\pi^2\langle r^2\rangle}{\lambda^2}\right) \tag{10.3}$$

where $\langle r^2 \rangle$ is the square of the displacement of the emitting or absorbing atom from its equilibrium position along the direction of the γ-ray momentum, averaged over the lifetime of the nuclear excited state; λ is the wavelength of the radiation. It can be seen from equation (10.3) that f is large when the scattering center is confined to a region small with respect to the wavelength of the radiation involved. $\langle r^2 \rangle$ decreases with increasing lattice binding energy; it also decreases as the temperature is lowered. In addition, f is a function of the angle of emission (or incidence) of the γ-ray with respect to crystalline or molecular axes if the binding is anisotropic. Hence the intensity of Mössbauer absorption in a single crystal may vary with the orientation of the crystal relative to the direction of the γ-ray beam.

The Debye–Waller factor has been calculated for a crystal in which the forces are harmonic, using the Debye model of a solid:

$$f = \exp\left\{ -\frac{3}{2}\frac{E_0^2}{2Mc^2} \cdot \frac{1}{k\theta}\left[1 + \frac{2}{3}\left(\frac{\pi T}{\theta}\right)^2 \right] \right\} \qquad (10.4)$$

in which θ is the Debye temperature, M is the atomic mass, k is the Boltzmann constant, and E_0 is the γ-ray energy. The recoil energy in the case of Fe-57 is 2×10^{-3} eV; this is well below the average vibrational energy at room temperature ($\sim 10^{-2}$ eV). The low recoil energy coupled with relatively high Debye temperatures for iron complexes (e.g., $\theta = 355°C$ for Fe metal (Gray, 1957)) makes Fe-57 particularly suitable for Mössbauer work. The Debye–Waller factor for Fe-57 in metallic iron is 0.7 at room temperature.

In the low temperature limit

$$f = \exp\left[-\frac{3}{2}\frac{E_0/2Mc^2}{k\theta} \right] \qquad (10.5)$$

It can be seen from equation (10.5) that if the free atom recoil energy is less than $k\theta$, which is the average energy of a lattice vibrational mode, a recoil-free event has a high probability of occurring. At 5°K the value of f in oxyhemoglobin has been found to be 0.83 (Gonser and Grant, 1965).

There is an additional feature of the Debye–Waller factor in cases where the Mössbauer nucleus is bound to a molecule. The probability of a recoilless event depends upon internal vibrational frequencies of the molecule (the optical branch of the phonon spectrum) as well as the vibrations of the molecules relative to one another (the acoustical branch of the phonon spectrum) (Herber and Wertheim, 1962). It is further of note that despite the large size of the hemoglobin molecule, the recoil energy due to absorption of a 14.4 keV photon is 2×10^{-6} eV, which is far greater than the line width.

10.3 APPARATUS AND ABSORBER

General Features: The experimental apparatus for the detection of Mössbauer resonance may differ widely depending on the nature of the experiments that are being performed; nevertheless a large class of experiments have certain features in common.   Figure 10.2 is a schematic diagram illustrating the important functional units required for the detection of Mössbauer absorption.   They are (1) radioactive source, (2) velocity drive, (3) absorber or sample under study, (4) detector, and (5) pulse sorting system.

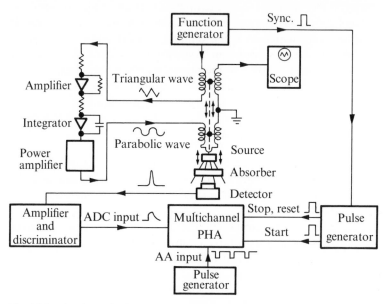

Fig. 10.2   A schematic diagram of the Mössbauer spectrometer used in this laboratory. A function generator provides a low frequency triangular voltage which is amplified and integrated. The resulting parabolic wave is used to drive a speaker on which is mounted the Mössbauer source. Since the speaker displacement is proportional to input voltage, source velocity is a triangular function in time. The detector generates pulses from γ-rays that penetrate the absorber, these pulses are amplified and fed to a discriminator with window set to accept pulses corresponding to the 14.4 keV γ-ray. These pulses are fed to a multi-channel PHA operating in the multiscalar mode, whose memory is being scanned synchronously with the triangular wave motion of the source. Synchronism is accomplished by introducing properly timed memory reset and start pulses into the PHA. These come from a pulse generator triggered at the beginning of every triangular wave period by the sync. pulse of the triangular wave generator.

The overall operation of the system may be described as follows; the radioactive source in the form of a thin foil produces a beam of highly homogeneous photons having an energy ε, of 14.4 keV.   The homogeneity, or line width ($\Delta\varepsilon$) is 4.55×10^{-9} eV, so that $\Delta\varepsilon/\varepsilon$ is less than 10^{-12}.   By mounting the source (or the absorber) on an accurately controlled vibrator the energy of the photons is shifted by means of the Doppler effect.   A velocity of 1 mm/sec corresponds to an energy change of 4.8×10^{-8} eV or more than 10 line widths.   In practice, there are certain broadening effects which are difficult to eliminate entirely and the line width is somewhat greater than that stated above.   Nevertheless velocities of a few mm/sec are usually sufficient for most experiments.

In this manner the sample is exposed to a beam of 14.4 keV photons which have a very narrow line width and whose central energy is swept over a number of line widths.   The absorption of these photons by the sample occurs only at certain Doppler velocities corresponding to certain photon energies.   The intensities of absorption and velocities at which absorption occurs depend upon the internal constitution of the sample, in particular the presence of Fe-57 nuclei and their interactions with electrons.   The function of the apparatus is to display such absorption curves.

1. *Radioactive source:* Sources for Mössbauer absorption experiments are commercially available.   They consist of thin foils of non-magnetic materials such as stainless steel, copper, or palladium, into which radioactive Co-57 has been allowed to diffuse.   The source shown in Fig. 10.2 was 20 mC of Co-57 diffused into palladium foil 0.001 in. thick (prepared by New England Nuclear Corporation, Boston).

2. *Velocity drive:* A wide variety of velocity drives exist.   The arrangement used here (Fig. 10.2) is one in which the source is mounted on the cone of a speaker and the speaker is driven so that the velocity increases and decreases linearly in time (symmetric triangular wave form) at 5 Hz.   Since the displacement of the speaker coil is quite closely proportional to the input voltage, it is necessary to provide a parabolic voltage in order to produce a linear velocity.   This is accomplished by integrating a triangular wave.   A function generator is employed to produce an accurate, low frequency triangular voltage.   This voltage is amplified, integrated, and applied to the speaker through a power amplifier.   In practice, it is necessary to employ considerable negative feedback to produce an accurately linear velocity. This is accomplished by coupling a second double voice coil speaker to the drive speaker with a rigid rod, and placing one coil of the second speaker in series with the input as shown schematically in Fig. 10.2.   The source is mounted on the rod connecting the two speakers.   Such a drive system is described by Cohen, *et al.* (1963).

3. *Absorber:* An important feature in Mössbauer experiments with heme proteins is the scarcity of iron in these molecules and in particular, the scarcity of Fe-57.   In hemoglobin, for instance, approximately one molecule in eleven contains a nucleus of Fe-57.   As a consequence, thick samples of hemoglobin are required; however, because of the absorption and scattering of 14.4 keV γ-rays by electronic processes, there exists an upper limit to the

thickness of the sample before the counting rate becomes impractically low. Samples of dry hemoglobin (and other heme proteins) usually have an optimum thickness in the region of one centimeter.   Other considerations regarding sample thickness, source strength, etc., are discussed by Boyle and Hall (1962).   One means of overcoming the problem of low density of iron is to enrich the heme protein in Fe-57 and this has been done by a number of workers, either by chemical replacement or by obtaining heme protein from an animal fed on a diet containing enriched Fe-57 (Gonser and Grant, 1965; Caughey, *et al.*, 1966; Lang and Marshall, 1966).   Also, from the standpoint of characterizing a sample it is often preferable to work with solutions; this causes a further reduction in the concentration of Fe-57 and, under certain conditions, makes enrichment essential to the observation of a resonance.

Another parameter, particularly important in the case of dilute iron systems such as heme proteins, is the sample temperature.   The Debye–Waller factor is temperature dependent; so are certain hyperfine interactions. In this spectrometer, for temperatures in the vicinity of 250°K, an ordinary refrigeration unit proves to be convenient.   It is important to eliminate vibration however.   For very low temperatures, a cryostat filled with liquid nitrogen or liquid helium is required; over a restricted range, the temperature can be varied by pumping on the coolant.   Samples are either immersed directly in the coolant, in which case the sample and coolant temperature are the same or they are mounted in a copper tube soldered crosswise into the tail of the cryostat.   The latter arrangement requires a direct measurement of the sample temperature.

4. *Detector:* The transmitted γ-ray beam, which includes 14.4 keV photons as well as photons of other energies is usually detected by a sodium iodide scintillator, photomultiplier, and pre-amplifier or a proportional counter and pre-amplifier.   Pulses from the pre-amplifier are applied to a linear amplifier and discriminator.   The latter has a voltage window which is set to accept pulses corresponding to the 14.4 keV photons while excluding pulses from all other regions of the spectrum.   The spectrometer in Fig. 10.2 uses a scintillation counter with a 0.5 mm NaI crystal.

5. *Pulse sorting system:* The object of the detection system in a Mössbauer absorption experiment is to determine the counting rate of photons transmitted through a sample as a function of photon energy.   The photon energy is varied by means of a Doppler shift which is achieved by vibrating the source, and the detection system is designed to measure the counting rate as a function of relative velocity between source and absorber.   If the transition energies of Fe-57 nuclei in the absorber lie within the energy range of the Doppler shifted photons emitted by the source, a resonant absorption spectrum will be observed.   A multi-channel pulse height analyzer (PHA) operating as a multiscalar can be used to sort out the scintillator pulses

ccording to the velocity of the source.   This is done by sweeping the PHA
1emory synchronously with the velocity sweep while feeding the discrimina-
)r pulses into the analyzer.   Thus, an incoming pulse is stored in a channel
ddress which corresponds uniquely to the phase of the pulse relative to the
riangular wave which drives the speaker system.   The memory of the PHA
sed in the spectrometer diagrammed in Fig. 10.2 is swept synchronously
vith the velocity sweep by means of two pulse generators.   One generator
n receiving a trigger (sync) pulse from the function generator signals the
tart of the triangular wave analyzer memory address to zero and then
riggers the start of the memory address advance.   An address advance (AA)
ulse generator then advances the analyzer memory address linearly in time
ntil a stop-reset pulse is received, resetting the analyzer memory to channel
ero.   The reset pulse is followed immediately by the start pulse which
nitiates the next cycle.

Since the source executes two velocity excursions, one at positive and
ne at negative acceleration and the memory of the pulse height analyzer is
canned synchronously with the triangular wave, once each period, two
dentical Mössbauer spectra are recorded in the memory.   The data presen-
ed in the figures are in each case the summation of these two spectra.   Sum-
ning the data in this manner cancels, to first order, the geometric effect on
ounting rate due to the small periodic displacement of the source with re-
pect to the detector.   In experiments with heme protein, where the total
umber of counts in each channel is high, the geometric effect is noticeable
n the separate spectra, but not after summation.

It is important to note that the intensity of the resonance is a function
f the counting rate.   This is due to a limitation both in the pulse detection
nd amplification systems, leading to a non-resonant 14 keV pulse back-
round.   In the spectrometer described here, the non-resonant 14 keV pulse
ackground contributed 27% to the total number of counts at a counting
ate, at the output of the discriminator, of 1500 per sec.   This counting rate
s used in all experiments.

0.4   HYPERFINE STRUCTURE

10.4.1   ELECTRIC MONOPOLE INTERACTION

This interaction is illustrated by the Mössbauer absorption in $K_3Fe(CN)_6$
hown in Fig. 10.3.   Absorption of the γ-beam is plotted as a function of γ-
ay energy in units of Doppler velocity.   The data in Fig. 10.3 were taken
vith both the source and absorber at 295°K.   The line has a width of
pproximately 0.05 cm/sec or 2.4×10^{-8} eV; this is about five times the
atural width of the 14.4 keV excited state of Fe-57.   Part of the additional

width arises from superposition of source and absorber level widths, another part is due to the finite thickness of source and absorber.

The quantity δ in Fig. 10.3 is called the isomer shift and is due to the electric monopole interaction between the nucleus and its surrounding electrons. If E_g is the energy of the nuclear ground state in the approximation that the nucleus is a point charge, then the true ground state energy of spherical nucleus with radius R_g and a uniform charge distribution is

$$E'_g = E_g + kR_g^2 e|\psi(0)|^2 \qquad (10.6)$$

where $e|\psi(0)|^2$ is the total electron charge density within the nuclear volume and k is a proportionality constant.

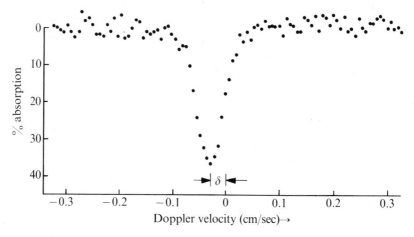

Fig. 10.3 The Mössbauer absorption of Fe-57 in potassium ferricyanide. Percent absorption is plotted against γ energy in units of Doppler velocity. The source is Co-57 diffused into a palladium matrix. The isomer shift, δ, is negative indicating that s-electron density is greater at Fe-57 nuclei in the absorber than it is at Fe-57 nuclei in the source.

Similarly, in the case of the excited state

$$E'_e = E_e + kR_e^2 e|\psi(0)|^2 \qquad (10.7)$$

The γ-ray emitted from the source nucleus therefore has an energy

$$E_\gamma = E_0 + ke|\psi(0)|_s^2(R_e^2 - R_g^2) \qquad (10.8)$$

where $E_0 = E_e - E_g$.

The energy E'_γ of the absorber nucleus can be written in a similar fashion:

$$E'_\gamma = E_0 + ke|\psi(0)|_A^2(R_e^2 - R_g^2) \qquad (10.9)$$

The condition for resonant absorption of the γ-ray is obtained by adding an energy δ, called the isomer shift, to E_γ such that

$$E_\gamma + \delta = E'_\gamma \qquad (10.10)$$

It follows that

$$\delta = ke[R_e^2 - R_g^2][|\psi(0)|_A^2 - |\psi(0)|_S^2]$$
$$= K\left(\frac{\delta R}{R}\right)[|\psi(0)|_A^2 - |\psi(0)|_S^2] \qquad (10.11)$$

where $\delta R = R_e - R_g$, and R is an average nuclear radius.   For Fe-57 K is positive and δR is negative (DeBenedetti, *et al.*, 1961; Walker, *et al.*, 1961).

The isomer shift is a measure of the difference in electron charge density over the nuclear volume of absorber nuclei as compared with source nuclei.   This charge density is due solely to electrons in *s*-orbitals.   Since δR is negative, a negative δ means that $|\psi(0)|_A^2$ is greater than $|\psi(0)|_S^2$, as is the case, for example, in Fig. 10.3.   The total electron density at the Fe-57 nucleus is greater in the cyanide complex (absorber) than in the palladium matrix (source).

Isomer shifts have been measured for a series of inorganic compounds containing iron in various valence states (DeBenedetti, *et al.*, 1961; Walker, *et al.*, 1961), with respect to a single source matrix and correlated in a semi-empirical fashion with theoretical values of total electron density at the nucleus.   In all $(3d)^n$ configurations, six *s*-state electrons contribute to the charge density at the nucleus; thus, at the absorber nucleus

$$|\psi(0)|^2 = \sum_{k=1}^{3} 2|\psi_{ks}(0)|^2 \qquad (10.12)$$

According to this relation the isomer shift for all $(3d)^n$ configurations is predicted to be a constant.   A considerable variation was found, however, among compounds with different $(3d)^n$ configurations, as well as among different compounds with the same $(3d)^n$ configuration.

The reason for the first type of variation may be understood on the basis of a partial penetration of 3*d*-orbitals into core orbitals.   Thus 3*d*-electrons may spend a fraction of their time inside closed shells; their presence there has the effect of partially shielding the nucleus and thereby modifying the core orbitals.   In particular, *s*-orbitals expand slightly, resulting in a reduction of $|\psi(0)|^2$.   From equation (10.11), with δR negative, we see that the net effect is to increase δ.   As the number of 3*d*-electrons is increased so is the isomer shift.   In Fig. 10.4, taken from Walker, *et al.* (1961), the values of $|\psi(0)|^2$ for several $(3d)^n$ configurations are shown on the left vertical scale.   The configurations of interest in heme protein are $(3d)^5$ and

$(3d)^6$ corresponding to Fe^{3+} and Fe^{2+} oxidation states respectively.   According to Fig. 10.4 it is expected that larger isomer shifts will generally occur in compounds having Fe^{2+} as compared with those having Fe^{3+}.   Numerical estimates indicate that isomer shifts in ionic ferrous compounds with respect to Co-57 in a palladium matrix will lie in the region of 0.1 cm/sec, whereas in

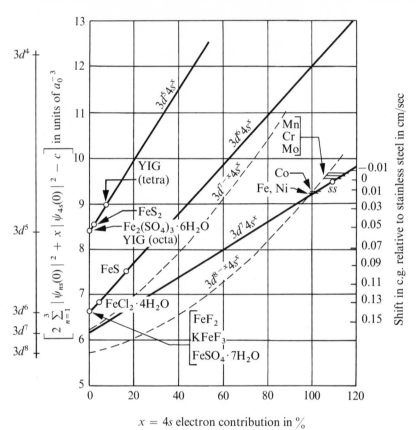

$x = 4s$ electron contribution in %

Fig. 10.4   A plot of isomer shift for various $3d$-electron configurations as a function of the fraction of one electron in the $4s$ shell. This interpretation of the isomer shift is due to Walker, *et al.* (1961). The figure is taken from their paper.

ionic ferric compounds the isomer shift will be approximately zero.   The absolute isomer shift values will depend upon source matrix but their differences will not.   For a convenient table relating isomer shift for one source matrix to another see Herber (1966).

The second type of variation in isomer shift, namely that within a single $(3d)^n$ configuration, is interpreted as a covalency effect.   By this it is meant that in the iron–ligand complex, for example, a ligand electron partially resides in the 4s-orbital of iron. $|\psi(0)|^2$ was therefore given the general form

$$|\psi(0)|^2 = \sum_{k=1}^{3} |\psi(0)|^2 + x|\psi_{4s}(0)|^2 \qquad (10.13)$$

where x is the fraction of 4s-electron contributed by the ligand to the iron. Theoretical values of $|\psi(0)|^2$ were plotted against x for the configurations $(3d)^n(4s)^x$ (Fig. 10.4, solid lines) and for configurations $(3d)^{n-x}(4s)^x$ (Fig. 10.4, dashed lines). Isomer shift data were related to this set of theoretical curves by taking the most ionic of each of the $(3d)^n$ compounds measured, assuming x to be zero in each case. Thus from a knowledge of the valence state of the iron in a given complex and the measured isomer shift it is possible on the basis of this model to determine with the aid of Fig. 10.4 what fraction of a 4s-electron has been donated by the ligands to the iron atom.

Not all iron compounds fit into this scheme. Ferro- and ferricyanide were found to have similar isomer shifts. There is now good evidence (Shulman and Sugano, 1965) that the ferrous and ferric ion in complex with cyanide, although differing formally in valency by one unit, have approximately the same number of d-electrons in their valence orbitals. There is apparently a 'back-donation' of approximately one more d-electron to the cyanide ligands in the case of ferrocyanide relative to ferricyanide.

Finally, it should be mentioned that the second-order Doppler effect also contributes to the isomer shift, particularly when source and absorber are not at the same temperature in which case a correction is required. This was first pointed out by Pound and Rebka (1959). The shift is very small however. In Fe metal it is less than the natural line width between 300 and 4°K (Pound and Rebka, 1960).

10.4.2   ELECTRIC QUADRUPOLE INTERACTION

An absorption spectrum for $FeSO_4 \cdot 7H_2O$ is shown in Fig. 10.5. The doublet is characteristic of the interaction between the quadrupole moment of the excited state of the nucleus and the gradient of the electric-field produced at the nucleus by the surrounding electrons. The quantity ΔE is called the quadrupole splitting. In the principal axis system of the ion–ligand complex, the quadrupole interaction takes the form

$$\mathscr{H}_Q = \frac{eQ}{6I(2I-1)} \left[V_{xx}(3I_x^2 - I^2) + V_{yy}(3I_y^2 - I^2) + V_{zz}(3I_z^2 - I^2) \right] \qquad (10.14)$$

where Q is the quadrupole moment of the nucleus, I_x, I_y, and I_z are components of the nuclear spin operator $\mathbf{I}$, and V_{xx}, V_{yy}, and V_{zz} are the diagonal elements of the electric field gradient tensor

$$V_{xx} = \partial^2 V/\partial x^2 = -\partial E_x/\partial x, \quad \text{etc.}$$

For $V_{xx} = V_{yy} = V_{zz}$ the interaction vanishes; this is the case when the distribution of charges surrounding the nucleus has either spherical or cubic symmetry.   If the symmetry is lower, say axial or rhombic, the components of the electric field gradient tensor are no longer identical and $\mathcal{H}_Q$ is not zero.

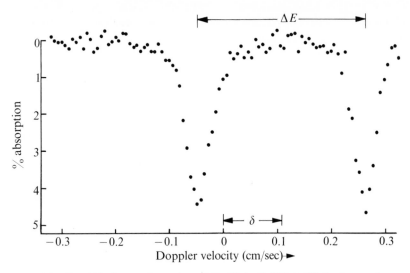

Fig. 10.5   The Mössbauer absorption of Fe-57 in $Fe(SO_4).6H_2O$ at room temperature. The source was Co-57 in palladium.

The interaction is also a function of nuclear spin; the nuclear state in question must have a spin greater than $\frac{1}{2}$ in order that the quadrupole interaction be non-vanishing. $\mathcal{H}_Q$ is usually written in a more compact form

$$\mathcal{H}_Q = \frac{e^2 qQ}{4I(2I - I)} \left[3I_z^2 - I^2 + \eta(I_x^2 - I_y^2) \right] \qquad (10.15)$$

where

$$eq = V_{zz} = -\frac{\partial E_z}{\partial z}$$

and

$$\eta = (V_{xx} - V_{yy})/V_{zz}$$

η is called the asymmetry parameter and eq is the field gradient along the major axis of symmetry evaluated at the nucleus which is placed at the origin of the coordinate system. If the ion–ligand complex has axial symmetry, $\eta = 0$ and the interaction energy is

$$\varepsilon_Q = \frac{e^2 qQ}{4I(2I - 1)}[3m_I{}^2 - I(I + 1)] \tag{10.16}$$

The nuclear spin of the ground state of Fe-57 is $\frac{1}{2}$ (Fig. 10.1), therefore $\varepsilon_Q = 0$ in the ground state. The nuclear spin in the 14.4 keV, first excited state is $\frac{3}{2}$ and it is therefore split in the presence of a field gradient. The quadrupole interaction energy for this case using equation (10.16) is given in Table 10.1 as a function of m_I.

Table 10.1

Nuclear state	I	m_I	ε_Q
Ground state	$\frac{1}{2}$	$\pm\frac{1}{2}$	0
14.4 keV, first excited state	$\frac{3}{2}$	$\pm\frac{3}{2}$	$+\frac{1}{4}e^2qQ$
		$\pm\frac{1}{2}$	$-\frac{1}{4}e^2qQ$

The quadrupole splitting of the first excited state is therefore

$$2|\varepsilon_Q| = \Delta E = \frac{1}{2}e^2qQ \tag{10.17}$$

The two transitions possible to the first excited state from the ground state lead to a doublet absorption spectrum such as the one shown in Fig. 10.5. In the case of rhombic symmetry, $\eta \neq 0$, and the expression for the quadrupole splitting is

$$\Delta E = \frac{e^2 qQ}{2}\left(1 + \frac{\eta^2}{3}\right)^{1/2} \tag{10.18}$$

Experimentally, the quantity that is measured is eqQ. For Fe-57, the value of Q, the quadrupole moment of the 14.4 keV state has been estimated (Ingalls, 1964) to be 0.29×10^{-24} cm^2, to within a factor of about 2.

The charges surrounding the nucleus, which are responsible for the field gradient eq, may be due to electrons on the surrounding ligands (i.e., the lattice') or to electrons in valence orbitals, or to both. The quadrupole splitting is therefore useful in obtaining a qualitative understanding of the local electronic environment of the nucleus. (For a detailed discussion of the quadrupole interaction for Fe-57 in hemoglobin see Weissbluth (1967).) For Fe surrounded by ligands as in heme proteins, both contributions to the quadrupole splitting need to be considered. Ingalls (1964) writes

$$q = (1 - R)q_v + (1 - \gamma_\infty)q_l$$
$$q\eta = (1 - R)(q\eta)_v + (1 - \gamma_\infty)(q\eta)_l \tag{10.19}$$

in which $(1 - R)$ and $(1 - \gamma_\infty)$ are Sternheimer factors which take into account the polarization of the inner core electrons by the valence and ligand charges respectively.

The valence contribution to the quadrupole interaction in iron comes from electrons occupying orbitals in the partially filled $3d$-shell. The ligand contribution will be due almost entirely to the nearest neighbors of the iron. In the case of heme protein they form a nearly octahedral complex of five nitrogens and a variable sixth ligand such as oxygen or water. In the ligand field approximation there are five degenerate $3d$-orbitals (d_{z^2}, $d_{x^2-y^2}$, d_{xy}, d_{zx}, d_{yz}) in the free ion which under the influence of an octahedral ligand field split into two groups, a two-fold (d_{z^2}, $d_{x^2-y^2}$) and a three-fold (d_{xy}, d_{zx}, d_{yz}) degenerate set with an energy splitting proportional to the strength of the octahedral field. For a positive central ion at the origin with negatively charged ligands situated on the axes of the coordinate system, the three-fold degenerate set lies lowest in energy. In a field of axial symmetry the degeneracy of these orbitals is further broken, and in a field of rhombic symmetry degeneracy is entirely lifted. The number of electrons in the five $3d$ orbitals depends upon the oxidation state of the iron (five electrons for Fe^{3+}, six electrons for Fe^{2+}). Their distribution depends upon the energy of the ligand field relative to the energy required to place two negatively charged electrons in the same orbital (correlation energy). This distribution ultimately determines the total spin of the iron–ligand complex. For example, if the ligand field is strong, the lowest energy state will be the state where electrons are paired in the three lowest orbitals. This in turn produces a low total spin. If the ligand field is weak, the electrons, rather than pairing up in the lowest orbitals will distribute themselves among all five orbitals with their spins parallel; the complex will therefore have a high total spin. This $3d$-electron distribution in turn determines the quadrupole interaction; spin and quadrupole splitting are therefore correlated in this model. For $3d$-electrons, q_v and $(q\eta)_v$ have the following values, in units of $\langle r^{-3}\rangle_{3d}$:

	d_{z^2}	$d_{x^2-y^2}$	d_{xy}	d_{zx}	d_{yz}
q_v	$-\frac{4}{7}$	$\frac{4}{7}$	$\frac{4}{7}$	$-\frac{2}{7}$	$-\frac{2}{7}$
$(q\eta)_v$	0	0	0	$-\frac{6}{7}$	$\frac{6}{7}$

The special cases of interest in heme proteins are Fe^{2+} ($S = 0, 2$) and Fe^{3+} ($S = \frac{1}{2}, \frac{5}{2}$). For $S = 0$, the orbitals d_{xy}, d_{zx}, and d_{yz} are each doubly occupied hence both q_v and $(q\eta)_v$ vanish. For $S = \frac{5}{2}$, each d-orbital is singly occupied and again both q_v and $(q\eta)_v$ vanish. For $S = 2$, the first five electrons occupy each of the d-orbitals giving no net contribution to q_v or $(q\eta)_v$; the sixth electron is in d_{xy} which, according to the interpretation of ESR experiments on metHb azide (Griffith, 1957; Kotani, 1961) lies lowest and is separated by approximately 1500 cm^{-1} from d_{zx}, the next higher orbital (d_{yz} is about 1000 cm^{-1} higher than d_{zx}). Assuming this is the case for the high spin ferrous derivative,

$$(S = 2) \qquad \begin{aligned} q_v &= \tfrac{4}{7}\langle r^{-3}\rangle_{3d} \\ (q\eta)_v &= 0 \end{aligned} \qquad (10.20)$$

Finally, for $S = \tfrac{1}{2}$, d_{xy} and d_{zx} are doubly occupied while d_{yz} is singly occupied. Hence

$$(S = \tfrac{1}{2}) \qquad \begin{aligned} q_v &= \tfrac{2}{7}\langle r^{-3}\rangle_{3d} \\ (q\eta)_v &= -\tfrac{6}{7}\langle r^{-3}\rangle_{3d} \end{aligned} \qquad (10.21)$$

which corresponds to a hole in d_{yz}.

The contribution from the ligands may be estimated in two ways: the first method requires a knowledge of the positions of the ligands and their charges. When these are known

$$\begin{aligned} q_l &= \sum_{i=1}^{N} Z_i \frac{3\cos^2\theta_i - 1}{r_i^{3}} \\ (q\eta)_l &= \sum_{i=1}^{N} Z_i \frac{3\sin^2\theta_i \cos 2\phi_i}{r_i^{3}} \end{aligned} \qquad (10.22)$$

where (r_i, θ_i, ϕ_i) are the coordinates and Z_i the charge on the ith ligand. The second method requires a knowledge of the orbital energies. It may be shown that

$$\begin{aligned} q_l &= \frac{14\delta}{3e^2\langle r^2\rangle_{3d}} \\ (q\eta)_l &= \frac{7\mu}{e^2\langle r^2\rangle_{3d}} \end{aligned} \qquad (10.23)$$

where δ and μ are the tetragonal and rhombic splitting respectively.

Despite large uncertainties in the values of the parameters which enter into the above equations, numerical estimates indicate that in those cases where both valence electrons and ligands contribute to the quadrupole splitting ($S = \tfrac{1}{2}, 2$), the magnitude of the splitting is 4–5 times greater than the splitting when only the ligands contribute ($S = 0, \tfrac{5}{2}$).

10.4.3   MAGNETIC DIPOLE INTERACTION

Figure 10.6 shows three Mössbauer absorption spectra of Fe-57; in the first (Fig. 10.6a) the matrix which contained Fe-57 was non-magnetic stainless

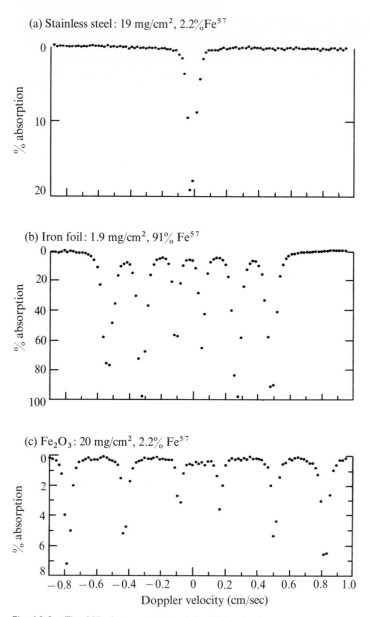

Fig. 10.6   The Mössbauer spectra of Fe-57 in the inorganic iron compounds stainless steel foil (5a), pure iron foil (enriched in Fe-57) (5b), and ferric oxide (5c). The latter two compounds show magnetic hyperfine structure indicating the presence of a strong magnetic field at the Fe-57 nucleus. The source was Co-57 in palladium.

.teel; in the second (Fig. 10.6b) the matrix was ferromagnetic iron, while the matrix in the third (Fig. 10.6c) was antiferromagnetic Fe_2O_3. The multiine spectrum in the last two (Fig. 10.6b, c) is due to interactions between the magnetic moment of the nucleus and the magnetic field produced by the electrons at the site of the nucleus. The interaction–Hamiltonian is

$$\mathcal{H}_m = -\mu_N \cdot \mathbf{H}_e$$
$$= -\gamma\hbar\mathbf{I} \cdot \mathbf{H} \qquad (10.24)$$

where μ_N and $\mathbf{I}$ are the nuclear magnetic moment and spin operators respectively, γ is the gyromagnetic ratio and $\mathbf{H}_e$ is given by

$$\mathbf{H}_e = -2\beta \sum_i \left[\left(\frac{\mathbf{l}_i}{r^3} - \frac{\mathbf{s}_i}{r^3} + 3\frac{\mathbf{r}(\mathbf{s}_i \cdot \mathbf{r})}{r^5} \right) + \frac{8\pi}{3}\mathbf{s}_i\,\delta(\mathbf{r}) \right] \qquad (10.25)$$

where $\mathbf{s}_i$ and $\mathbf{l}_i$ are the one electron spin and orbital angular momentum operators respectively. The expectation value of $\mathbf{H}_e$ is the internal magnetic field at the nucleus due to the surrounding electrons. The first three terms in (10.25) make up the dipolar field due to orbital and spin angular momenta; the last term is the Fermi contact interaction. In the case of iron complexes the dipolar field has contributions both from unpaired electrons in $3d$-orbitals and from unpaired electrons on the ligands. Both contributions are small compared to the Fermi term (Wertheim, 1964) which arises from the penetration of the nuclear volume by electrons in s-orbitals of the ion. (See detailed discussion of the internal magnetic field, for example, by Freeman and Watson, 1962; Marshall and Johnson, 1962; and Wertheim, 1964.)

Electrons with orbital angular momentum (non s-state electrons) do not directly contribute to the contact term; however they are responsible for an indirect interaction through the phenomenon of 'core polarization'. In the case of Fe-57, the exchange interaction between unpaired $3d$-electrons and inner shell electrons due to the interpenetration of their orbitals, results in a small net polarization (unpairing) of the inner shell s-electrons. The unpaired electrons couple with the nuclear spin to produce the observed splittings.

Since the contact term is the dominant term, $\mathcal{H}_m$ can be written to good approximation as

$$\mathcal{H}_m = a\mathbf{I} \cdot \mathbf{S} \qquad (10.26)$$

where $\mathbf{S}$ is the total electron spin of the ion and

$$a = \tfrac{16}{3}\pi\beta\gamma\hbar|\psi(0)|^2 \qquad (10.27)$$

For simplicity an isotropic interaction has been assumed although this in general need not be the case. The magnetic energy to first order is

$$\varepsilon_m = am_I m_s \qquad (10.28)$$

This approximation is suitable for describing magnetically ordered systems where the exchange interaction, $J\mathbf{S}_i \cdot \mathbf{S}_j$, between electron spins on atoms i and j breaks the magnetic degeneracy of the ground state with an energy in general much larger than kT at room temperature. Because of this the ground state consists of a single m_S magnetic substate. In the case of Fe-57 $I_e = \frac{3}{2}$ and $I_g = \frac{1}{2}$, therefore from equation (10.28), the excited nucleus has four equally spaced energies while the ground state nucleus has two. Since Mössbauer experiments involve transitions between two nuclear states, the value of the magnetic hyperfine coupling parameter, a, may be different in the two states. For Fe-57 the data of Kistner and Sunyar (1960) give

$$|a| = 0.245 \text{ cm/sec}$$
$$a/a^* = -1.77$$

where a and a^* are splitting parameters for ground state and excited state respectively.

The selection rules for the nuclear transitions are $\Delta m_I = 0, \pm 1$ resulting in six line Mössbauer spectra of the type shown in Figs. 10.6b and 10.6c. In Fe_2O_3 (Fig. 10.6c) there is evidence of an isomer shift and quadrupole splitting in addition to the magnetic interaction. The picture is more complex in the case of paramagnetic systems where there is no exchange interaction present. In such cases, it is necessary to consider an exact solution to the Hamiltonian (10.26) where a, because of an anisotropic crystalline field environment is a tensor quantity.

The spin-lattice relaxation time for electrons is a critical factor in determining whether magnetic hyperfine interactions can occur. If the spin-lattice relaxation time τ_R is short compared with a time of the order of $\hbar/a$, the characteristic time for magnetic hyperfine interactions, the internal field, H_e, will average to zero and there will be no splitting. This is not the case with magnetically ordered materials below their Curie temperature; this is, however, the case with paramagnetic iron compounds at ordinary temperatures. For example, both $K_3Fe(CN)_6$ and $FeSO_4 \cdot 6H_2O$ are paramagnetic, but their Mössbauer absorption spectra (Figs. 10.3 and 10.5) give no evidence of magnetic hyperfine interactions. Wertheim (1964) has shown that under conditions which provide a sufficiently long spin-lattice relaxation time, magnetic hyperfine structure in a paramagnetic iron system is observed. It should be observed that the above considerations hold provided the lifetime of the nuclear excited state is long compared with $\hbar/a$; this is the case for Fe-57.

Two mechanisms contribute to τ_R: One is the spin–spin interaction among paramagnetic species or the exchange interaction in the case of magnetically ordered materials, and the second is the spin–lattice interaction. The former is negligible in heme proteins because of the large separations $(\sim 30$ Å) among the hemes. The second process (spin lattice relaxation) couples spins with the lattice by means of spin–orbit interactions. In systems with no orbital angular momentum the process is inefficient and leads to relatively long $(10^{-8}\text{-}10^{-9}$ sec) relaxation times which increase as the temperature is lowered. In anticipation of certain experimental results, one might therefore expect that magnetic hyperfine interactions would be observable in high spin ferric hemoglobin (an orbital singlet), particularly at low temperatures and this has been found to be the case. In the remaining two cases—low spin ferric and high spin ferrous—relaxation times are expected to be shorter. If they are comparable to the nuclear Larmor precession period, the magnetic hyperfine interaction is likely to manifest itself in a general broadening of the Mössbauer spectrum, otherwise no magnetic *hfs* will be visible. In general the latter situation is found to hold.

In high spin ferric hemoglobin the zero field splitting, as deduced from ESR experiments, obeys a spin–Hamiltonian of the form DS_z^2 (Weissbluth, 1967). Recent measurements by infrared absorption (Feher and Richards, 1966) yield $D = 6.95$ cm^{-1}; therefore, at temperatures above 60°K all three Kramers doublets $(|\pm\frac{1}{2}\rangle, |\pm\frac{3}{2}\rangle$, and $|\pm\frac{5}{2}\rangle)$ will be populated, whereas below 20°K most of the population will reside in the $|\pm\frac{1}{2}\rangle$ doublet. (See Bearden, *et al.*, 1965; Caughey, *et al.*, 1966; Lang and Marshall, 1966, for discussions of this effect.) The qualitative description of the magnetic hyperfine interaction will now be as follows: As the temperature is reduced from room temperature the spin–lattice relaxation time increases and the chances for resolv-

Table 10.2 *Theoretical isomer shifts, quadrupole splittings, and magnetic hyperfine interactions*

	Fe^{2+}		Fe^{3+}	
	$S = 0$	$S = 2$	$S = \frac{1}{2}$	$S = \frac{5}{2}$
Isomer shift	Large	Large	Small	Small
Quadrupole splitting	Small	Large	Large	Small
Magnetic hyperfine interaction	Small	Small or large	Small[a]	Large[b]

[a] The relaxation time of electronic spins is expected to be short in comparison with the nuclear Larmor precession time.

[b] At temperatures of 20–60°K.

ing the magnetic hyperfine interaction improve. Bearing in mind that the effective magnetic field at the nucleus is proportional to S_z, it is seen that above 60°K (approximately) all three Kramers doublets will contribute. However, at about 20°K and lower only the $|\pm\frac{1}{2}\rangle$ doublet contributes; the effective magnetic field at the nucleus is consequently reduced and the magnetic hyperfine interaction becomes smaller. A further effect has been pointed out by Blume (1965); he notes that effective magnetic fields perpendicular to the four-fold symmetry axis induce transitions among the magnetic substates of the nucleus, thereby altering their lifetimes (and their widths). This effect is shown to lead to asymmetric broadening. The consequences of the above consideration are summarized in Table 10.2.

10.5   MÖSSBAUER SPECTRA OF HEME PROTEINS

10.5.1   INTRODUCTION

The parameters that characterize Mössbauer spectra have been discussed in sections 10.2 and 10.4 along with certain underlying theoretical ideas. The elements of the Mössbauer spectrometer and characteristics of heme protein absorbers have been discussed in section 10.3. Here we summarize certain Mössbauer data obtained in this and other laboratories on heme protein systems and discuss these data in the light of the above theoretical ideas.

10.5.2   EXPERIMENTAL METHODS

A considerable body of Mössbauer data now exists on heme protein (Gonser, et al., 1963, 1964; Craig and Sutin, 1963; Maling and Weissbluth, 1964; Gonser and Grant, 1965; Caughey, et al., 1966; Lang and Marshall, 1966). This data has been obtained mainly from samples enriched in Fe-57; it is however feasible under certain conditions to obtain satisfactory spectra with unenriched samples of ferrous hemoglobin derivatives in concentrated (30%) solution and powder samples of ferric hemoglobin derivatives above 60°K. Below about 60°K ferric hemoglobin and myoglobin spectra exhibit marked broadening due to the appearance of the magnetic hyperfine interaction. This causes a considerable loss in signal amplitude despite the favorable effect of the Debye–Waller factor. In most cases where the magnetic hyperfine interaction is fully expressed, enrichment seems essential (Lang and Marshall, 1966).

Data on isomer shift and quadrupole splitting as a function of protein moiety, temperature sixth position ligand, and oxidation state are summarized in Table 10.3. The examples of spectra shown in Fig. 10.7 were obtained in this laboratory with unenriched samples using the spectrometer described in section 10.3. This data was obtained with a Co-57:Pd source and isomer shift data from other groups represented in Table 10.3 have been corrected to this source matrix (Herber, 1966). The isomer shift relative to Pd at room temperature for Fe-57 (91% enrichment) in Fe foil 0.0001 in. thick was -0.020 ± 0.003 cm/sec, and the line width of each of the inner pair of lines was 0.033 ± 0.002 cm/sec. The isomer shift at room temperature for both

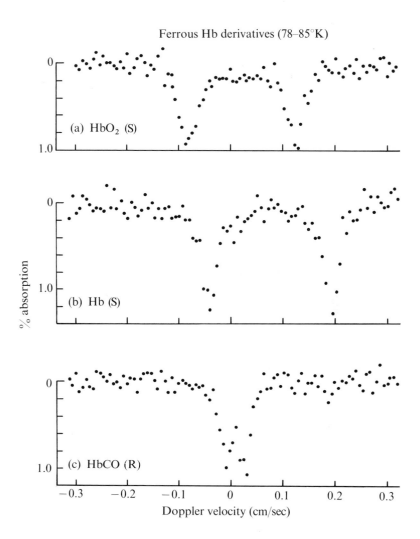

Fig. 10.7   Mössbauer spectra at 78–85°K in (a) oxyhemoglobin (30% solution), (b) deoxyhemoglobin (30% solution) and (c) carbon monoxide hemoglobin (rabbit reticulocytes).

Table 10.3 *Isomer shifts and quadrupole splittings of heme-proteins*

Protein[a]	Species	Type[b]	Form of sample[c]	Temperature (°K)	Isomer shift[d] (cm/sec)	Quadrupole splitting (cm/sec)
1. HbO$_2$[e]	human	A	C	85	$+0.012 \pm 0.010$	0.216 ± 0.010
	human	A	S	85	$+0.022$	0.214
	human	$A + D + F + S$	C	84	$+0.015$	0.214
	rabbit	—	R	80	$+0.020$	0.220
	horse	—	C	77	$+0.014 \pm 0.005$	0.216 ± 0.005
	horse	—	C	4.2	$+0.011$	0.226
HbO$_2$[f]	rat	—	S	195	0.000 ± 0.005	0.189 ± 0.005
	rat	—	S	77	$+0.006$	0.219
	rat	—	S	1.2	$+0.004$	0.224
HbO$_2$[g]	rat	—	C	5	$+0.010 \pm 0.005$	0.225 ± 0.005
2. Hb[e]	human	A	P	150	$+0.072 \pm 0.010$	0.209 ± 0.010
	human	A	P	100	$+0.077$	0.220
	human	A	S	85	$+0.087$	0.243
	human	$A + D + F + S$	C	84	$+0.080$	0.223
	human	$A + D + F + S$	C	32	$+0.085$	0.233
	rabbit	—	C	80—85	$+0.085$	0.225
	rabbit	—	S	78—80	$+0.082$	0.237
	rabbit	—	S	10	$+0.085$	0.250
Hb[f]	rat	—	S	195	$+0.070 \pm 0.005$	0.240 ± 0.005
	rat	—	S	4	$+0.071 \pm 0.005$	0.240 ± 0.005
Hb[g]	rat	—	C	5	$+0.077 \pm 0.005$	0.24 ± 0.01
3. HbCO[e]	human	A	P	297	$+0.010 \pm 0.010$	0.040 ± 0.010
	rabbit	—	R	78	$+0.008$	0.033
	rabbit	—	R	10	$+0.008$	0.037
HbCO[f]	rat	—	S	195	-0.002 ± 0.005	0.036 ± 0.005
	rat	—	S	4	$+0.006 \pm 0.005$	0.036 ± 0.005
HbCO[g]	human	A	C	5	$+0.011 \pm 0.003$	0.034 ± 0.005
4. MetHb[e]	human	A	P	297	-0.002 ± 0.010	0.196 ± 0.010
	human	$F + S$	S	78	$+0.007$	0.207
	human	—	P	297	-0.005	0.203
	rabbit	—	P	297	$+0.006$	0.201

Compound	Source	Type[b]	Form[c]	Temp (K)	Δ	δ
MetHb[f]	porcine	—	P	297	+0.002	0.208
	unknown	—	P (denatured)	297	−0.002	0.208
	human	—	P (denatured)	297	−0.001	0.203
5. MetHbF[e]	rat	A	S	195	+0.002*	0.203*
	human	—	P	297	0.000 ± 0.005	0.200 + 0.005
MetHbF[f]	rat	—	S	4	0.000 ± 0.010	0.200 ± 0.10
6. MetHbCN[e]	human	A	P	297	—	~0.03
	human	—	P	250	0.000	0.122
	human	—	S	—	0.000	0.130
	human	—	S	297	0.003	0.140
	human	—	S	253	no resonance observed	
7. MetHbCN[f]	rat	—	S	195	+0.000	0.130
MetHbOH[f]	rat	A	S	195	−0.003 ± 0.005	0.139 ± 0.005
		—	S	77	−0.002	0.157
8. MetHbN₃[e]	human	—	P	297	−0.00	0.19
MetHbN₃[f]	rat	A	S	195	+0.006 ± 0.010	0.201 ± 0.010
9. MetMb[e]	sperm whale	—	P	297	−0.005 ± 0.005	0.230 ± 0.005
MetMb[h]	sperm whale	—	P	298	+0.010 ± 0.010	0.206 ± 0.010
	sperm whale	—	P	228	−0.010 ± 0.002	0.196 ± 0.002
	sperm whale	—	P	77	−0.010	0.202
10. Ferrous[e] cytochrome c	equine	heart	P	297	−0.004	0.204
	equine	heart	P	297	+0.032 ± 0.010	0.127 ± 0.010
11. Ferric[e] cytochrome c	equine	heart	P	297	+0.005	0.201
			P	77	+0.007 ± 0.005	0.205 ± 0.007

* Average values
[a] Compounds preceded by the prefix 'met' are ferric; all others are ferrous.
[b] Type A hemoglobin is normal human hemoglobin; all others are mutant varieties (C. Baglioni, 1963).
[c] C—red cells; R—reticulocytes; S—aqueous solution containing 30% of the protein (by weight); P—lyophilized powder.
[d] Isomer shifts are relative to Co-57 in palladium.
[e] This laboratory.
[f] Data from Lang and Marshall (1966).
[g] Data from Gonser and Grant (1965).
[h] Data from Caughey, et al. (1966).

310 stainless steel (0.001 in. foil) and $K_3Fe(CN)_6$ was -0.025 ± 0.003 cm/ sec. Unless otherwise noted, the protein mass in powder samples was 0.5 g/cm^2; samples in other forms (solution, frozen cells) contained 0.2 g/cm^2 of protein.

Hemoglobin and myoglobin derivatives were usually identified by measuring the extinction coefficient at an absorption maximum or by measuring ratios of two prominent absorption maxima, and comparing these values with published data. Extinction coefficients were measured at room temperature both by comparing the optical density of a protein solution with that of the alkaline pyridine hemochromogen of oxyhemoglobin, and by drying and weighing the protein in a given volume of the solution. The samples are described below; details of their preparation are to be found elsewhere (Perini, et al., 1966).

Extractions of oxyhemoglobin were carried out according to the methods of Drabkin (1946, 1949). Deoxyhemoglobin was prepared from solutions of oxyhemoglobin derived from either normal human red cells or from rabbit reticulocytes. The preparation was carried out by a combination of reduced pressure and nitrogen flushing with the residual oxygen removed by the addition of a small amount of sodium dithionite. Carbonmonoxyhemoglobin was prepared by saturating solutions of deoxyhemoglobin with carbon monoxide gas for 20 min. The acid form of normal human methemoglobin and a mixed mutant sample of methemoglobin consisting of types S and F were prepared from their respective oxyhemoglobins by oxidation with sodium nitrite following, with modification, the procedure of Keilin and Hartree (1951). Acid denatured human metHb was prepared by precipitation of metHb at pH 3. Commercial samples of salt-free lyophilized canine, equine, and porcine metHb were obtained from Mann Research Laboratories, New York. Bovine metHb and an unknown species of metHb denatured for protease assay were obtained from Nutritional Biochemical Corporation, Cleveland. Sperm whale metMb was obtained from Mann Research Laboratories, New York, as a salt-free lyophilized powder. The three methemoglobin derivatives were prepared from metHb according to the methods of Keilin and Hartree (1951); metmyoglobin azide was prepared from metMb following Stryer, et al. (1964)

In the heme protein experiments where resonances are extremely weak ($\sim 1\%$) it was important to check for resonances due to impurity amounts of iron in material other than the absorber in the beam path. The γ-ray beam, in addition to penetrating the sample, passed through a series of mylar windows having a combined thickness of 0.008–0.010 in. and a beryllium window 0.005 in. thick. In experiments where the sample was immersed in the coolant the beam traversed, in addition to the window material, 0.2 cm of coolant in the liquid nitrogen experiments and up to 1.5 cm of coolant in the liquid helium experiments. A weak absorption line was always observed in the absence of a sample; it was 0.1% in amplitude, 0.04 cm/sec broad and had no isomer shift.

10.5.3 EXPERIMENTAL RESULTS

Oxyhemoglobin $[HbO_2(Fe^{2+})]$ has been examined in several different forms: normal human oxyhemoglobin (type A) in red cells and in solution; mutant oxyhemoglobin (type $S + D$—51%, type $A + F$—49%) (Baglioni, 1963) in red cells, rabbit oxyhemoglobin in reticulocytes, and rat oxyhemoglobin in cells and in frozen solution. The Mössbauer spectra consist in every case of a symmetric doublet whose quadrupole splitting and isomer shift were independent of the form of the sample and the type and species of protein. Intensity of the spectrum increased with decreasing temperature due to the Debye–Waller factor. Gonser and Grant (1965) have found the Debye–Waller factor for oxyhemoglobin at 5°K to be 0.83. The quadrupole splitting has been found to be temperature dependent (Gonser and Grant, 1965; Lang and Marshall, 1966); the sign of the quadrupole splitting has been estimated to be negative (Lang and Marshall, 1966), and there is an absence of magnetic hyperfine structure at low temperatures, consistent with the fact that oxyhemoglobin is diamagnetic ($S = 0$).

Deoxyhemoglobin $[Hb(Fe^{2+})]$ has been examined in several different forms and from several different species: normal human deoxyhemoglobin as a lyophilized powder and in frozen solution, cells of mutant human hemoglobin and cells and frozen solutions of rat and rabbit deoxyhemoglobin. The spectra of deoxyhemoglobin consists of a symmetric doublet independent of species and form, whose splitting is slightly temperature dependent. An example is given in Fig. 10.7b. The spectrum has a large positive isomer shift relative to HbO_2, a quadrupole splitting slightly larger than that of oxyhemoglobin, and a line width that is independent of temperature down to 4°K.

Carbonmonoxyhemoglobin $[HbCO(Fe^{2+})]$: normal human, rabbit, and rat carbonmonoxyhemoglobin have been examined in frozen solution. A symmetric doublet was observed, with splitting and isomer shift independent of temperature and species. The isomer shift was approximately that of oxyhemoglobin; however, the quadrupole splitting was smaller than that of oxyhemoglobin by a factor of 5.5. Line widths were independent of temperature. An example of the HbCo spectrum is shown in Fig. 10.7c.

Methemoglobin $[metHb(Fe^{3+})]$ and metmyoglobin $[metMb(Fe^{3+})]$: samples of rabbit, canine, equine, porcine, human, and denatured methemoglobin have been examined as lyophilized powders, as have a mixed human mutant hemoglobin ($F + S$). Human and rat methemoglobin have been examined in frozen solution. Sperm whale metmyoglobin has been examined as a lyophilized powder. Isomer shift and quadrupole splitting were approximately the same as those of oxyhemoglobin, and independent of species, type, and hydration.

Unlike the Fe^{2+} derivatives marked changes in the spectra of metHb and metMb were observed at low temperatures. Figure 10.8 illustrates the effect of reduced temperature on the spectra of methemoglobin as a lyophilized powder. This same behavior is noted for methemoglobin in solution (Lang and Marshall, 1966). The appearance of asymmetry in both solution and powder spectra is associated with an unequal, temperature dependent broadening of the two components of the quadrupole doublet. Component areas were computed for both hemoglobin and myoglobin spectra and were found to be the same. Lang and Marshall (1966) show the presence of resolved magnetic hyperfine structure at $4°K$.

Methemoglobin fluoride [metHbF(Fe^{3+})]: methemoglobin fluoride has been examined as a frozen solution and as a dry powder. Solution spectra at 195, 77, 4, and $1.2°K$ showed the presence of unresolved hyperfine structure (Lang and Marshall, 1966). MetHbF is a high spin complex in solution (Table 10.4) and in order to explain the $77°K$ spectrum it was necessary to include contributions from the three Kramers doublets. By applying a strong magnetic field these workers were able to increase spin–lattice relaxation time sufficiently at $4°K$ to resolve completely a six line magnetic hyperfine spectrum. The powder spectrum resembles that of methemoglobin and metmyoglobin both as a powder and in solution.

Methemoglobin cyanide [metHbCN(Fe^{3+})]: methemoglobin cyanide has been examined as a frozen solution and as a dry powder. Isomer shift in each case was the same as that of methemoglobin; quadrupole splitting in each case was about two-thirds that of methemoglobin. The spectrum of the cyanide complex shows the same broadening and asymmetry as that of methemoglobin at liquid nitrogen temperatures (due to the appearance of the magnetic hyperfine interaction). At $4°K$ however the magnetic hyperfine structure is much more well resolved than that of methemoglobin (Lang and Marshall, 1966). The spectrum of methemoglobin as a dry powder shows essentially the same behavior as that of the solution spectra (Fig. 10.9) including well resolved structure at $4°K$ (Fig. 10.10). Resolution of the powder spectrum is poor because the sample contains the natural abundance of Fe-57; however the main features of the powder spectrum match quite well those of the solution spectrum of Lang and Marshall.

Methemoglobin azide [metHbN$_3$(Fe^{3+})]: methemoglobin azide has been examined as a frozen solution and as a dry powder. Isomer shift in both cases is the same as that of methemoglobin. Quadrupole splitting of the powder spectrum is the same as that of methemoglobin but is slightly

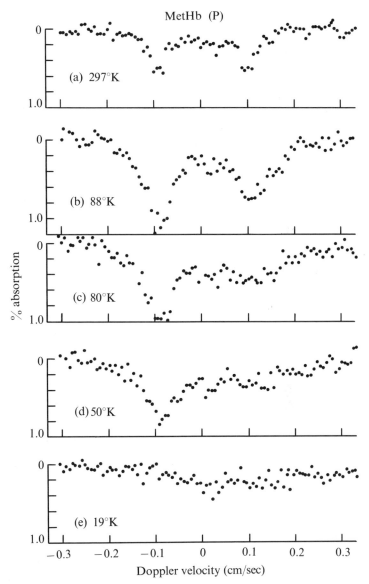

Fig. 10.8   Human methemoglobin in the form of a lyophilized powder at (a) 29°K, (b) 88°K, (c) 80°K, (d) 50°K, and (e) 19°K.

greater in frozen solution spectrum.   At 4°K the spectrum of methemoglobin azide in solution shows resolved magnetic hyperfine structure (Lang and Marshall, 1966).

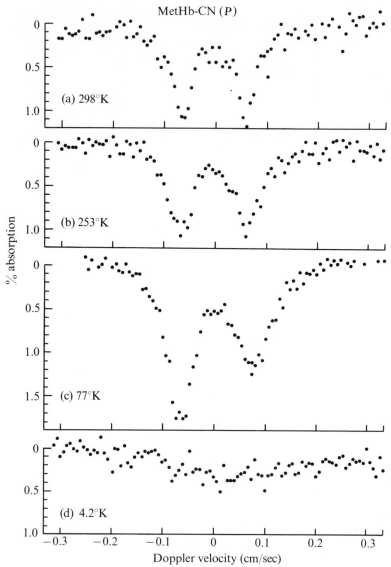

Fig. 10.9   Human methemoglobin cyanide in the form of a lyophilized powder at (a) 298°K, (b) 253°K, (c) 77°K, and (d) 4.2°K.

Cytochrome c: horseheart cytochrome c has been examined in both oxidized and reduced form as a dry powder. The spectrum of ferricyto-chrome c is identical to that of methemoglobin (Fig. 10.11a). Ferrocyto-chrome c however produces a spectrum different from that of (ferro)

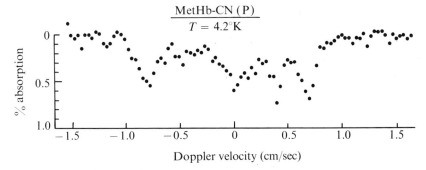

Fig. 10.10   Human methemoglobin cyanide in the form of a lyophilized powder at 4.2°K; the velocity excursion is ±1.5 cm/sec. The concentration of iron is 2.2% by weight.

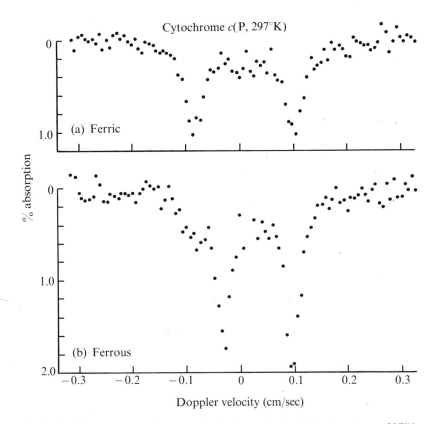

Fig. 10.11   Horseheart cytochrome c in the form of a lyophilized powder at 297°K: (a) ferric, and (b) ferrous.

hemoglobin (Fig. 10.11b). The quadrupole splitting is about 40% smaller (it resembles that of methbCN) and the isomer shift is intermediate between that of HbO_2 and Hb (Table 10.3). Preliminary low temperature studies show that the spectrum of ferricytochrome c broadens in a manner similar to that of methemoglobin while the line width of the spectrum of ferrocytochrome c is independent of temperature, resembling the ferrous hemoglobin derivatives in this respect.

10.5.4   DISCUSSION

Some general conclusions may be drawn from an examination of the various Mössbauer data in Table 10.3: (1) the spectra are insensitive to the species from which the hemoglobin was derived despite differences in amino acid composition. Also, various types of human hemoglobin, which may differ drastically in their physiological behavior, nevertheless produce the same Mössbauer spectrum. (2) The spectra are unaffected by the number of subunits per molecule as evidenced by the similarity of the spectra of methemoglobin, metmyoglobin, and oxidized cytochrome c. (3) Both native and denatured methemoglobin produce the same spectrum. On the assumption that denaturation alters the tertiary structure of the protein, the data suggest that the Mössbauer spectra are independent of tertiary structure. These results may be taken as an indication that Mössbauer absorption, in the heme-proteins that have been examined, probes an electronic environment which is common to all these molecules. This would mean that in the interpretation of the various Mössbauer spectra it is probably justifiable to ignore factors like amino acid composition and tertiary structure and to base the interpretation entirely on the properties of the heme group (together with the fifth and sixth ligands).

The asymmetric broadening of the spectra of the ferric derivatives methHb, metMb, methbCN, and ferric cytochrome c as the temperature is reduced to that of liquid nitrogen is due to the appearance of the magnetic h.f. interaction. Similar asymmetries observed in the quadrupole doublets from tin (Goldanskii, et al., 1962), iron-organic compounds other than hemoglobin (King, et al., 1964) and deoxyHb (Gonser and Grant, 1965) have been attributed to an anisotropic Debye–Waller factor. An anisotropic Debye–Waller factor would lead both to a difference in integrated intensities of the two components of a quadrupole doublet and to a decreasing anisotropy with decreasing temperature. (See Wertheim, 1964, for a discussion of this effect.) This mechanism fails in both respects to account for the effect observed in the above compounds. This effect is within 10% entirely a broadening of one component with respect to the other, and the broadening increases with decreasing temperature until at sufficiently low temperature magnetic h.f. is visible in most cases.   For discussions of the magnetic h.f. interaction in these and other systems see Wertheim, 1964; Wickman, 1964; Blume, 1965; Lang and Marshall, 1966; Bradford and Marshall, 1966.

Most of the heme-proteins studied had isomer shifts lying between zero and ± 0.015 cm/sec.   These included the ferric derivatives—metHb, metMb, metHbF, metHbN$_3$, metHbCN, and oxidized cytochrome c—as well as the ferrous derivatives, HbCO and HbO$_2$.   Only deoxyhemoglobin and reduced cytochrome c lay outside the above region.   These (at the lowest temperatures measured) had isomer shifts of $+0.085$ and $+0.032$ cm/ sec respectively.   All the compounds that have been examined showed evidence of a quadrupole interaction which for the majority of derivatives was large and surprisingly constant.   Quadrupole splittings for most of the derivatives lay within 15 or 20% of one another.   The only exceptions to this were metHbCN and reduced cytochrome c with splittings approximately two-thirds that of the mean of the majority group; HbCO had a very small quadrupole splitting—about a fifth of that in most other compounds.

It is useful to attempt an interpretation of the Mössbauer spectra of the various compounds in the light of the theoretical ideas discussed in section 10.4, although it is recognized that these ideas may be vastly oversimplified.   Nevertheless such interpretations are necessary to indicate in

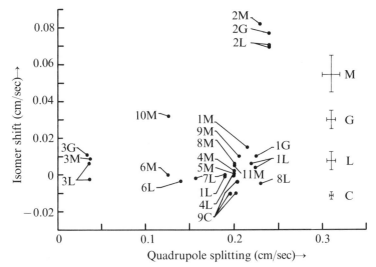

Fig. 10.12   Isomer shift vs. quadrupole splitting for the data in Table 10.3. M: this laboratory, the points represent average values; G: Gonser and Grant (1965); L: Lang and Marshall (1966); C: Caughey, et al. (1966). The numbers correspond to those in Table 10.4: (1) HbO$_2$, (2) Hb, (3) HbCO, (4) MetHb, (5) MetHbF, (6) MetHbCN, (7) MetHbOH, (8) MetHbN$_3$, (9) MetMb, (10) ferrous cytochrome c, (11) ferric cytochrome c.

which directions greater theoretical sophistication may be necessary. For clarity the data of Table 10.3 have been plotted in Fig. 10.12 in the form of isomer shift (I.S.) versus quadrupole splittings (Q.S.)   It appears from Fig. 10.12 that most compounds are located in one of three regions: (a) large I.S. –large Q.S., (b) small I.S.–large Q.S. and (c) small I.S.–small Q.S.

Table 10.4   *Effective Bohr magneton numbers for hemoglobin derivatives and cytochrome c*

Protein	Form[a]	% Hydration by weight	n_{eff} per heme	Ref.[b]
HbO$_2$	S	100	0	1
HbCO	S	100	0	1
Hb	S	100	5.5	1
	P	0	3.0	5
metHb	S	100	5.8, 5.6, 5.8	2, 3, 5
	P	45	6.0	5
	P	32	5.0	5
	P	21	4.0	5
	P	0	2.7, 3.0	5, 4
metHbF	S	100	5.9, 5.8	2, 3
	P	0	4.5	4
metHbN$_3$	S	100	2.4	3
	P	—	3.1	4
metHbCN	S	100	2.5	2, 3
	P	—	1.9	4
Mb	S	100	5.5	7
metMb	S	100	5.7, 5.9, 5.7	3, 7, 8
Ferrous cytochrome *c*	S	100	0.8	6
	P	0	2.7	6
Ferric cytochrome *c*	S	100	2.8	6
	P	0	4.1	6

[a] *S*: Solution; *P*: Power.
[b] (1) Pauling and Coryell (1936); (2) Coryell, *et al.*, (1937); (3) Scheler, *et al.*, (1957); (4) Schoffa, *et al.*, (1959); (5) Havemann and Haberditzl (1959); (6) Lumry, *et al.*, (1962); (7) Taylor, (1939); (8) Theorell and Ehrenberg (1951).

(a) Large I.S.—Large Q.S.: There is only one compound in this region—deoxyhemoglobin.   The prediction based on Table 10.2 is that Hb in whatever form—powder, solution, cells—is a ferrous high-spin ($S = 2$) compound, in agreement with the usual chemical assignment.   However, the data on magnetic susceptibility (Table 10.4) distinguish quite clearly between solutions and powders; the former correspond to high spin while the latter have a susceptibility corresponding to an intermediate value of spin ($S = 1$). Whether this is actually the case or whether the powders are mixtures of high and low spin compounds, as seems to be the case for the metHb hydroxide (George, et al., 1964), is not known. The lack of magnetic hyperfine interaction is not inconsistent with the description of the compound as ferrous (either high or low spin).

(b) Small I.S.–Large Q.S.: Most of the compounds that have been studied lie in this region. It includes oxyhemoglobin, methemoglobin, methemoglobin fluoride, methemoglobin hydroxide, methemoglobin azide, metmyoglobin, and ferric cytochrome c. On the basis of Table 10.2 these would all be ferric, low spin ($S = \frac{1}{2}$) compounds and should show no magnetic hyperfine interaction down to the lowest temperatures.

To find oxyhemoglobin among this group is surprising since the susceptibility data clearly indicate that $S = 0$. The low temperature spectra which show no magnetic hyperfine interaction are inconclusive since, according to Table 10.2, the lack of magnetic hyperfine interaction is consistent with both $S = 0$ and $S = \frac{1}{2}$. It appears, then, that we have only the Mössbauer and the susceptibility data which, seemingly, are in contradiction. However, it should be noted that a measurement of the susceptibility in effect determines the magnetic moment of the molecular complex as a whole whereas the Mössbauer spectrum seems to be sensitive only to the local region in the vicinity of the iron atom. As pointed out by Weiss (1964), on the basis of totally different considerations, there may well be a transfer of an electron from Fe to O_2. If we assume this to take place from a filled t_2-shell, without any further electronic rearrangements, an appropriate description of the iron would then be Fe^{3+} with $S = \frac{1}{2}$. At the same time the oxygen molecule would become O_2^-, also with $S = \frac{1}{2}$.

In this connection, recall that Shulman and Sugano (1965), in a molecular orbital analysis of the iron-group cyanides, conclude that approximately one more d-electron is back-donated to the ligand in the case of ferrocyanide than in the case of ferricyanide leaving the effective charge on the ion within the ion–ligand complex the same in the two cases.

Methemoglobin and metmyoglobin are generally assumed to be ferric high spin ($S = \frac{5}{2}$) compounds. The Mössbauer data and Table 10.2 suggest that they are indeed ferric but of low spin ($S = \frac{1}{2}$). To discuss these compounds we must distinguish between powder and solution spectra. It has been suggested (Caughey, et al., 1966) that in the process of drying the spin changes from $\frac{5}{2}$ to $\frac{1}{2}$. Magnetic susceptibility measurements on powders (Table 10.4) support this hypothesis. However, the low temperature Mössbauer spectra show ample evidence of magnetic hyperfine interaction (Lang and Marshall, 1966) which, according to Table 10.2 is inconsistent with $S = \frac{1}{2}$. In solution there seems to be a clear contradiction between the Mössbauer data, which suggest $S = \frac{1}{2}$, and the measurements of magnetic susceptibility which indicate $S = \frac{5}{2}$ (Table 10.4). The low temperature behavior is more nearly consistent with $S = \frac{5}{2}$. Lang and Marshall have investigated this problem; they invoke a certain amount of covalency and are able to obtain a reasonable value of the quadrupole splitting as well as a fit of the low temperature spectrum by means of one parameter.

Methemoglobin fluoride in solution is a ferric, high spin ($S = \frac{5}{2}$) compound, as deduced from both electron spin resonance (Gibson, $et\ al.$, 1958) and magnetic susceptibility data (Table 10.4) measurements. Lang and Marshall (1966), by application of an external magnetic field, were able to deduce a small quadrupole splitting (0.03 cm/sec) at 4°K—a result consistent with high spin. Moreover they obtain a value for D, the zero-field splitting constant, of 7 cm^{-1} which is remarkably close to the value obtained from infrared absorption measurements (Feher and Richards, 1966). The magnetic susceptibility of the powder (Table 10.4) is substantially smaller than that of the solution; this suggests that methemoglobin fluoride in powder, as in the case of deoxyhemoglobin, may be a mixture of high and low spin compounds. The Mössbauer data favor the assignment of $S = \frac{1}{2}$ to the powder form.

For methemoglobin azide, data from magnetic susceptibility, electron spin resonance, and Mössbauer spectra are all consistent with the description of the compound as ferric, low spin ($S = \frac{1}{2}$).

Ferric cytochrome c, as a powder at room temperature and at 4°K, produces Mössbauer spectra identical with those of methemoglobin. On this basis alone the assignment would be $S = \frac{1}{2}$. The magnetic susceptibility data (Table 10.4) lie at a value intermediate between that for high and low spin compounds; hence the assignment is neither supported nor contradicted by the susceptibility data. It is to be noted that in contrast to methemoglobin, the data on magnetic susceptibility show that dry cytochrome c (both ferric and ferrous) has a higher susceptibility than the dissolved or hydrated form.

(c) Small I.S.—Small Q.S.: Of the compounds that have been examined only carbon monoxide hemoglobin has both a small isomer shift and a small quadrupole splitting. According to Table 10.2, the compound would be described as ferric, high spin ($S = \frac{5}{2}$), in clear contradiction to the measurements of magnetic susceptibility (Table 10.4) which indicate that $S = 0$. The low temperature Mössbauer spectra show no magnetic hyperfine structure, which throws the weight of the evidence in favor of $S = 0$. The situation using the ligand field model is therefore anomalous.

Magnetic susceptibility measurements on methemoglobin cyanide indicate that the compound is ferric, low spin ($S = \frac{1}{2}$). The small isomer shift is consistent with the ferric assignment but the quadrupole splitting is somewhat low for a system in which $S = \frac{1}{2}$. Moreover, a well-defined magnetic hyperfine structure is observed at $4°K$—a feature not ordinarily expected when $S = \frac{1}{2}$. Ferrous cytochrome c has a quadrupole splitting approximately equal to that of methemoglobin cyanide but the isomer shift is substantially greater as might occur for a mixture of ferric and ferrous compounds.

10.5.5 CONCLUSIONS

Conclusions based on the examination of isomer shifts, quadrupole splittings, magnetic hyperfine interactions, magnetic susceptibility measurements, and electron spin resonance data appear to be consistent with the ligand field model for some, but by no means all, of the hemoglobin derivatives that have been studied. The resolution of these inconsistencies therefore requires a more sophisticated model than the one presented above, probably one that includes the concept of covalency in a more precise fashion.† Despite the difficulties in the theoretical interpretation of Mössbauer data the experiment is useful as a diagnostic technique used semi-empirically in conjunction with other physical and chemical methods. There is a clear distinction between spectra of certain heme protein derivatives and it can therefore be used in a manner analogous to that of optical absorption. Disadvantages of the experiment are, however, (i) the Mössbauer isotope, Fe-57 is low in abundance; without enrichment relatively massive samples (of the order of 500 mg of heme protein) are required, (ii) enrichment is essential if one is to study magnetic h.f.s, and (iii) the Mössbauer sample must be a solid, a frozen liquid, or a liquid of sufficiently high viscosity. A unique advantage on the other hand is the fact that the experiment is specific to certain nuclei. In a manner similar to that of the ESR experiment the technique probes only the local environment of a specific atom. This can be of great value in the case of a Mössbauer atom such as iron which plays a central role in the function of the molecule to which it is bound. Unfortunately iron (Fe-57) is almost unique among Mössbauer atoms in this respect.

† A theoretical estimate by Weissbluth and Maling (1967) of the relative magnitudes of the quadrupole splittings for certain hemoglobin derivatives (including the three ferrous hemoglobins discussed) based on recent molecular orbital (M.O.) calculations by Zerner, *et al.* (1966) on model iron-porphyrin complexes has produced a more favorable correlation with the data than have estimates based on the ligand field model. Although there are significant structural differences between the model compounds on which the M.O. calculation is based on the one hand and the heme in complex with globin as we understand it on the other, the M.O. model has succeeded in resolving inconsistencies in the ferrous hemoglobin derivative quadrupole data left unresolved by the ligand field approach. This success is probably due to the fact that the M.O. model automatically takes account of covalency in the ion–ligand bond.

ACKNOWLEDGEMENTS

We are grateful to Drs. B. Gerstl, D. Croll, and E. Movitt who provided us with blood samples containing mutant hemoglobin. We also wish to acknowledge the expert assistance, in various phases of the experiments performed in this laboratory, of Messrs. T. Rodehorst, O. Bezrukov (exchange scholar, University of Leningrad), D. Dexter, Marc Weissbluth, Miss C. Nardini and Miss Pui-Chu Chan.

This work was supported by National Science Foundation Grants GB 1409 and 3994.

REFERENCES

Abragam, A., 1964, *L'Effect Mössbauer* (New York: Gordon and Breach Inc.).

Baglioni, C., 1963, in *Molecular Genetics*, Ed., J. H. Taylor (New York: Academic Press), Part I, 405.

Bearden, A. J., 1964, *Proc. 3rd Int. Conf. Mössbauer Effect, Rev. mod. Phys.,* **36**, 333.

Bearden, A. J., Moss, T. H., Caughey, W. S., and Beaudreau, C. A., 1965, *Proc. natn. Acad. Sci. U.S.A.*, **53**, 1246.

Blume, M., 1965, *Phys. Rev. Lett.*, **14**, 96.

Boyle, A. J. F., and Hall, H. E., 1962, *Rep. Prog. Phys.*, **25**, 441.

Bradford, E., and Marshall, W., 1966, *Proc. phys. Soc.*, **87**, 731.

Caughey, W. S., Fujimoto, W. Y., Bearden, A. J., and Moss, T. H., 1966, *Biochem. J.*, **5**, 1255.

Cohen, R. L., McMullin, P. G., and Wertheim, G. K., 1963, *Rev. scient. Instrum.*, **34**, 671.

Compton, D. M. J., and Schoen, A. H., 1962, *Proc. 2nd Int. Conf. Mössbauer Effect*, Ed. D. M. J. Compton and H. A. Schoen (New York: Wiley).

Coryell, C. D., Stitt, F., and Pauling, L., 1937, *J. Am. chem. Soc.*, **39**, 633.

Craig, P. P., and Sutin, N., 1963, *Brookhaven Nat. Lab. Rep.* 7391.

De Benedetti, S., Lang, G., and Ingalls, R., 1961, *Phys. Rev. Lett.*, **6**, 60.

Drabkin, D. L., 1946, *J. biol. Chem.*, **164**, 703.

Drabkin, D. L., 1949, *Archs Biochem.*, **21**, 224.

Feher, G., and Richards, P. L., *International Conference on Magnetic Resonance*, Stockholm, June 1966.

Frauenfelder, H., 1962, *The Mössbauer Effect* (New York: W. A. Benjamin).

Freeman, A. J., and Watson, R. E., 1962, *Proc. 2nd Int. Conf. Mössbauer Effect*, Ed. D. M. J. Compton and A. H. Schoen (New York: Wiley).

George, P., Beetlestone, J., and Griffith, J. S., 1964, *Rev. mod. Phys.*, **36**, 441.

Gibson, J. F., Ingram, D. J. E., and Schonland, D., 1958, *Discuss. Faraday Soc.*, **26**, 72.

Goldanskii, V. I., Gorodinskii, G. M., Karyagin, S. V., Korytko, L. A., Krizhanskii, L. M., Makarov, E. F., Suzdalev, I. P., and Khrakov, V. V., 1962, *Dokl. Akad. Nauk. SSSR*, **147**, 127.
Gonser, U., and Grant, R. W., 1965, *Biophys. J.*, **5**, 823.
Gonser, U., Grant, R. W., and Kregzde, J., 1963, *Appl. Phys. Lett.*, **3**, 189; 1964, *Science*, N.Y., **143**, 690.
Gray, D. E., 1957, *Am. Inst. Phys. Handbook*, Ed. D. E. Gray (New York: McGraw-Hill Book Company, Inc.).
Griffith, J. S., 1957, *Nature*, Lond., **180**, 30.
Havemann, R., and Haberditzl, W., 1959, *Z. phys. Chem.*, **210**.
Herber, R. H., 1966, *Ann. Rev. phys. Chem.*, **17**, 261.
Herber, R. H., and Wertheim, G. K., 1962, *Proc. 2nd Int. Conf. Mössbauer Effect*, Ed. D. M. J. Compton and A. H. Schoen (New York: Wiley).
Ingalls, R., 1964, *Phys. Rev.*, **133**, A787.
Keilin, D. L., and Hartree, E. F., 1951, *Biol. J.*, **49**, 88.
Kendrew, J. C., 1963, *Science, N.Y.*, **139**, 1259.
King, R. B., Herber, R. H., and Wertheim, G. K., 1964, *Inorg. Chem.*, **3**, 101.
Kistner, O. C., and Sunyar, A. W., 1960, *Phys. Rev. Lett.*, **4**, 412.
Kotani, M., 1961, *Prog. theor. Phys.*, *Osaka*, Suppl. **17**, 8.
Lang, G., and Marshall, W., 1966, *Proc. phys. Soc.*, **87**, 3.
Lumry, R., Solbakken, A., Sullivan, J., and Reyerson, L. H., 1962, *J. Am. chem. Soc.*, **84**, 142.
Maling, J. E., and Weissbluth, M., 1964, *Electronic Aspects of Biochemistry*, Ed. B. Pullman (New York: Academic Press).
Margoliash, E., 1966, *Adv. Protein Chem.*, **21**, 113.
Marshall, W., and Johnson, C. E., 1962, *J. Phys. Radium*, Paris, **23**, 733.
Mössbauer, R. L., 1958, *Z. Phys.*, **151**, 124.
Mössbauer, R. L., 1959, *Z. Naturf.*, **14a**, 211.
Mössbauer, R. L., 1962, *A. Rev. nucl. Sci.*, **12**, 123.
Muir, A. H., Ando, K. J., and Coogan, H. M., 1966, *Mössbauer Effect Data Index*, 1958–65 (Interscience, John Wiley and Sons, N.Y.).
Pauling, L., and Coryell, C. D., 1936, *Proc. natn. Acad. Sci., U.S.A.*, **22**, 210.
Perini, F., Maling, J. E., and Weissbluth, M., *BL Report 171*, Biophysics Laboratory, Stanford University, 1966.
Perutz, M. F., 1963, *Science*, N.Y., **140**, 863.
Pound, R. V., and Rebka, G. A., Jr., 1959, *Phys. Rev. Lett.*, **3**, 440; 1960, ibid., **4**, 274.
Scheler, W., Schoffa, G., and Jung, F., 1957, *Biochem. Z.*, **329**, 232.
Schoffa, G., Scheler, W., Ristau, O., and Jung, F., 1959, *Acta biol. med. germ.*, **3**, 65.
Shulman, R. G., and Sugano, S., 1965, *J. chem. Phys.*, **42**, 39.

Stryer, L., Kendrew, J. C., and Watson, H. C., 1964, *J. molec. Biol.*, **8**, 96.
Taylor, D. S., 1939, *J. Am. chem. Soc.*, **61**, 2150.
Theorell, H., and Ehrenberg, A., 1951, *Acta chem. scand.*, **5**, 823.
Walker, L. R., Wertheim, G. K., and Jaccarino, V., 1961, *Phys. Rev. Lett.*, **6**, 98.
Weiss, J. J., 1964, *Nature, Lond.*, **202**, 83.
Weissbluth, M., 1967, *Structure and Bonding*, **2**, 1 (New York: Springer Verlag).
Weissbluth, M., and Maling, J. E., 1967, *J. chem. Phys.*, **47**, 4166.
Wertheim, G. K., 1964, *Mössbauer Effect* (New York: Academic Press).
Wickman, H. H., 1964, Ph.D. thesis, Univ. of Calif., Berkeley, (unpublished).
Zerner, M., Gouterman, M., and Kobayashi, H., 1966, *Theo. Chim. Acta*, **6**, 363.

CHAPTER ELEVEN

LASERS

Robert C. Smith

Department of Electronics, The University, Southampton, England

11.1   INTRODUCTION

Immediately after the announcement from Hughes Aircraft Company of the first laser (Maiman, 1960), there was much talk of the possibilities of lasers as death rays.   In the following six years the laser has not emerged as a viable weapon but the idea of the 'laser beam death ray' is now part of popular mythology.   One result of this discussion was that biologists and medical research workers were quick to realize the potential of laser light for the selective destruction or modification of small regions of living things.   The early work was carried out while laser technology was developing and was not as thorough as one would wish.   Some of the first claims have remained unsubstantiated but at least three applications are now well established. Two of these are clinical—the laser retinal photo-coagulator for eye surgery, and the use of high energy lasers in the treatment of skin disease.   The other application is in biology and concerns the use of focussed laser beams for the destruction, etc., of micron diameter regions in single cells.

My qualifications for writing this chapter are that I have been working in the laser field for the last five years and that I once did some research in medical physics.   I will therefore give a physicist's view of lasers in medicine; and the main part of this chapter will be concerned with the laser device and instrumentation.   At the end I will discuss some of the results of biological experiments but here any opinion I express should be treated with extreme caution.   Much of laser theory has been taken from electronics (lasers with masers are covered by the generic term Quantum Electronics) so you must be prepared for talk of feedback, oscillators, and so on.

The next section is the longest and is concerned with the laser, the fundamental principles behind its operation, devices, materials and nonlinear devices such as harmonic generators.   Sections after that cover instrumentation for biological experiments and the interaction of laser radiation with materials.   In the final section some medical and biological applications will be discussed.

11.2   LASERS

11.2.1   FUNDAMENTALS

Although readers of this book will have heard many 'simple' explanations of the operation of a laser, I will again very briefly cover the basic ideas but with the principal aim of getting you used to my laser vocabulary.

To continue on well trod ground, lasers depend for their operation upon stimulated emission of radiation.   With reference to Fig. 11.1, atoms in level 2 can make two kinds of radiative transition to level 1.   They can either fall spontaneously emitting photons randomly during the radiative lifetime or they can be stimulated to emit by the presence of light at the transition wavelength (frequency).   The process of stimulated emission is the exact reverse of 'stimulated' absorption by which light power is lost at the transition wavelength in raising atoms from level 1 to level 2. These two competing processes have equal probability for transitions between energy states. Since each energy level may correspond to a number of states, the light beam will gain more power by stimulated emission than it loses by absorption if

$$n_2/g_2 > n_1/g_1$$

where n_1 and n_2 are numbers of atoms, per unit volume, in levels 1 and 2, and

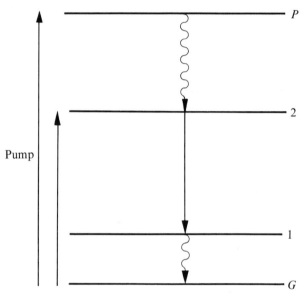

Fig. 11.1   Basic energy diagram: 1 and 2–laser levels, G–ground level, P–level reached by pumping.

g_1 and g_2 are degeneracies of levels 1 and 2. We then say that there is a population inversion. Here now is a light amplifier by which light, of the transition wavelength, can be increased in power. The gain of the amplifier (length l') is

$$G = \exp\left[\sigma_{12}g_1(n_2/g_2 - n_1/g_1)l'\right]$$

where σ_{12} is the transition cross-section, normally defined in terms of the absorption coefficient ($n_2 = 0$)

$$\alpha = \sigma_{12}n_1$$

The skill of the laser physicist lies in creating a population inversion.

The need is to excite atoms preferentially into level 2.   A wide variety of such 'pumping' techniques have been devised and they will be discussed in a little more detail later when talking about specific laser materials.   Essentially, atoms are pumped either direct from the ground level into level 2 or into a higher level, from which they decay into level 2.   Also it must be obvious that the gain is at a maximum if level 1 is unpopulated.   For this to happen level 1 must be many kT above the ground level and have a rapid coupling, possibly non-radiative, to ground.

The most important property of the laser amplifier is that it faithfully reproduces the light wave fed into it.   At first this might seem a little surprising; however, it comes from the equivalence of absorption and stimulated emission.   Figure 11.2(a) shows the decrease of a light wave in an absorbing material and, as expected, the form of the wave is retained while its amplitude gets smaller.   Stimulated emission is represented in Fig. 11.2(b);

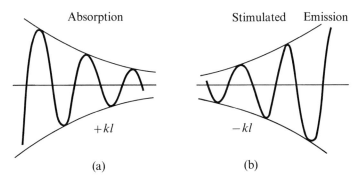

Fig. 11.2   Absorption and stimulated emission.

now the wave increases in size but again its shape is unchanged.   It is this coherent amplification which makes a light oscillator possible when the amplifier is combined with a resonant cavity.

An amplifier can be turned into an oscillator by the addition of a positive feedback loop with a loop gain greater than unity.   The frequency of oscillation is fixed by the combined characteristic of the feedback line and amplifier gain curve.   At light frequencies we obviously cannot use wires to make the feedback connection and we have to resort to a resonant cavity formed by two parallel mirrors, as in Fig. 11.3(a).   For this 'circuit', positive feedback is maximum when there is a standing wave between the mirrors. The simplest condition for a standing wave is

$$l = q\lambda/2$$

where λ is wavelength of oscillation and q is an integer.   There is a series of

standing waves corresponding to different values of q, and in laser terminology they are called axial modes. Oscillation is only possible for those
modes which fall within the transition bandwidth and where the amplifier
gain is greater than the total loss from the mirrors, etc. (see Fig. 11.3(b)).
The oscillation draws power from the atomic population to make the gain
at a mode frequency exactly equal to the loss.   The number of modes which

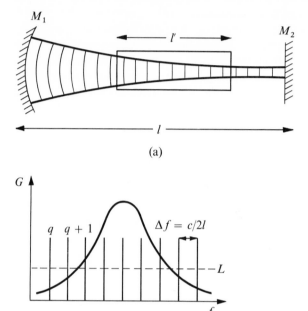

Fig. 11.3   (a) Standing waves in an optical resonant cavity.
(b) Axial modes within the laser gain curve (width $\triangle f$).

oscillate depends upon the physical mechanism which determines the transition bandwidth.   If the line is homogeneous, as in lifetime broadening,
power can be transferred from one part of the gain curve to another.   Oscillation is then on one mode, nearest to the peak of the line, the whole gain curve
being reduced to make $G = L$.   With an inhomogeneous line, there is no
transfer of power between frequencies and all modes for which $G > L$
oscillate, cutting holes in the gain curve to the depth of the loss line.   In both
cases the purity of the frequency for the individual modes is mainly a function
of the mirror spacing (l).   The oscillation always has a bandwidth many
times smaller than that from conventional light sources and it is said to be
time coherent.

When considering the standing waves which the cavity can support, we obviously oversimplified since we neglected variation of the light field in planes perpendicular to the axis of the cavity.   Patterns containing nodes and anti-nodes of intensity are also formed in these planes.   Diffraction theory can be used to find the transverse form of the standing wave (Boyd and Gordon, 1961).   A diffraction integral is constructed to describe the field set up on a mirror M_2 by that on M_1 and then back on M_1 from M_2 as

$$E_1(x, y) = \iint_{-a}^{+a} \frac{ik}{2\pi\rho} e^{-ik\rho} E_1(x, y) \, dx \, dy$$

where $E_1(x, y)$ is field distribution on M_1, dimension $2a \times 2a$, $k = 2\pi/\lambda$, and ρ is the distance of the round trip from the source field to diffraction field.

This integral equation is then solved for $E_1(x, y)$.   For resonant cavities made of one plane and one spherical mirror, there are solutions

$$E_1(x, y) = E_0 \cdot H_m(\sqrt{2} \, x/W) \cdot H_n(\sqrt{2} \, y/W) \cdot \exp\left[-(x^2 + y^2)/W^2\right]$$

($H_m(\sqrt{2} \, x/W)$, $H_n(\sqrt{2} \, y/W)$ are Hermite polynomials; W is the spot radius).

These functions are termed transverse modes and, when combined with the axial modes, are given the label TEM_{mnq}, where m and n are the numbers of nodes along the x and y directions.   For the lowest order transverse mode, TEM_{00q}, $H_0(x) = H_0(y) = 1$ and the standing wave has a surface of constant phase across both mirrors.   A very useful property of these 'Gaussian' modes is that they do not change their form through diffraction.   The angular radiation pattern for the laser is then given by the mode equation but replacing x, y, and W by θ_x, θ_y, and Φ where

$$\Phi = \frac{\lambda}{W\pi}$$

As an example, the total angular spread of the light from a 0.5 μ laser operating in a TEM_{00q} mode of 6 mm diameter is 10^{-4} radians (0.36 min of arc). The transverse modes are space coherent in a laser since the field at one point of the mirror can be calculated exactly from that at another point.

The condition

$$G > L$$

where L is the total cavity loss, tells us how difficult it is to make a particular laser oscillate.   The gain G is proportional to the population inversion and therefore more pumping is required the higher the loss.   The level of pumping for oscillation to commence is called the threshold pump.   Contributions to the loss come from mirrors with reflectivities less than 100%, unwanted reflections from windows and ends of laser rods, scattering from dust, etc., and diffraction spread missing the mirrors.   In some lasers, using solid materials for the amplifier, the gain can be greater than 10^3 to 10^4 and very large losses can be accepted. Gains of only a few per cent are obtained with some gas lasers and then great care has to be observed to keep the losses to a minimum.   Multi-layer dielectric mirrors are now available with re-flectivities greater than 99%.   The reflection loss from windows, etc., can be removed by setting them at Brewster's angle to the light beam.   There is then no loss for light polarized in the plane of incidence.   A result of using Brewster-angle components is that the laser oscillation is linearly polarized.

We have now covered all the background material we need and are in a position to examine in detail the range of laser devices available.

11.2.2   DEVICES

There are five distinct ways of operating a laser.   Four of these devices are oscillators, with a light amplifier between two mirrors.   The fifth device, the super-radiant laser, is essentially a source of amplified noise.   The four oscillators will be described first and in order of increasing power—decreasing pulse duration.   In the simplest oscillator, output is obtained for as long as the amplifier is pumped to a gain larger than the cavity losses.   Pulsed outputs with peak powers much greater than from the simple laser can be produced by control of the oscillation with a modulator placed inside the cavity.   The other three oscillators are concerned with various schemes of modulation.

A.   *CONTINUOUS AND PULSED PUMPING* (Yariv and Gordon, 1963)

Elementary electronics tells us that if we want a wave with a frequency purity of a few Hz the wave must have a duration of at least one second.   For ex-periments then which use the temporal coherence of laser light it is essential to have a laser with a continuous output.   To run a laser continuously implies pumping it continuously above threshold.   Then, provided there are no saturation effects the output power is proportional to the excess pump power.   Practical considerations such as cooling and mirror strength re-strict continuous powers to a few thousand watts.   To obtain high powers, without exceeding average ratings, lasers are frequently pumped with pulses of a low duty cycle.   The pulse energy rather than power is often given for such lasers.

Oscillation in certain of these lasers can be unstable.   Then, instead of getting a steady output for the duration of the pump, it breaks into a sequence of short pulses (Collins, *et al.*, 1960).   An example of such a 'relaxation oscillation' is shown in Fig. 11.4.

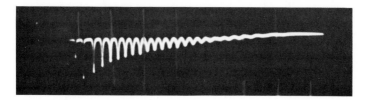

Fig. 11.4   Unstable output from a laser consisting of a ruby rod and two concave mirrors. The laser was pumped with a pulse of 400 μsec duration. Light power is downwards; sweep 30 μsec/div.

B. *Q-SWITCHING* (Missio and Seeber, 1965)

If the atoms have a long lifetime in the upper laser level the technique of Q-switching can be used to give high power pulses.   A shutter in the cavity inhibits oscillation while pumping produces a large population in the upper level.   Since there is no feedback the population inversion n_i (gain) can be made much larger than before.   When the shutter is opened a low loss (high Q-factor) cavity is presented to a high gain amplifier and the light intensity inside the cavity builds up very quickly.   The dynamics of this process are presented in Fig. 11.5(a).   With a large value of the starting inversion ratio n_i/n_{th}, nearly all the stored inversion is converted to light in a few nanoseconds $(10^{-9}$ sec).   The pulse then decays away with the damping time of the cavity, $2l/cL \simeq 10$ nsec.   Pulses only 10–20 nsec long can be created in this way with powers many orders of magnitude greater than without Q-switching.

Various shutters are used depending upon the particular application of the laser.   Rotation of one of the mirrors is a simple method for getting shutter action.   With a 24,000 r.p.m. motor, the two mirrors are sufficiently parallel for oscillation only during one microsecond of each revolution.   A small laser using this type of switch can be seen in the photograph, Fig. 11.6. Kerr and Pockels electro-optic modulators can also be used as shutters and have the advantage of an accurately timed output.   A very ingenious scheme uses a bleachable dye for the shutter.   A cell is placed in the cavity containing a solution of a dye which absorbs the laser wavelength and the dye concentration is arranged so that there is only a small transmission.   The laser has then to be pumped to a high population inversion before laser action can begin.   Once this happens however the dye molecules, on absorbing laser light, are raised to an excited state.   In this state they no longer absorb at the laser wavelength and the transmission of the cell has jumped to 100%.

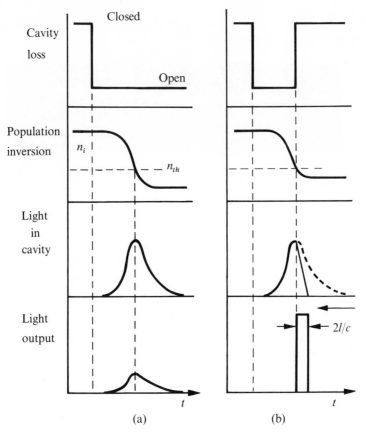

Fig. 11.5   Time variation of laser oscillation with (a) Q-switching, (b) PTM. n_i–population inversion before shutter is opened, n_{th}–population inversion for threshold of oscillation.

C. *PULSE TRANSMISSION MODE (PTM)* (Vuylsteke, 1963)

This device is a modification of Q-switching described above.   It is possible to produce a much shorter pulse if the output is taken from the Q-switch loss rather than from one of the mirrors.   Its operation will be described with reference to a Kerr cell modulator as shown schematically in Fig. 11.7.   The transmission direction of the polarizer is set at 45° to the optic axes of the $\lambda/4$ plate and Kerr cell.   When there is no field across the cell, the $\lambda/4$ retardation, coupled with the mirror, rotates through 90° the linearly polarized light from the polarizer.   This light is rejected from the cavity by the polarizer, and the mirror is therefore blocked.   The shutter can be opened by applying a voltage to one plate of the Kerr cell so that a retardation of

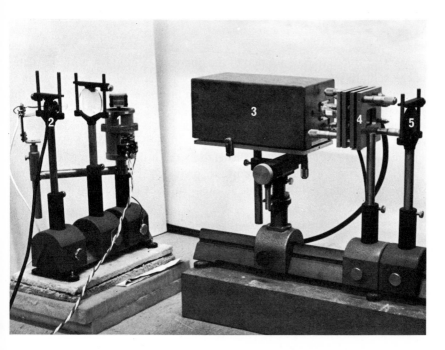

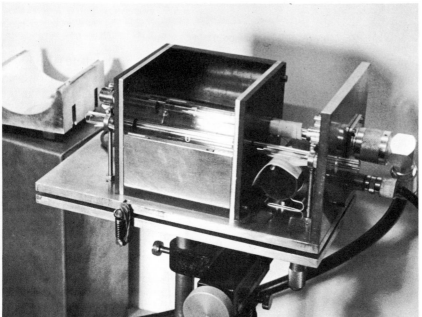

Fig. 11.6   (a) A small neodymium: glass Q-switched laser using a spinning reflector: 1–prism on motor (to maintain alignment in a vertical plane a total internal reflection right-angle prism is used with its apex horizontal), 2–optical arrangement for timing prism, 3–amplifier head, 4–fixed mirror, 5–infrared filter. (b) Exposed amplifier head: 6–glass laser rod, 7–flash tube.

$-\lambda/4$ is produced to balance that of the polarizer.   Initially, both the plates
of the cell are set at this voltage so there is no net field.   The operation is
then as in Fig. 11.5(b).   A large population inversion is established with the
shutter closed.   Then by shorting one of the plates to earth the shutter is
opened and normal Q-switched build-up takes place between the two totally
reflecting mirrors.   At the peak of the oscillation the second electrode is
shorted to earth.   The effect of this is to force all the light out of the cavity
via the polarizer.   It can be seen that, provided the Kerr cell is switched
sufficiently quickly, all the light is emitted from the laser cavity in its transit
time, $2l/c \simeq 1$ nsec.

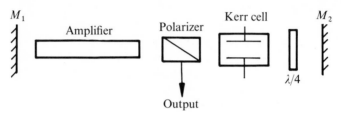

Fig. 11.7   Kerr cell PTM laser.

D. *MODE LOCKING* (Di Domenico, 1964)

Normally for a laser running on a number of axial modes there is no phase
relationship between the various waves at different frequencies.   However,
it is possible to lock the phases of these waves by means of a modulator in the
cavity driven at the frequency difference between the modes.   In this way a
coherent field spectrum is produced as in Fig. 11.8(a).   It can be shown that
this spectrum corresponds to a train of pulses as given in Fig. 11.8(b).   (The
reverse process is likely to be more familiar—proving that a train of pulses
with period $2l/c$ gives a frequency spectrum of bands separated by $c/2l$.)   The
really important result of this technique is that light pulses are obtained with
a width of only $2l/(cN)$, where N is the number of modes which are phase-

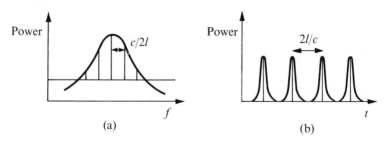

Fig. 11.8   Mode locking, (a) frequency spectrum, (b) pulse train.

locked. N can easily have a value of 100 and with $2l/c = 10^{-9}$ sec pulses of only 10^{-11} sec duration are possible.   Such pulses would only be 3 mm long!   Mode locking can be applied to continuous and pulse pumped lasers and to Q-switched lasers giving a considerable pulse power enhancement from the reduced pulse duration.

E. SUPER-RADIANCE

Laser gain is always accompanied by spontaneous emission at the transition wavelength.   In fact, the transitions with high cross-sections are just those which have short radiative lifetimes.   With a high gain amplifier there can be sufficient amplification of the spontaneous emission to produce a powerful output.   This amplified 'noise' has some of the properties of coherent laser light and is termed super-radiance.   Thus if the amplifier is long and narrow a super-radiant beam will be formed with a beam spread given by the acceptance angle of the amplifier.   Also the spontaneous emission is amplified by a narrow-band amplifier and, if the gain is high, there can be significant frequency narrowing around the peak of the gain.   This frequency narrowing is restricted by saturation of the amplifier.

Super-radiance has been demonstrated in all types of laser.   The experiments of Roess (1964) on a liquid nitrogen cooled ruby amplifier are a good illustration of the properties of super-radiance.

11.2.3   MATERIALS

A. GASES

Experiments have shown that many kinds of atoms, molecules, and ions undergo a population inversion in the gas phase leading to laser action. Gases are very attractive as laser media from the wide range of possible wavelengths and for their optical homogeneity.   The population inversion is normally produced by an electric discharge run in the gas.   There are two kinds of gas laser which do not use discharge pumping; the caesium laser which is pumped optically (as in Fig. 11.1) and the photo-dissociation laser, where a population inversion appears in one of the radical products of the dissociation.

The best known gas laser (Javan, 1961; White and Rigden, 1962) uses a mixture of helium and neon atoms and has one of its output wavelengths at 0.6328 μ.   The mechanism of pumping to a population inversion is as follows.   Electrons in the discharge excite helium atoms to one of two metastable states.   The energies of the two states are very close to two neon levels and energy can be transferred when a metastable helium atom collides with an unexcited neon atom.   Obviously there must be more helium than neon atoms and ratios of around 10:1 are used with a total pressure of a few torr.   The output power from this laser is restricted to less than one watt continuous by electrons pumping neon atoms into the lower laser level. Laser action has been obtained on the atoms of a number of other elements in continuous and/or pulsed discharges.

Lasers using ions of the inert gases neon, argon, krypton, and xenon (Paananen, 1966a) give large continuous powers in the ultraviolet and visible.   The argon ion (A^+) laser is the most highly developed and powers of up to 58 W have been obtained on a range of wavelengths between 0.4880 and 0.5145 μ.   For oscillation on a single transition, a prism is placed in the laser cavity so that through dispersion the mirrors are optically parallel for only a narrow wavelength band.   Pumping proceeds by electron impact on ions in the ground and metastable levels and an inversion is set up between pairs of levels where the lower level has a shorter lifetime than the upper. Very high current densities are required for efficient operation with typically 10–100 amps in a tube with a bore of a few millimeters.   At these currents the inside surface of the tube is quickly damaged; magnetic field containment and tubes of ceramic or metal sections are being developed to overcome this problem.   A typical medium power argon laser is shown in Fig. 11.9. Continuous coherent ultraviolet radiation can be obtained from singly

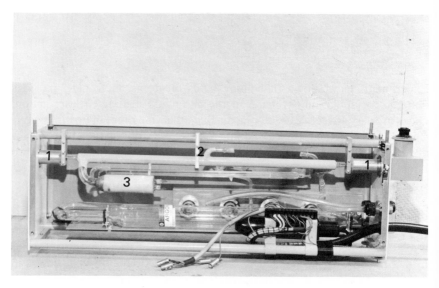

Fig. 11.9   Argon ion laser: 1 mirrors and Brewster-angle windows, 2 discharge tube with water cooling jacket, 3 cathode. (Courtesy Laser Associates.)

ionized neon and doubly ionized krypton and xenon. The neon laser (Paananen, 1966b) gives 30 mW c.w. on lines at 0.3324 μ and 0.3378 μ

Molecules can also be used in gas lasers with outputs covering the whole of the infrared (Garrett, 1965). The population inversion occurs between the various vibrational and rotational levels. The longest laser wavelength, 676 μ, comes from pulsed lasers with molecules containing CN groups. 676 μ, or 0.68 mm, lies just inside the microwave region but the laser powers of 1 W are larger than what is available from electron tubes. Very high efficiencies are possible for the conversion of electrical energy to light (Patel, et al., 1965). Carbon dioxide lasers have been made with efficiencies as large as 15% and continuous powers up to 1100 W. Laser power of this magnitude really brings the 'death ray' a step nearer. This laser gives a number of wavelengths around 10.6 μ due to various rotational levels. The carbon dioxide laser has been Q-switched for 50 kW of peak power (Kovacs, et al., 1966).

Oscillation on pure single modes is possible with gas lasers with as much as half of the total available power obtained on the lowest order mode, TEM_{00q}.

B. OPTICALLY PUMPED DIELECTRIC SOLIDS

Lasers from this group have been widely used in biological and medical experiments since they give by far the largest pulse energy (5000 J) and peak power (10,000 MW). They can be run continuously but the powers obtained are smaller than those from gas lasers.

The amplifying element is a transparent dielectric crystal or glass, doped with 1% or so of a transition metal or rare earth. The dopant is incorporated into the crystal (or glass) as a positive ion and the bonding between the ion and the lattice has a strong effect on the optical spectrum. Again a large range of crystals with different dopings have been shown to exhibit laser action but only two types have been developed to the point of being really useful. There are a number of lasers (Johnson, 1964) which use neodymium (Nd^{3+}) in crystals, calcium tungstate, and yttrium aluminum garnet (YAG), and in glasses of various base compositions. The principal output is at about 1.06 μ. Since there are a number of different hosts for this ion there is some flexibility of choice depending upon the application. Thus Nd^{3+} : glass is widely used in large lasers since it is comparatively cheap and has good optical quality. Nd^{3+} : YAG is excellent for continuous pumping and Nd^{3+} : calcium tungstate is a compromise between glass and YAG. The second type of material widely used is pink ruby (0.05% Cr^{3+} in aluminum oxide). Ruby was part of the very first laser (Maiman, 1961; Maiman, et al., 1961) and has continued in use for a number of years. It has a serious disadvantage in that the lower laser level is also the ground level; a much stronger pump is then required since more than half the ions have to be put into level 2 for a population inversion. It is still used in very high power lasers since it does not damage as easily as Nd^{3+} : glass. There are two output wavelengths 0.6943 μ and 0.6929 μ and oscillation is on the long wavelength unless a filter is used in the cavity.

These lasers are pumped with incoherent light. The energy transfer processes which take place are the same as for fluorescence—spontaneous emission from level 2. The best materials have a broad absorption band so that white light can be used for pumping and also a large fluorescent quantum efficiency. The laser solid is normally cut into a cylindrical rod and the light from a cylindrical lamp is coupled to it by a reflector in the shape of an elliptical cylinder. For continuous pumping the lamp is a capillary discharge tube—xenon for neodymium lasers and mercury for ruby. One kW lamps are required to maintain oscillation and both the lamp and laser have to be water cooled. The larger lasers are pulse pumped with the light from a xenon flash tube. An electrical energy between 10 and 10,000 J is stored in a capacitor bank and then discharged through the tube in times of 100 μsec to 10 msec. It goes almost without saying that this amount of electrical energy can do far more biological damage than any laser.

All modes of device operation have been demonstrated with solid lasers. Continuously pumped Nd^{3+} : YAG lasers (Geusic, et al., 1964) have given powers in excess of 20 W. Once thermal equilibrium is reached oscillation can take place on a single stable mode. Pulse pumped lasers are sources of very large pulses of energy. Systems giving as much as 5000 J in single 1 msec pulses have been reported and there are surely even larger ones hidden behind security fences. Up to 10,000 MW (10 GW) in 20 nsec pulses is possible with Q-switching. In terms of damage to the laser, ruby is best but even with ruby, only tens of pulses are obtained before the rod is unusable. Very recently, PTM has been put into practice (Ernest, et al., 1966) and gave 3 nsec pulses of 30 MW. Even shorter pulses have generated by mode locking. Pulses of down to 2×10^{-13} sec have been claimed (Stetser and De Maria, 1966) for a laser of Nd^{3+} with a special dye as the modulator. The big problem is, how do you measure a pulse only 10 microns long?

C. *SEMICONDUCTORS* (Rediker, 1965)

This group is the least important for biological work since they give only low powers of rather incoherent radiation. Semiconductor lasers are however being used in many communications projects and the hazards of eye damage may need to be assessed.

The laser transition takes place between the bottom of the conduction band and the top of the valence band. The band positions are dependent upon doping and temperature so that the laser wavelength can be tuned over quite a wide range. The laser can be in the form of a p-n junction diode and pumped by a forward current. Electrons and holes are then injected into the junction and recombination of these produces light with a frequency corresponding to the band gap. The size of the laser is obviously that of the junctions, the ends of which are cleaved parallel to form a cavity. Since the cross-section of the junction may be only 5 μ × 100 μ the beam spread is very large. Gallium arsenide is the only semiconductor commercially available as a laser diode. The output wavelength from this semiconductor is between 0.8 and 0.9 μ depending upon temperature. Heating of the junction limits the maximum powers to 11 W c.w. when the diode is at 4.2°K and 10 W in 50 nsec pulses at 300°K. They are the most efficient of all the lasers and up to 60% of the input electrical power can be converted to light.

Bulk semiconductors have been pumped with light and high energy electron beams. The shortest wavelengths from a solid state laser have been obtained in this way with 0.3291–0.3425 μ from zinc sulphide pumped by an electron beam (Hurwitz, 1966).

11.2.4 NON-LINEAR OPTICS

Since the output wavelength (frequency) of a laser is fixed by the spectrum transition a different amplifying material is essentially required for every wavelength. The optical band is very wide and it is impossible to cover it completely with lasers. In electronics/radio/microwaves however, we are well used to generating new frequencies by modulation (for side-bands), mixing and harmonic conversion. All these processes use some kind of non-linear component, normally a diode. At the field strengths from high power lasers many optical materials go non-linear and the above techniques can then be employed to extend the range of coherent frequencies. There are two classes of optical non-linearity: non-linear polarizability and Raman scattering. The first of these can be used for mixing and harmonic generation, and the second is similar to modulation, with the side-band separation a molecular vibration or rotation frequency.

A. *MIXING, HARMONIC GENERATION, PARAMETRIC OSCILLATION*
(Franken and Ward, 1963)

$$D = E + 4\pi P$$

describes the displacement produced by an electric field E. P is the polarization set up in the dielectric medium by movement of electrons and ions.

If we include non-linear terms, P can be written

$$P = X_1 E + X_2 E^2 + X_3 E^3 + \cdots$$

where X_1, X_2, X_3, etc., are susceptibilities.   With an incident field $E_0 \sin \omega t$ the linear polarization

$$P_1 = X_1 E_0 \sin \omega t$$

re-radiates at the same frequency.   However

$$P_2 = X_2 E_0^2 \sin^2 \omega t$$

$$= X_2 \frac{E_0^2}{2} (1 - \cos 2\omega t)$$

and the second harmonic (2ω) is generated.   With two driving fields at different frequencies (ω_1, ω_2) this quadratic polarization can be used for sum ($\omega_1 + \omega_2$) and difference ($\omega_1 - \omega_2$) mixing.   Similarly, the term E^3 can give the third harmonic of the fundamental field.   There are symmetry restrictions on materials for the various processes; for example, crystals for second harmonic generation must be of those classes which exhibit piezo-electricity.

For maximum efficiency it is obviously essential that the harmonic or mixed wave remains in phase with the driving waves over the length of the crystal.   Unfortunately normal dispersion gives different refractive indices and velocities for the various waves.   In certain cases, an 'index-match' can be made by using the birefringence of the crystal.   This is possible when the polarization of the non-linear field is in a different direction to that of the driving field.   As an example, Fig. 11.10 shows the situation for harmonic doubling from 1.06 to 0.53 μ in the crystal lithium niobate (Miller, et al., 1965).   The fundamental field is polarized as an ordinary wave and its refractive index has a spherical surface.   In contrast, the harmonic field is extra-ordinary with an ellipsoidal surface.   For the fundamental wavelength of 1.06 μ the crystal birefringence is exactly equal to the dispersion so that the two index surfaces touch at 90° to the optic axis.   This gives an index-match for light travelling in this direction and much enhanced harmonic conversion efficiencies.

The non-linear susceptibilities are really very small and power densities of megawatts per cm² are needed for useful amounts of conversion. Such powers are no real problem though, with Q-switched lasers, and a wide range of non-linear devices have been demonstrated.   Harmonic generation with lithium niobate was discussed above, 25% conversion from 2 MW of 1.06 μ is practical.   With higher powers, larger conversion efficiencies are obtained and 60% conversion from 0.6943 to 0.3472 μ has been reported.

Two stages of second harmonic generation from 1.06 μ have been used to produce 35 kW of power at 0.265 μ (Killick, *et al.*, 1966).   In early experiments (Terhune, *et al.*, 1963) on third harmonic generation from a ruby laser in calcite, a conversion energy of $3 \times 10^{-3}\%$ to 0.2314 μ was measured but there has been no further development since then.   Harmonic generators

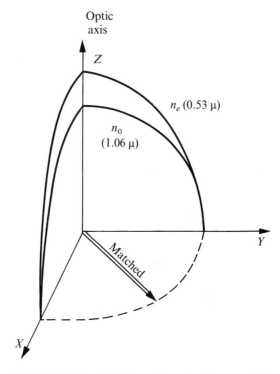

Fig. 11.10   Refractive index surfaces for phase-matched second harmonic generation in uniaxial lithium niobate.

give very substantial powers in the near ultraviolet which can be used for the destruction of photolytically sensitive tissue.   Provided suitable non-linear crystals can be found it should be possible to produce coherent radiation in the far ultraviolet with the powerful ultraviolet lasers now becoming available.

Mixers are most useful as sources of coherent radiation in the middle and far infrared.   An example (Hanna, *et al.*) uses a Q-switched ruby laser, giving simultaneously 0.6943 and 0.6929 μ, and quartz for 1 W at 338 μ. Some tuning of the difference wavelength is possible since it is very sensitive to the laser wavelengths.

Both mixers and harmonic generators are particular examples of a wider range of 'parametric' devices. Parametric amplifiers may be familiar from their wide use as low noise pre-amplifiers for microwaves. In the parametric terminology, a sum mixer is an up-converter. The reverse process for down-conversion can be used to construct a coherent oscillator which can be tuned over a very wide range of wavelengths. The basic non-linear equation

$$\omega_1 = \omega_2 + \omega_3$$

describes energy conservation. Then for up-conversion we go from the right-hand side of the equation to the left. Down-conversion goes from left to right, a single frequency 'pump' generating two waves termed the signal and idler. In practice, this means that if a non-linear crystal is pumped at ω_1 then there is a gain at ω_2 and ω_3. Oscillation can also be obtained at ω_2 and ω_3 if the parametric amplifier is placed in a cavity resonant at both frequencies. No values have been set for ω_2 and ω_3 (except that they satisfy the energy equation) and in principle they can take up any frequency. The restrictions of phase-matching

$$k_1 = k_2 + k_3 \quad (k = 2\pi n/\lambda)$$

limit the frequency range but it can still be very wide.

Successful parametric oscillators have been built using lithium niobate (Giordmaine and Miller, 1965, 1966) and potassium di-hydrogen phosphate (KDP) as the non-linear crystal. Both are pumped with the second harmonic from a neodymium laser and the wavelengths of the idler and signal lie between 0.97 and 1.15 μ. These oscillations can be continuously tuned over the whole of the working range and they should have very wide applications where the interaction is with a narrow absorption band. The present oscillators are pulsed but there are real hopes for continuous operation in the near future.

B. RAMAN LASERS (Bloembergen, 1965)

Raman scattering of light from molecules is well known from molecular spectroscopy. A light wave, on being scattered by the molecule, loses or gains the energy of quantized molecular vibration or rotation. The longer scattered wavelength is called Stokes radiation and the shorter anti-Stokes. Laser powers greater than 10 MW/cm^2 can drive the scattering coherently to give stimulated Raman radiation with conversion efficiencies in excess of 10%. Stimulated Stokes radiation can be obtained with a solid or a cell, containing a liquid or gas, placed in the laser cavity. The anti-Stokes process involves loss of energy from the molecules and for high efficiencies this has to be replaced with a Stokes process.   Stimulated anti-Stokes radiation is therefore always accompanied by Stokes radiation.   The Raman material has then to be at the focus of a lens to allow vector matching of the phase velocities of the three waves present.

Table 11.1 lists some of the frequency shifts.   In very efficient Raman materials, such as benzene, the Stokes radiation itself can act as the exciting field and produce a further shift.   In this way, four to five Stokes lines are formed, each an integral number of molecular frequencies from the laser line. A wide range of coherent frequencies are made available in the red and near infrared by a suitable Raman material and a ruby or Nd^{3+} : glass Q-switched

Table 11.1   *Raman frequency shifts (cm^{-1})*

Deuterated benzene	944
Benzene	990
Toluene	1004
Nitrobenzene	1344
l-bromonaphthalene	1368
Cyclohexane	2852
Benzene	3064
Hydrogen	4150

laser.   Molecular hydrogen has a particularly large shift (4150 cm^{-1}) and the second Stokes line from a neodymium laser (Martin and Thomas) is well into the infrared at 8.8 μ.   By second harmonic generation and mixing, a range of wavelengths can also be produced in the ultraviolet and visible (Martin, *et al.*, 1965).   Table 11.2 lists the characteristics of a number of different types of laser.

11.3   INSTRUMENTATION

11.3.1   ENERGY TRANSFER

To date, nearly all the applications of lasers in medicine and biology have been concerned with the effects, normally damaging, of coherent radiation on living matter.   For the irradiation of external surfaces then, the laser beam falls direct on the surface and the energy density is controlled with filters and lenses.   This is perhaps a good point to advise caution in using the transmission factor of filters as measured at low powers.   At the power densities of lasers, particularly Q-switched, etc., the filter may bleach to give unexpected transmission.   Irradiation of internal surfaces can sometimes be accomplished by the use of a light pipe, typically made of some flexible plastic.   The light beam can be trapped inside the polished rod by total internal reflection and steered around corners to the surface of interest.   Fiber

Table 11.2 *Characteristics of popular lasers* (April 1967)

Material	Wavelength(s) (μ)	Operation	Power or energy Maximum	Power or energy Convenient	Other information
Gas lasers					
Ne^{3+}	0.2358	Continuous			
Nitrogen	0.3371	Pulsed	500 kW	50 kW	Super-radiant
A^+	0.4880, 0.5145, etc.	Continuous	58 W	1 W	
Helium–neon	0.6328, 1.152, 3.39	Continuous	0.9 W	25 mW	
Carbon dioxide (+ nitrogen, helium)	10.6	Continuous Q-switched	1.1 kW 50 kW	100 W —	Efficiency > 15%
Cyanogen	337	Continuous Pulsed	1 W 10 W	— 1 W	
Dielectric solids					
Ruby	0.6929, 0.6943	Continuous Pulsed Q-switched	1 W 5000 J 20 GW	— 50 J 50 MW	
Nd^{3+}:YAG	1.06	Continuous	50 W	1 W	Also high repetition rate Q-switched
Nd^{3+}:glass	1.06	Pulsed Q-switched	5000 J 5 GW	50 J 50 MW	
Non-linear devices					
Calcite	0.2314	Q-switched	30 kW	—	3rd harmonic of 0.6943
A.D.P. twice	0.2650	Q-switched	35 kW	—	4th harmonic of 1.06 μ
K.D.P.	0.3472	Q-switched	3 MW	500 kW	2nd harmonic of 0.6943
Lithium niobate	0.5300	Q-switched	—	500 kW	2nd harmonic of 1.06 μ
Lithium niobate	0.37–1.92	Q-switched	1 kW	—	Parametric oscillator, 0.53 μ pump
Molecular hydrogen	8.8	Q-switched	10 W	—	2nd Stokes of 1.06 μ
Quartz	338	Q-switched	1 W	—	Difference 0.6929 μ and 0.6943 μ

optics (bundles of low refractive index fibers with high index cladding) are attractive since they are very flexible but at the moment none are available which will transmit energies above a few joules. Bulk material can be partly irradiated by forcing into it a light pipe or fiber optic like a hypodermic. One of the most valuable characteristics of laser light is that it can be focussed into a very small area.   We can consider this property to come from either the space coherence or the narrow beam spread since we cannot have one without the other.   The size of the focal spot can be calculated very simply from the angular spread of the laser beam

Diameter of spot = focal length of lens × beam spread.

If we again take, as example, our 0.5 μ, 6 mm diameter beam with a 1 cm aberration-free lens, a spot of diameter $10^4 \times 10^{-4} = 1$ μ would be formed. The pattern of intensity across the spot from the TEM_{00q} mode is Gaussian. The spot produced with high energy/power dielectric solid lasers is again often Gaussian but now due to the randomness of the angular radiation pattern from these lasers rather than a real mode.   Since the beam spreads are much larger, the spot diameters are then one hundred times those for a gas laser.   Of course the spot size can be reduced with an aperture some-where in the optical system but only with a loss of energy.   An example of the use of an aperture is given in the ruby laser microscope (Fig. 11.11) to be discussed in the next section.

At the power densities from Q-switched lasers many optical materials are damaged, particularly when the laser beam is focussed.   The breakdown strengths of a few useful materials are given in Table 11.3.   Breakdown in these particular materials is most likely due to either large electric or ultra-sonic fields but the types of mechanisms of damage will be discussed in more detail later in this chapter.

The comments above are applicable to a wide range of laser appara-tus.   In the following three sections I will briefly describe three particular instruments in the hope that they will serve to illustrate design principles.

Table 11.3   *Breakdown strengths of optic materials*

Fused silica	4.7×10^{11} W/cm^2
Borosilicate glass	0.6–4.5×10^{10} W/cm^2
Pink ruby	10^9 W/cm^2
Air (spark)	1–5×10^{10} W/cm^2

A. *LASER MICROSCOPE* (Peppers, 1965)

The most convenient way to irradiate small areas is by introducing the laser beam into the optics of a microscope.   The main advantage of the method is that the same instrument can be used for examination of the impact area and positioning of the laser beam.   The technique was first used by Bessis and his collaborators for destruction of parts of individual cells.

Figure 11.11 shows the functional diagram of a commercial instru-ment.   The laser is coupled to the microscope by a dichroic mirror and focussed by a lens into the image plane.   The multi-layer dichroic mirror has a large reflectivity for 0.6943 μ but is transparent to most of the visible spectrum.   A camera can therefore be placed beyond the laser coupler.   A binocular eyepiece can be used for visual examination when the sliding prism is in place.   The size of the focal spot can be varied by changing the aperture between lenses L_1 and L_2 or by using different objectives.   Spot diameters between 1 and 8 μ can be produced with a 63 × objective.   The laser output is 0–500 mJ in a 150 μsec pulse.

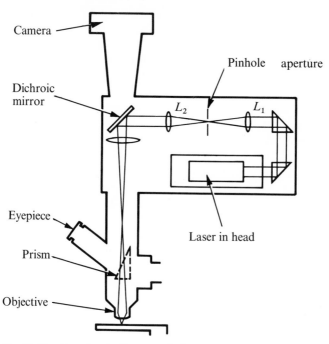

Fig. 11.11   Functional diagram of the TRG model 513 laser microscope.

B. *LASER RETINAL PHOTO-COAGULATOR* (Koester, *et al.*, 1962; Kapany, *et al.*, 1965)

The earliest clinical application of lasers was for eye surgery.   Here the eye lens can be used to focus the energy onto the retina.   Figure 11.12 gives the layout of an instrument which combines the functions of a photo-coagulator and ophthalmoscope.   The retina can be examined via lens L_1 under the illumination from the source S.   Both the laser and illuminator are coupled to the eye by mirror M_1. M_2 is a dichroic mirror.   An image of the cross-

wires is projected onto the retina to assist in setting the laser target.   The
center region of the cross-wires is removed to allow the laser beam to pass
unattenuated.   The size of the focussed spot can be varied by moving L_2.

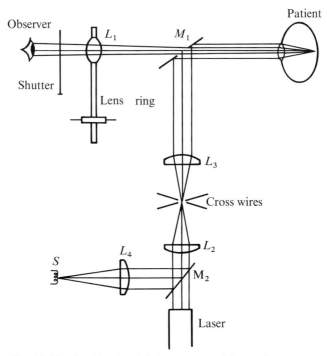

Fig. 11.12   Combined ophthalmoscope and laser photo-coagulator.

C. *LASER MICROPROBE* (Franken, 1962)

When a laser beam strikes a small area of material some of it is vaporized.
By passing the vapor through a pair of charged electrodes an arc can be set
up with a spectrum characteristic of the vaporized substance.   This is the
basis of the laser microprobe invented at the Jarrell Ash Company.   Normally a microscope is used for irradiation and monitoring.   Only 10^{-7} g of
material are needed for photographic or photoelectric spectroscopy and,
with such small quantities, *in vivo* spectroscopy is possible for the first time.
A microscopic map of atomic concentrations can also be made by repeated
shots on different parts of a sample.

The microprobe has been used to determine concentrations of elements in teeth (enamel, dentin healthy, and carious, cementum, etc.) (Sherman, *et al.*, 1965) and bones from dogs and human infants (Lithwick, *et al.*).

The concentration can be used to trace physiological functions and, for instance, titanium was found to vary widely in the two tissues.

11.3.2 DOSIMETRY (Nowak, et al., 1964)

Quantitative experiments on the biological effectiveness of laser radiation require accurate knowledge of the energy absorbed, or failing that, the energy incident on the sample.   The first of these is difficult to obtain except for very simple systems.   There is no direct method of dosimetry as with hard X-rays or γ-rays.   A 'rule of thumb' can be given for complex materials under reasonably high energy densities—that between 30 and 100% of the incident energy will be absorbed.   For better control we must resort to measuring the energy before absorption and then an accuracy of 5% is possible.

The pulsed energies to be measured lie in the range 10^{-3}–10^4 J and continuous powers 10^{-2}–10^3 W.   All these energies/powers can be handled calorimetrically and the same instrument used for a number of wavelengths, although more than one calorimeter may be required to cover the 10^7 energy range.   The problem is to avoid evaporation of the absorbing surfaces which would give an artificially low reading.   For this reason, the absorber is preferably made of polished metal so that only a few per cent of laser energy is absorbed at each reflection.   There are two geometries where the light undergoes a large number of reflections before it escapes.   The first of these (Bruce and Collett, 1965) is a thin hollow sphere with a small hole into which the laser beam is focussed.   The second (Killick, et al., 1966) is an open-ended cone which, for the correct cone angles, operates like a Mendenhall wedge with very little radiation re-emitted.   In both calorimeters, the temperature rise is measured with a number of thermo-couples in series.   An alternative approach is the liquid calorimeter (Damon and Flynn, 1963).   This consists of a cell containing a solution of a stable colored compound which absorbs at the laser wavelength.   The concentration of the dye is chosen so that the absorbed energy is spread fairly evenly through the cell.   The energy can again be determined from the temperature rise, or from the increase in volume.   Liquid calorimeters can obviously only be used for a limited range of laser wavelengths.

In addition to the difficulty of the very short pulse duration, measurement of Q-switched powers present new problems from breakdown and non-linearities in detectors.   The simplest technique is to use a vacuum photo diode to record the pulse shape and to compare the integral of this signal to the energy measured in a calorimeter.   Satisfactory results can be obtained in this way for powers up to 100 MW.   There are no instruments available for general use with larger powers and this represents a problem area in laser technology.   One promising scheme uses the d.c. term in the quadratic non-linear polarization (Bass, *et al.*, 1965).   Examination of the equations given earlier will show that such optical rectification is possible in piezo-electric crystals.   There is negligible loss of light since the instrument consists of a transparent crystal with two plates between which the beam passes.

11.4   REACTION OF RADIATION WITH MATTER

In this section I will describe the mechanisms by which light is absorbed by materials and then go on to say what the energy does to the material.

11.4.1   LINEAR ABSORPTION

The most familiar mechanism by which light is absorbed in non-metals is through raising a molecule into an excited state.   In linear absorption one photon is lost for each molecule excited.   The molecules get rid of their excitation energy in one of three ways; they can fluoresce, they can decompose into smaller molecules, or the energy can increase the temperature of the molecule and its surroundings.   The material must obviously have an absorption band at the laser wavelength for large absorption.   Most biological materials scatter light and so the path length for absorption is effectively increased.   Weak bands and the tails of strong bands may then absorb significant amounts of light.   The absorption wavelengths for a few biologically interesting substances are given in Table 11.4.

Table 11.4 *Absorption bands (μ)*

Serum albumen (protein)	<0.24 (coagulation)
	0.28 (denatures)
Nucleic acids	0.265
Vitamin A	0.32
Hemoglobin	0.55
Retina	0.4–0.7
Chlorophyll	0.645
Flesh	>1.1
Water	>22

Light can also be absorbed by free electrons as in metals and plasmas. As will be discussed later, plasmas can occur at the surfaces of materials under intense illumination and in laser sparks.   These plasmas are virtually opaque to light giving a very hot plasma very close to the irradiated sample.

At the light powers from lasers a large population may be maintained in the excited state of the molecule.   If there is a further band, with the correct spacing above the first level, then there may be further excitation with the absorption of a second photon.   In this way, an infrared laser may excite a molecule into an ultraviolet absorption band, and the result could be unexpected decomposition of the molecule.   The amount of second absorption is proportional to the square of the light intensity.

11.4.2   TWO-PHOTON ABSORPTION (Kleinman, 1962)

Again, with laser powers, the normal linear absorption behavior can be modified.   At very high fluxes, two photons can be absorbed simultaneously to span one energy gap twice the size of the photon energy.   This effect is sometimes described by inventing a virtual level halfway between the real energy levels.   The two-photon absorption is then similar to absorption via a real level.   The fundamental difference, of course, is that there is no real level and the material will be transparent at the laser wavelength but absorb strongly into an ultraviolet band.   This effect is very important at the power densities from Q-switched lasers.

For linear absorption

$$dI = -\alpha_1 I \, dx, \quad \text{i.e.} \quad I = I_0 \exp\left[-\alpha_1 x\right]$$

(where I is light intensity, x is linear dimension of absorber, and α_1 is absorption coefficient.   Two-photon absorption increases as the square of the light intensity, so

$$dI = -\alpha_2 I^2 \, dx$$

and we can define an effective linear absorption coefficient

$$\alpha_1 = I\alpha_2$$

which obviously depends on laser power.

11.4.3   THERMAL EFFECTS

Consider what happens when a laser density of 100 J/cm^2 falls on a medium with the thermal properties of water and an absorption coefficient of 20 cm^{-1} (2 mm^{-1}).   We will assume that the laser pulse is only a few msec long so that heat conduction can be neglected.   A very simple calculation then shows that the first tenth of a millimeter of surface would be raised in temperature by 500°C or that it would all be converted to super-heated steam.   The energy density of 100 J/cm^2 will also ignite wood.   A temperature rise of only 50°C can do considerable damage to physiological systems and this can be obtained with 10 J/cm^2.   By focussing, much higher energy densities are possible—1 mJ into a 1 μ diameter spot gives 10^5 J/cm^2, and it goes without saying what tremendous thermal damage can be done then.

The detailed behavior of the hot spot is very complex. If a lot of vapor is produced this may itself absorb laser power to become sufficiently hot to be a plasma. The intense evaporation can correspond to a back pressure of many atmospheres. The spot may then go unstable and large amounts of liquid be ejected in addition to the vapor.

11.4.4   PHOTO-CHEMICAL EFFECTS

Individual molecules can be destroyed if the absorbed frequency corresponds to an energy greater than that for dissociation of a chemical bond. These effects are very important when irradiating with ultraviolet light. For example, proteins are denatured by light of a wavelength less than 0.3 μ. Photo-chemical damage can also be produced by two-photon absorption from red and infrared laser light.

11.4.5   SHOCK WAVES

In the discussion of thermal effects, I mentioned the large back pressure from the evaporation. This pressure can be even larger if the absorption takes place some distance from the surface and the gas is trapped (see Fig. 11.13).

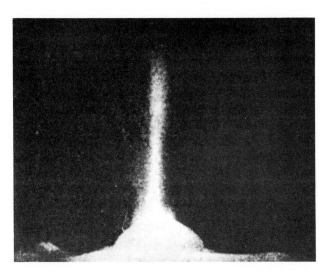

Fig. 11.13   Distension of abdominal skin of mouse, irradiated with 60 J. (From Fine, et al., 1965, Federation Proceedings, Supplement 14, pp. S–35–S–45).

The high pressure zone is created in less than a msec and as a result a shock wave may be generated.   Fine, *et al.* (1965) have reported an experiment in which a mouse was killed by a pulse of 100 J falling on the forehead.   A post-mortem examination showed extensive brain damage on the opposite side of the skull which could only have been produced by a shock wave.

Laser radiation can also generate ultrasonic energy directly by Brillouin scattering (Bruma, *et al.*, 1965).   This is very similar to Raman scattering except that the coupled vibration is simply an acoustic wave.   The Stokes radiation can be stimulated and the excess energy appears in the ultrasonic wave.

11.4.6   DIELECTRIC BREAKDOWN

When a Q-switched laser is focussed, the optical electric field at the focus can be sufficiently large to break down air or any other material there. A small plasma 'fire-ball' is formed, Fig. 11.14, with a temperature in excess of $30,000°K$.   Electrical breakdown in solids and liquids will produce ions and electrons and there will follow chemical reactions similar to those from ionizing radiations.

11.5   APPLICATIONS IN MEDICINE AND BIOLOGY

11.5.1   CELL SURGERY

The ability to focus laser light to a very small spot was first exploited by Bessis, *et al.* (1962) in the destruction of small areas of single cells.   The technique is complementary to the ultraviolet microbeam, previously developed, since it uses red or infrared light and does its damage in less than a msec.   The short exposure makes it possible to study dynamically the immediate effects of the damage.   Cell surgery has been applied to the nucleus, cytoplasm, and cell wall.   Fig. 11.15 shows the results of an experiment using red blood cells.   In the last case, the cell had to be injected with a vital blue or green dye since the wall is rather transparent (Saks and Roth, 1963).   Bessis and Ter-Pogossian (1965) have studied the behavior of a population of red and white cells after the wall of one red cell had been opened with a laser.   They found that the white cells rapidly cannibalized the remains of the red cell.   One very interesting possibility is that of producing genetic aberrations by irradiation of chromosomes.

11.5.2   EYE SURGERY

The lens of the eye can focus a laser beam in exactly the same way as a microscope objective.   If the eye is relaxed, this results in a very large energy

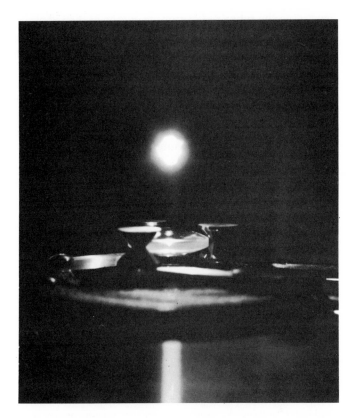

Fig. 11.14   Spark in air from focussed Q-switched laser beam. (Courtesy Lasers Section, Royal Aircraft Establishment, Ministry of Technology, U.K.)

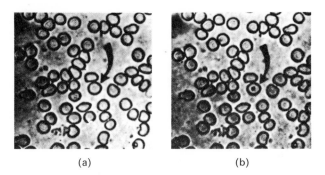

(a)   (b)

Fig. 11.15   2 μ damage spots in dry 7 μ human red blood cells; (a) before irradiation, (b) after irradiation. (From Peppers, 1965, *Appl. Optics*, **4**, 555–8.)

density on the retina.   Laser wavelengths in the visible or near infrared are transmitted by the optics of the eye and the laser energy absorbed by the retina.   This absorbed energy will produce a lesion of the retina as shown by the early experiments of Zaret, *et al.* (1961) on rabbits.

The lesions have a surgical use since they can induce a kind of 'spot weld' between the retina and choroid.   This effect has been known for a number of years (Meyer–Schwickerath, 1960) and exploited in the repair of detached retinas by photo-coagulation.   In the past, a continuous xenon arc has been used as the light source, entailing exposures over several seconds

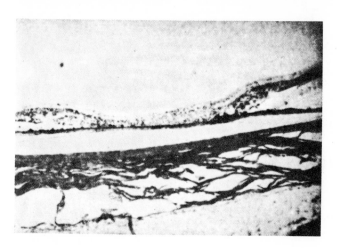

Fig. 11.16   Histological section showing satisfactory weld be-tween retina and fundus in a rabbit eye. (From Kapany, Silbertrust, and Peppers, 1965, *Appl. Optics*, **4**, 517–22.)

and an anesthetic for the patient.   Laser welds (see Fig. 11.16) can be pro-duced in milliseconds with the patient prepared as for a normal fundus examination.   The laser energy has to be controlled very closely since an excess will cut right through the choroid and cause hemorrhage.   If any-thing, the laser weld is too small and the optics are therefore sometimes de-focussed or a number of welds made.   At least three industrial companies are now marketing laser retinal photo-coagulators.   The laser can be suffi-ciently small to be placed in the handle of a conventional ophthalmoscope. Laser photo-coagulation is now widely used (Zweng and Flocks, 1965) and more than 500 patients have been treated in this way.   Preliminary work is also under way for the use of it against eye cancers.   In one such operation, the tumor was prevented from spreading by means of an encircling ring of laser lesions.

11.5.3   LASER SCALPEL

Lasers may possibly replace the scalpel in certain types of surgery. The laser beam is focussed to a point or line and cutting is by the thermal damage of the tissue. One attractive property of this 'laser knife' is that it is obviously completely sterile. Continuous argon lasers are particularly suitable (Hoye and Minton, 1965) since their output wavelengths are strongly absorbed by hemoglobin, a constituent of all soft tissue. One successful operation has already been performed (Brown) for the removal of a tumor from a man's thigh. A 2 W argon laser was used and the beam directed to the cutting point by a concave mirror on a gimbal mount. There was no hemorrhage since the light beam cauterized the small blood vessels as it cut them. This bloodless surgery may be of great value in dealing with the liver, spleen, and brain.

Dental surgery (Lancet Staff, 1964) also offers scope for the laser both in the destruction of caries and in the fusing of refractory materials into cavities. Preliminary experiments have used 90 J of energy in 1 msec pulses. There is also a suggestion that enamel could be reglazed with laser radiation.

11.5.4   SKIN SURGERY (Goldman, 1965)

The simplest type of laser surgery is that of the skin. Growths such as warts have been successfully excised by a focussed laser beam. Some progress has also been obtained in the removal of large colored regions such as angiomas and tattoos. It seems certain that the laser will become a standard piece of dermatological equipment.

11.5.5   CANCER

Like all new approaches to this dreadful disease the laser has been hailed as a panacea. There has indeed been a certain success but mainly with laboratory animals (McGuff, 1965). Figure 11.17 shows, as an example, the effect of laser radiation on a human melanoma transplanted to a hamster. The cheek pouches of a hamster are very suitable for such experiments since access is simple and there are two of them, one for the test and one for the control. A ruby laser pulse between 60 and 380 J produced the result shown. There was no sign of cancer cells after about 20 days. Autogenous tumors of hamster origin behaved rather differently and the laser had very little effect on them. Eight human patients with various malignant conditions have also been treated with a laser (Goldman, et al., 1965). To help the tumor destruction an injection of Evans-blue dye was made prior to the treatment. The results obtained were rather inconclusive and much more work is required.

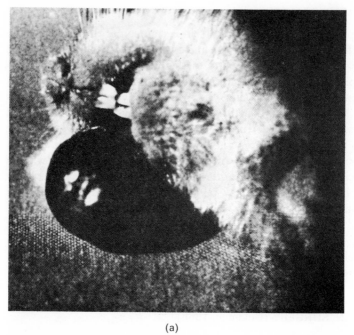

(a)

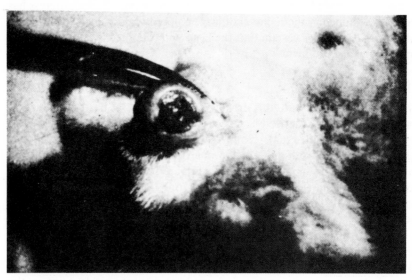

(b)

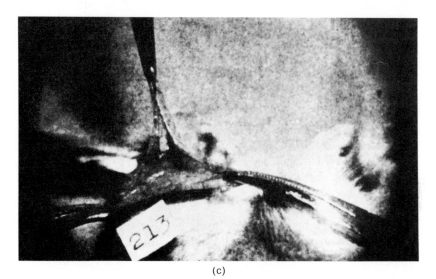

(c)

Fig. 11.17   Laser treatment of human melanoma on hamster cheek pouch; (a) post laser day 2, (b) 6, (c) 36—pouch grossly free of tumor. (From McGuff, *Surgical Application of Laser*, 1966, Chap. 4, Thomas: Springfield, Ill.)

11.5.6   FREE RADICALS, ETC.

The existence of free radicals in biological systems, as demonstrated by electron spin resonance spectroscopy, is discussed with much detail in chapters 3–7.   As described there, large concentrations of free radicals can be produced by irradiation with ultraviolet light or ionizing radiation.   Some preliminary experiments (Derr, *et al.*, 1964, 1965) have been carried out to see if the high energies from ruby lasers can give free radicals in biological materials.   The samples were irradiated with 100 J and then stored in solid carbon dioxide.   Enzyme collagenase and mouse tissues of white skin, abdominal wall, intestine, and spleen gave no spectrum before or after irradiation.   Liver and a melanoma contained radicals but these did not change with irradiation.   An increase in radical concentration was found for black skin and the enzyme homolysin, radical concentrations in the range 1–8 $\times$ 10^{15} spins/g being produced.   In the former case it is very likely the melanin which is causing the radicals.

A number of other experiments have been performed using more conventional biochemical techniques.   One such experiment (Ingelman, *et al.*, 1965) used enzyme activity as a test of a radiation effect from a ruby laser.

Peroxidase showed evidence of inactivation but dehydrogenase, catalase, amylase, lysozyme, and trypsin were unaffected. Similar experiments using focussed light demonstrated two-photon absorption in biological materials (Rounds, *et al.*, 1966). Cell suspensions of mouse and chick fibroblasts were undamaged by 8 impacts of 10 J but were killed by one shot of 80 J.

11.5.7   SAFETY

Scientists and engineers working with lasers are exposed to a very real hazard in the form of eye damage. The focussing action of the eye, which was used in eye surgery, can also give dangerous energy densities in the event of un-expected exposures. An energy density on the eye of only 10^{-6} J/cm^2 can produce lesions of the retina. To my knowledge, there have been at least five accidents, three of which were very serious since the light beam was focussed onto the fovea centralis.

Several organizations have examined the question of safety and drawn up a number of rules (Weston, 1964). Essentially these are

(i) Never look direct, or via a specular reflector, into a laser beam. It is not safe to use a filter since it may bleach.

(ii) When not wearing safety spectacles, do not look at a laser beam on a scattering surface for energy densities greater than 0.3 J/cm^2 or con-tinuous power densities greater than 30 W/cm^2.

(iii) Use safety spectacles wherever possible. For 0.6943 μ and 1.06 μ, Schott filter glass BG 18 has a very high attentuation. The safest system is, wherever possible, to totally enclose the experimental apparatus.

In addition to the eye hazard, care should be taken to avoid large energies on exposed skin. Energy densities above 30 J/cm^2 will cause burns of increasing degree and there may be long term effects such as the development of skin cancer.

We cannot take too much care at this stage of laser technology until concrete evidence is available firmly delineating safety limits. The tragic history of the first twenty years of radiology should be a sufficient warning.

11.6   CONCLUDING REMARKS

It seems certain that the laser will have growing usefulness in the parallel fields of biology and medicine. Laser technology has now attained some stability and it is possible to see what powers, energies, etc., will be available for the next few years, and at what wavelengths. It is a good time to start assessing the role of lasers in biological work. There are however two words of warning.   The first is that laser light has *no* magical properties; it is simply *coherent* electromagnetic radiation with a power and frequency larger than those to which we are accustomed.   Second, the use of lasers in medicine and biology is a *joint* effort between the physicist and biological scientist and each must apply to the work the full professional standards of his discipline.

REFERENCES

Bass, M., Franken, P. A., and Ward, J. F., 1965, *Phys. Rev.*, **138**, A534–A542.

Bessis, M. F., Gires, G., Mayer, G., and Nomsarski, G., 1962, *C. r. hebd. Séanc. Acad. Sci.*, Paris, **255**, 1010–2.

Bessis, M. F., and Ter-Pogossian, M. M., 1965, *Ann. N.Y. Acad. Sci.*, **122**, 689–94.

Bloembergen, N., 1965, *Nonlinear Optics* (New York: W. A. Benjamin, Inc.)

Boyd, G. D., and Gordon, J. P., 1961, *Bell Syst. Tech. J.*, **40**, 489–508.

Brown, T. E., unpublished.

Bruce, C. W., and Collett, E. H., 1965, *Pulsed Laser Instrumentation* (U.S. Govt. Research Report, AD–618031).

Bruma, M., Velghe, M., and Amor, L., 1965, *C. r. hebd. Séanc. Acad. Sci.*, Paris, **260**, 1357–60.

Collins, R. J., Nelson, D. F., Schawlow, A. L., Bond, W., Garrett, C. G. B., and Kaiser, W., 1960, *Phys. Rev. Lett.*, **5**, 303–5.

Damon, E. K., and Flynn, J. T., 1963, *Appl. Optics*, **2**, 163–4.

Derr, V. E., Klein, E., and Fine, S., 1964, *Appl. Optics*, **3**, 786–7; 1965, *Fedn. Am. Socs. exp. Biol.*, Part 3, Suppl. **14**, S99–S103.

Di Domenico, M., 1964, *J. appl. Phys.*, **35**, 2870–6.

Ernest, J., Michou, M., and Debrie, J., 1966, *Phys. Lett.*, **22**, 147–9.

Fine, S., Klein, E., Nowak, W., Scott, R. E., Laor, Y., Simpson, L., Crissey, J., Donoghue, J., and Deer, V. E., 1965, *Fedn. Proc. Fedn. Am. Socs. exp. Biol.*, Part 3, Suppl. **14**, S35–S45.

Franken, P. A., 1962, *Int. Sci. and Technol.*, **10**, 62–8.

Franken, P. A., and Ward, J. F., 1963, *Rev. mod. Phys.*, **35**, 23–39.

Garrett, C. G. B., 1965, *Int. Sci. and Technol.*, **39**, 39–44.

Geusic, J. H., Marcos, H. M., and Van Uitert, L. G., 1964, *Appl. Phys. Lett.*, **4**, 182–4.

Giordmaine, J. A., and Miller, R. C., 1965, *Phys. Rev. Lett.*, **14**, 973–6; 1966, *Appl. Phys. Lett.*, **9**, 298–300.

Goldman, L., 1965, *Dermatology Digest*, **4**, 47–9.

Goldman, L., Wilson, R., Hornby, P., and Meyer, R., 1965, *Cancer*, **18**, 533–45.

Hanna, D. C., Gambling, W. A., and Smith, R. C., unpublished.

Hoye, R., and Minton, J. P., 1965, *Surg. Forum*, **16**, 93–5.

Hurwitz, C. E., 1966, *Appl. Phys. Lett.*, **9**, 116–8.

Ingelman, J. M., Rotte, T. C., Schecter, E., and Blaney, D. J., 1965, *Ann. N.Y. Acad. Sci.*, **122**, 790–801.

Javan, A., 1961, *Advances in Quantum Electronics* (New York: Columbia University Press), pp. 18–27.

Johnson, L. F., 1964, *Quantum Electronics* III (New York: Columbia University Press), pp. 1021–35.

Kapany, N. S., Silbertrust, N., and Peppers, N. A., 1965, *Appl. Optics*, **4**, 517–22.

Killick, D. E., Bateman, D. A., Brown, D. R., Moss, T. S., and De La Perelle, E. T., 1966, *Infrared Phys.*, **6**, 85–109.

Killick, D. E., Channing, D. A., and Bateman, D. A., 1966, *Royal Aircraft Establishment Technical Memo Rad.* 761.

Kleinman, D. A., 1962, *Phys. Rev.*, **125**, 87–8.

Koester, C. J., Snitzer, E., Campbell, C. J., and Rittler, M. C., 1962, *J. opt. Soc. Am.*, **52**, 607.

Kovacs, M. A., Flynn, G. W., and Javan, A., 1966, *Appl. Phys. Lett.*, **8**, 62–3.

Lancet Staff, 1964, *Lancet*, **1964** II, 949.

Lithwick, N. H., Healy, M. K., and Cohen, J., unpublished.

Maiman, T. H., 1960, *Br. Commun. Electron.*, **7**, 674–5; 1961, *Phys. Rev.*, **123**, 1145–50.

Maiman, T. H., Hoskins, R. H., D'Haenens, I. J., Asawa, C. K., and Evtukov, V., 1961, *Phys. Rev.*, **123**, 1151–7.

Martin, M. D., and Thomas, E. L., unpublished.

Martin, M. D., Thomas, E. L., and Wright, J. K., 1965, *Phys. Lett.*, **15**, 136–7.

McGuff, P. E., Deterling, R. A., Gottlieb, L. S., Fahimi, H. D., Bushnell, D., and Roeber, F., 1965, *Fedn. Proc. Fedn. Am. Socs. exp. Biol.*, Part 3, Suppl. **14**, S150–S154.

Meyer-Schwickerath, G., 1960, *Light Coagulation* (St. Louis: C. V. Mosby Co.)

Miller, R. C., Boyd, G. D., and Savage, A., 1965, *Appl. Phys. Lett.*, **6**, 77–9.

Missio, D. V., and Seeber, K. N., 1965, *Microwaves*, **4**, 40–51.

Nowak, W. B., Fine, S., Klein, E., Hergenrother, K., and Hansen, W. P., 1964, *Life Sci.*, **3**, 1475–81.

Paananen, R., 1966a, *IEEE Spectrum*, **3**, 88–99; 1966b, *Appl. Phys. Lett.*, **9**, 34–5.

Patel, C. K. N., Tien, P. K., and McFee, J. H., 1965, *Appl. Phys. Lett.*, **7**, 290–2.

Peppers, N. A., 1965, *Appl. Optics*, **4**, 555–8.

Rediker, R. H., 1965, *Physics To-day*, **18**, 42–50.

Roess, D., 1964, *Proc IEEE*, **52**, 853.

Rounds, D. E., Olson, R. S., and Johnson, F. M., 1966, *IEEE Jnl. Quantum Electron.*, **QE2**, p. xxi.

Saks, N. M., and Roth, C. A., 1963, *Science*, **141**, 46–7.

Sherman, D. S., Ruben, M. P., and Goldman, H. M., 1965, *Ann. N.Y. Acad. Sci.*, **122**, 767–72.

Stetser, D. A., and De Maria, A. J., 1966, *Appl. Phys. Lett.*, **9**, 118–20.

Terhune, R. W., Maker, P. D., and Savage, C. M., 1963, *Appl. Phys. Lett.*, **2**, 54–5.

Vuylsteke, A. A., 1963, *J. appl. Phys.*, **34**, 1615–22.

Weston, B. A., 1964, *Laser Systems–Code of Practice* (London: Ministry of Aviation).

White, A. D., and Rigden, J. D., 1962, *Proc. Inst. Radio Engrs.*, **50**, 1697.

Yariv, A., and Gordon, J. P., 1963, *Proc. IEEE*, **51**, 4–29.

Zaret, M. M., Breinin, G. M., Schmidt, H., Ripps, H., and Siegel, I. M., 1961, *Science*, **134**, 1525–6.

Zweng, H. C., and Flocks, M., 1965, *Fedn. Proc. Fedn. Am. Socs. exp. Biol.*, Part 3, Suppl. **14**, S65–S70.

BIBLIOGRAPHY

Birnbaum, G., *Optical Masers*, Academic Press Inc., New York, 1964.

Heavens, O. S., *Optical Masers*, Methuen and Co. Ltd., London, 1964.

Lengyell, B. A., *Lasers*, John Wiley and Sons Inc., New York, 1962.

Lengyell, B. A., *Introduction to Laser Physics*, John Wiley and Sons Inc., New York, 1966.

Levine, A. K., Ed., *Lasers—A Series of Advances*, Vol. I, Edward Arnold (Publishers) Ltd., London, 1966.

Smith, W. V., and Sorokin, P. P., *The Laser*, McGraw-Hill Book Company Inc., New York, 1966.

Troup, G., *Masers and Lasers*, 2nd Ed., Methuen and Co. Ltd., London, 1963.

Applied Optics: Laser retinal photocoagulation, *Appl. Optics*, **4**, No. 5, May 1965.

Fine, S., Klein, E., and Scott, R. E., Laser irradiation of biological systems, *IEEE Spectrum*, **1**, pp. 81–95, April 1964.

Litwin, M. S., and Earle, K. M., Eds. 'Proceedings of the First Annual Conference on Biologic Effects of Laser Radiation', *Fedn Proc. Fedn Am. Socs exp. Biol.*, Part 3, Suppl. 14, January-February 1965.

McGuff, P. E., *Surgical Applications of Laser*, Charles C. Thomas, Springfield, Illinois, 1966.

New York Academy of Sciences, 'The Laser', *Ann. N.Y. Acad. Sci.*, **122**, Article 2, May 28, 1965.

AUTHOR INDEX

Numbers in *italics* refer to the pages on which references are listed at the end of each chapter.

SUBJECT INDEX